Musculoskeletal Disorders and Diseases: Biomechanical Modeling in Sport, Health, Rehabilitation and Ergonomics

Musculoskeletal Disorders and Diseases: Biomechanical Modeling in Sport, Health, Rehabilitation and Ergonomics

Guest Editor

Philippe Gorce

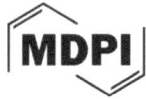

Basel • Beijing • Wuhan • Barcelona • Belgrade • Novi Sad • Cluj • Manchester

Guest Editor
Philippe Gorce
International Institute of
Biomechanics and
Occupational Ergonomics
Toulon University
Toulon
France

Editorial Office
MDPI AG
Grosspeteranlage 5
4052 Basel, Switzerland

This is a reprint of the Special Issue, published open access by the journal *Bioengineering* (ISSN 2306-5354), freely accessible at: https://www.mdpi.com/journal/bioengineering/special_issues/679QA5L9B0.

For citation purposes, cite each article independently as indicated on the article page online and as indicated below:

Lastname, A.A.; Lastname, B.B. Article Title. *Journal Name* **Year**, *Volume Number*, Page Range.

ISBN 978-3-7258-3845-5 (Hbk)
ISBN 978-3-7258-3846-2 (PDF)
https://doi.org/10.3390/books978-3-7258-3846-2

© 2025 by the authors. Articles in this book are Open Access and distributed under the Creative Commons Attribution (CC BY) license. The book as a whole is distributed by MDPI under the terms and conditions of the Creative Commons Attribution-NonCommercial-NoDerivs (CC BY-NC-ND) license (https://creativecommons.org/licenses/by-nc-nd/4.0/).

Contents

About the Editor vii

Philippe Gorce
Musculoskeletal Disorders and Diseases: Biomechanical Modeling in Sport, Health, Rehabilitation and Ergonomics
Reprinted from: *Bioengineering* **2025**, *12*, 300, https://doi.org/10.3390/bioengineering12030300 . 1

Qian Xiang, Shijie Guo, Jiaxin Wang, Kazunobu Hashimoto, Yong Liu and Lei Liu
Modeling and Analysis of Foot Function in Human Gait Using a Two-Degrees-of-Freedom Inverted Pendulum Model with an Arced Foot
Reprinted from: *Bioengineering* **2023**, *10*, 1344, https://doi.org/10.3390/bioengineering10121344 . 4

Anthony C. Goo, Curt A. Laubscher, Douglas A. Wajda and Jerzy T. Sawicki
Preliminary Virtual Constraint-Based Control Evaluation on a Pediatric Lower-Limb Exoskeleton
Reprinted from: *Bioengineering* **2024**, *11*, 590, https://doi.org/10.3390/bioengineering11060590 . 21

Xin Han, Norihiro Nishida, Minoru Morita, Takashi Sakai and Zhongwei Jiang
Compensation Method for Missing and Misidentified Skeletons in Nursing Care Action Assessment by Improving Spatial Temporal Graph Convolutional Networks
Reprinted from: *Bioengineering* **2024**, *11*, 127, https://doi.org/10.3390/bioengineering11020127 . 37

Philippe Gorce and Julien Jacquier-Bret
Musculoskeletal Disorder Risk Assessment during the Tennis Serve: Performance and Prevention
Reprinted from: *Bioengineering* **2024**, *11*, 974, https://doi.org/10.3390/bioengineering11100974 . 54

Yile Wang, Liu Xu, Hanhui Jiang, Lin Yu, Hanzhang Wu and Qichang Mei
Biomechanical Effects of the Badminton Split-Step on Forecourt Lunging Footwork
Reprinted from: *Bioengineering* **2024**, *11*, 501, https://doi.org/10.3390/bioengineering11050501 . 77

Chih-Kuan Wu, Yin-Chou Lin, Ya-Lin Chen, Yi-Ping Chao and Tsung-Hsun Hsieh
The Influence of Dynamic Taping on Landing Biomechanics after Fatigue in Young Football Athletes: A Randomized, Sham-Controlled Crossover Trial
Reprinted from: *Bioengineering* **2024**, *11*, 631, https://doi.org/10.3390/bioengineering11060631 . 93

Wei Liu, Liu Xu, Haidan Wu, Yile Wang, Hanhui Jiang, Zixiang Gao, et al.
Bilateral Asymmetries of Plantar Pressure and Foot Balance During Walking, Running, and Turning Gait in Typically Developing Children
Reprinted from: *Bioengineering* **2025**, *12*, 151, https://doi.org/10.3390/bioengineering12020151 . 105

**Enrique Hernandez-Laredo, Ángel Gabriel Estévez-Pedraza,
Laura Mercedes Santiago-Fuentes and Lorena Parra-Rodríguez**
Optimizing Fall Risk Diagnosis in Older Adults Using a Bayesian Classifier and Simulated Annealing
Reprinted from: *Bioengineering* **2024**, *11*, 908, https://doi.org/10.3390/bioengineering11090908 . 118

Yi-Lang Chen and Ying-Hua Liao
Differential Back Muscle Flexion–Relaxation Phenomenon in Constrained versus Unconstrained Leg Postures
Reprinted from: *Bioengineering* **2024**, *11*, 736, https://doi.org/10.3390/bioengineering11070736 . 136

Michael Weiser, Lindsay Stoy, Valerie Lallo, Sriram Balasubramanian and Anita Singh
The Efficacy of Body-Weight Supported Treadmill Training and Neurotrophin-Releasing
Scaffold in Minimizing Bone Loss Following Spinal Cord Injury
Reprinted from: *Bioengineering* **2024**, *11*, 819, https://doi.org/10.3390/bioengineering11080819 . **149**

About the Editor

Philippe Gorce

Philippe Gorce is a Professor of Biomechanics and Ergonomics at the University of Toulon. Since 2021, he has acted as Director of the International Institute of Biomechanics and Occupational Ergonomics and has led and established several research laboratories. He is a Director and member of many established committees at universities and private agencies, and serves as president or deputy director and/or member of the board of directors of several international scientific societies. Since 1994, he has published more than 230 scientific articles in peer-reviewed journals and has presented papers at over 200 international conferences. Over the last 25 years, he has received a number of research awards as the principal investigator of research projects, and in collaboration with partners from across the globe. He serves as an EBM of many notable journals spanning from biomechanics to ergonomics, sports, biomedical engineering, healthcare, bioengineering, occupational health, disability, biorobotics, and robotics. He has served as a reviewer for many international journals and private/public grant agencies. He has also supervised more than 35 PhDs and 55 students, including those studying for their bachelor's and master's.

His research interests mostly concern musculoskeletal disorders and the relative effects of working conditions, motor impairments, diseases, and aging in the context of global and public health, healthcare professions, rehabilitation, disability, industrial engineering, and sport. Specifically, his work pertains to the following topics: work-related musculoskeletal disorders, risk factors, risk assessment, prevalence, occupational ergonomics, dynamic and kinematic motion analysis, posture, biomechanical modeling and simulation, motion analysis, muscle modeling, muscular fatigue, safety, occupational health, sport performance, active living, sport medicine, intelligent wheelchairs, and neuro- or biorobotics.

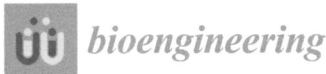

Editorial

Musculoskeletal Disorders and Diseases: Biomechanical Modeling in Sport, Health, Rehabilitation and Ergonomics

Philippe Gorce [1,2]

1 International Institute of Biomechanics and Occupational Ergonomics, 83418 Hyères, France; gorce@univ-tln.fr
2 University of Toulon, CS60584, 83041 Toulon, France

Citation: Gorce, P. Musculoskeletal Disorders and Diseases: Biomechanical Modeling in Sport, Health, Rehabilitation and Ergonomics. *Bioengineering* 2025, 12, 300. https://doi.org/10.3390/bioengineering12030300

Received: 11 March 2025
Accepted: 13 March 2025
Published: 16 March 2025

Citation: Gorce, P. Musculoskeletal Disorders and Diseases: Biomechanical Modeling in Sport, Health, Rehabilitation and Ergonomics. *Bioengineering* 2025, 12, 300. https://doi.org/10.3390/bioengineering12030300

Copyright: © 2025 by the author. Licensee MDPI, Basel, Switzerland. This article is an open access article distributed under the terms and conditions of the Creative Commons Attribution (CC BY) license (https://creativecommons.org/licenses/by/4.0/).

Protecting people at work and at leisure, and improving their quality of life, is one of the major challenges faced in this century. From this perspective, understanding the mechanisms that lead to the development of musculoskeletal disorders and diseases is a major multidisciplinary scientific challenge. This Special Issue is dedicated to recent advances in biomechanical modeling research used to explore and understand the musculoskeletal system (macro- and microscopic). Computational techniques, biomechanical computation tools and numerical tools enable us to quantify and qualify the most important parameters (biomechanical, physiological, biological or environmental) involved in the onset, prevention and reduction in the effects of musculoskeletal disorders and/or the development of musculoskeletal diseases. They can be used as a complement to experimental protocols, clinical studies, process design, ergonomics, etc., to study, evaluate and understand various situations in life, such as repeated movements in the workplace, evaluation of leisure-time physical activities, analysis of sporting gestures to assess performance, the design of new equipment to compensate for a motor impairment, the proposal of new recommendations in a clinical setting, etc. We support all articles promoting the latest research in the fields of sport, health, rehabilitation and ergonomics that contribute to improving people's health and quality of life.

The Special Issue "Musculoskeletal disorders and diseases: biomechanical modeling in sport, health, rehabilitation and ergonomics" brings together ten high-quality publications focusing on new advances and applications in the prevention and understanding of musculoskeletal disorders and diseases.

In this context, the use of biomechanical gait models represents an original approach. Xiang et al. utilized a two-degree-of-freedom inverted pendulum gait model with a roll factor to identify different gait styles [1]. Goo et al. exploited a "virtual controller" for pediatric gait rehabilitation. In their work, the authors experimentally compare this virtual controller with a conventional position-tracking controller associated with a questionnaire [2]. The study of ergonomic risks and postures is also helping to expand knowledge of the risk factors and prevalence of musculoskeletal disorders. Han et al. propose a "skeletal compensation" method using convolutional networks of enhanced spatio-temporal graphs to assess MSD risk in healthcare workers. The proposed method is compared with other postural assessment methods and qualified using the REBA score [3]. The study of MSD risks in sport is also the subject of more recent research. For example, Gorce et al. studied the risks of MSD during the tennis serve to protect athletes while maintaining performance. Using the ergonomic Rapid Entire Body Assessment (REBA) tool at each time step and a 3D kinematic analysis of joint angles, the authors assessed the impact of slow and fast serves on the risk of MSD [4]. Wang et al. investigate the biomechanical impact of the split-step technique on forehand and backhand lunges in badminton on injury risk. The results highlight the potential of split-stepping (reduced ground reaction forces, reduced knee flexion on ground contact, etc.) in swing techniques, performance improvement and injury reduction [5]. The use of technical or therapeutic means makes it possible to propose solutions and recommendations to reduce injuries or pathologies of the musculoskeletal system. The application of dynamic taping to prevent the risk of cruciate ligament injury in fatigued soccer athletes has been studied by Wu et al. Dynamic taping, particularly using the spiral technique, appears to attenuate defective landing biomechanics and offer protective benefits [6]. Studying the impact of gait asymmetry on the stability and coordination of dynamic movements also contributes to a better understanding of the mechanisms that lead to the onset of MSD. Liu et al. have shown that early identification of loading patterns enables the development of targeted interventions to prevent foot pathology in children [7]. Fall prevention is also a field that contributes to better identification and diagnosis of musculoskeletal diseases and disorders. Hernandez-Laredo et al. have proposed a fall risk classification method using a Bayesian approach and the simulated annealing algorithm [8]. Analysis of the flexion–relaxation phenomenon of back muscles is important in the development of musculoskeletal disorders. In this context, Chen et al. have explored the influence of leg posture control on the activity of certain muscles, along with the value of such information in the design of prevention protocols [9]. Finally, animal studies have been found to contribute to a better understanding of the causes of bone loss, which increases the risk of fractures and morbidity. Weiser et al. reported on the effects of a combined treatment strategy (neurotrophin transplantation and bodyweight treadmill training) on bone loss in animals with T9–T19 spinal cord injury [10].

In summary, the publications in this Special Issue mark a significant step forward in the field of musculoskeletal disorders and diseases in the workplace and during leisure time, with the aim of improving people's quality of life. We would like to express our sincere gratitude to all the authors and reviewers who contributed to this Special Issue, and to the *Bioengineering* magazine team for their invaluable help and support.

Funding: This research received no external funding.

Conflicts of Interest: The author declares no conflicts of interest.

References

1. Xiang, Q.S.; Guo, S.; Wang, J.; Hashimoto, K.; Liu, Y.; Liu, L. Modeling and Analysis of Foot Function in Human Gait Using a Two-Degrees-of-Freedom Inverted Pendulum Model with an Arced Foot. *Bioengineering* **2023**, *10*, 1344. [CrossRef] [PubMed]
2. Goo, C.; Laubscher, C.A.; Wajda, D.A.; Sawicki, T.J. Preliminary Virtual Constraint-Based Control Evaluation on a Pediatric Lower-Limb Exoskeleton. *Bioengineering* **2024**, *11*, 590. [CrossRef] [PubMed]
3. Han, X.; Nishida, N.; Morita, M.; Sakai, T.; Jiang, Z. Compensation Method for Missing and Misidentified Skeletons in Nursing Care Action Assessment by Improving Spatial Temporal Graph Convolutional Networks. *Bioengineering* **2024**, *11*, 127. [CrossRef] [PubMed]
4. Gorce, P.; Jacquier-Bret, J. Musculoskeletal Disorder Risk Assessment during the Tennis Serve: Performance and Prevention. *Bioengineering* **2024**, *11*, 974. [CrossRef] [PubMed]
5. Wang, Y.; Xu, L.; Jiang, H.; Yu, L.; Wu, H.; Mei, Q. Biomechanical Effects of the Badminton Split-Step on Forecourt Lunging Footwork. *Bioengineering* **2024**, *11*, 501. [CrossRef] [PubMed]
6. Wu, C.K.; Lin, Y.C.; Chen, Y.L.; Chao, Y.P.; Hsieh, T.Y. The Influence of Dynamic Taping on Landing Biomechanics after Fatigue in Young Football Athletes: A Randomized, Sham-Controlled Crossover Trial. *Bioengineering* **2024**, *11*, 631. [CrossRef] [PubMed]
7. Liu, W.; Xu, L.; Wu, H.; Wang, Y.; Jiang, H.; Gao, Z.; Jánosi, E.; Fekete, G.; Mei, Q.; Gu, Y. Bilateral Asymmetries of Plantar Pressure and Foot Balance During Walking, Running, and Turning Gait in Typically Developing Children. *Bioengineering* **2025**, *12*, 151. [CrossRef] [PubMed]
8. Hernandez-Laredo, E.; Estévez-Pedraza, A.G.; Santiago-Fuentes, L.M.; Parra-Rodríguez, L. Optimizing Fall Risk Diagnosis in Older Adults Using a Bayesian Classifier and Simulated Annealing. *Bioengineering* **2024**, *11*, 908. [CrossRef] [PubMed]

9. Chen, Y.L.; Liao, Y.H. Differential Back Muscle Flexion–Relaxation Phenomenon in Constrained versus Unconstrained Leg Postures. *Bioengineering* **2024**, *11*, 736. [CrossRef] [PubMed]
10. Weiser, M.; Stoy, L.; Lallo, V.; Balasubramanian, S.; Singh, A. The Efficacy of Body-Weight Supported Treadmill Training and Neurotrophin-Releasing Scaffold in Minimizing Bone Loss Following Spinal Cord Injury. *Bioengineering* **2024**, *11*, 819. [CrossRef] [PubMed]

Disclaimer/Publisher's Note: The statements, opinions and data contained in all publications are solely those of the individual author(s) and contributor(s) and not of MDPI and/or the editor(s). MDPI and/or the editor(s) disclaim responsibility for any injury to people or property resulting from any ideas, methods, instructions or products referred to in the content.

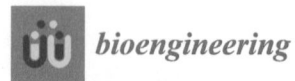

Article

Modeling and Analysis of Foot Function in Human Gait Using a Two-Degrees-of-Freedom Inverted Pendulum Model with an Arced Foot

Qian Xiang [1,2,3], Shijie Guo [1,2,3,*], Jiaxin Wang [1,2,3], Kazunobu Hashimoto [2], Yong Liu [1,2,3] and Lei Liu [1,2,3]

1. Engineering Research Center of the Ministry of Education for Intelligent Rehabilitation Equipment and Detection Technologies, Hebei University of Technology, Tianjin 300401, China; 201811201005@stu.hebut.edu.cn (Q.X.); wangjx@hebut.edu.cn (J.W.); 202131205130@stu.hebut.edu.cn (Y.L.); 202131205073@stu.hebut.edu.cn (L.L.)
2. The Hebei Key Laboratory of Robot Sensing and Human-Robot Interaction, Hebei University of Technology, Tianjin 300401, China; kazu_h@muf.biglobe.ne.jp
3. School of Mechanical Engineering, Hebei University of Technology, Tianjin 300401, China
* Correspondence: guoshijie@hebut.edu.cn

Abstract: Gait models are important for the design and control of lower limb exoskeletons. The inverted pendulum model has advantages in simplicity and computational efficiency, but it also has the limitations of oversimplification and lack of realism. This paper proposes a two-degrees-of-freedom (DOF) inverted pendulum walking model by considering the knee joints for describing the characteristics of human gait. A new parameter, roll factor, is defined to express foot function in the model, and the relationships between the roll factor and gait parameters are investigated. Experiments were conducted to verify the model by testing seven healthy adults at different walking speeds. The results demonstrate that the roll factor has a strong relationship with other gait kinematics parameters, so it can be used as a simple parameter for expressing gait kinematics. In addition, the roll factor can be used to identify walking styles with high accuracy, including small broken step walking at 99.57%, inefficient walking at 98.14%, and normal walking at 99.43%.

Keywords: human gait; walking model; inverted pendulum model; roll factor

1. Introduction

Walking is an important mode of transportation for people [1–6]. Thus, many kinds of lower limb exoskeletons that can assist in people's walking have been developed [7–14]. However, the design of the exoskeletons mostly depends on the experience of engineers due to the lack of a reasonable gait model of a human body that can be used to analyze the gait characteristics of the coupled system composed of the exoskeleton and the wearer [15–18].

Modeling human walking is complex because it is a system with multiple joints, involving multiple muscles with different functions, as well as intermittent impulsive contact with the environment. The research on the kinematics and dynamics of human gait can be divided into two categories according to the different applications of the model: biomechanics gait analysis and robotics analysis [19]. The former typically uses a musculoskeletal model to investigate the details of human gait physiology, involving a large number of variables [20–23]. The latter analyzes human gait from a mechanical perspective, treating the human body as a rigid body, in order to establish a model that can be used for exoskeleton design [24,25].

Based on the energy conversion between dynamic potential energy during walking, human gait is usually approximated as a gait with an inverted pendulum model. Cavagna et al. [26] first proposed a one-degree-of-freedom (DOF) inverted pendulum model. The 1-DOF inverted pendulum is the simplest mechanical model and has been expanded in many versions (by adding springs, dampers, and telescopic actuators) [27–36] as the research foundation, making the model more accurate in expressing human walking. The most representative one is the 1-DOF inverted pendulum proposed by Gard et al. [37] based on a rocker foot, a human wheel-like gait can be characterized by the roll factor. This model is widely used in the study of leg mechanics [38–42]. However, the disadvantages of these models are the same as those of the 1-DOF inverted pendulum model, which is simple and difficult to generate a natural and realistic gait.

In order to better reflect human walking, more segments and joints have been added to the model. The model with multiple degrees of freedom has been extensively studied, which are multi-link models [43–47]. In the earliest of these, Hanavan et al. proposed a mathematical model with 15 links connected via spherical joints [44], but it is too complicated for practical use. Although both Hurmuzlu et al. [45], Ishigaki et al. [46], and Borisov et al. [47] have made models physiologically much closer to real human walking, they still cannot avoid complex calculations. High complexity and too many calculation parameters increase the calculation time and lead to poor comfort of the exoskeleton.

This paper establishes a kinematic model with simple parameters that can effectively express human walking characteristics for the design and motion planning of lower-limb-assisted exoskeletons. A kinematic analysis is conducted on the model, and expressions for the model parameters are derived. The relationship between model parameters and important gait parameters is studied, and the correctness of the model is verified. High-precision recognition of walking mode is performed using the model parameters. Finally, the application of the model parameters in the design of lower-limb-assisted exoskeletons is introduced.

2. Methods

2.1. Gait Model

Gard's inverted pendulum model [37] is shown in Figure 1A, in which a virtual leg with length L_V is introduced, and the foot is modeled as a rocker with radius r. The ratio of the length of the virtual leg to that of the real leg is called the roll factor and can be expressed as

$$\rho_G = 1/(1 - r/L) \tag{1}$$

where ρ_G represents the roll factor of the rocker-based inverted pendulum model proposed by Gard, and L represents the length of the leg. However, Gard's model ignores the knee joints, making it unsuitable for the design of lower limb exoskeletons.

Considering the importance of the knee joint and the arced foot in human walking, we expand Gard's model to a 2-DOF model as shown in Figure 1B. The human foot structure has the structure suitable for bipedal walking. As shown in Figure 1C, the ankle joint is located approximately a quarter of the foot length from the heel [48,49]. Humans can progress forward effectively by using the foot functions of heel-rocker, ankle-rocker, forefoot-rocker, and toe-rocker, which produce a wheel-like rolling motion under the foot [50]. Based on the foot's structure and function, we model the foot as an unsymmetrical rocker to make the model more practical than Gard's model (see Figure 1B). The center of mass (COM) is regarded as the intersection point of the two legs. From the kinematic analysis of the model, the roll factor can be expressed as

$$\rho = 1 + f/(S_l - f) \tag{2}$$

where f represents the foot length, and S_l represents the step length (see Figure 1D).

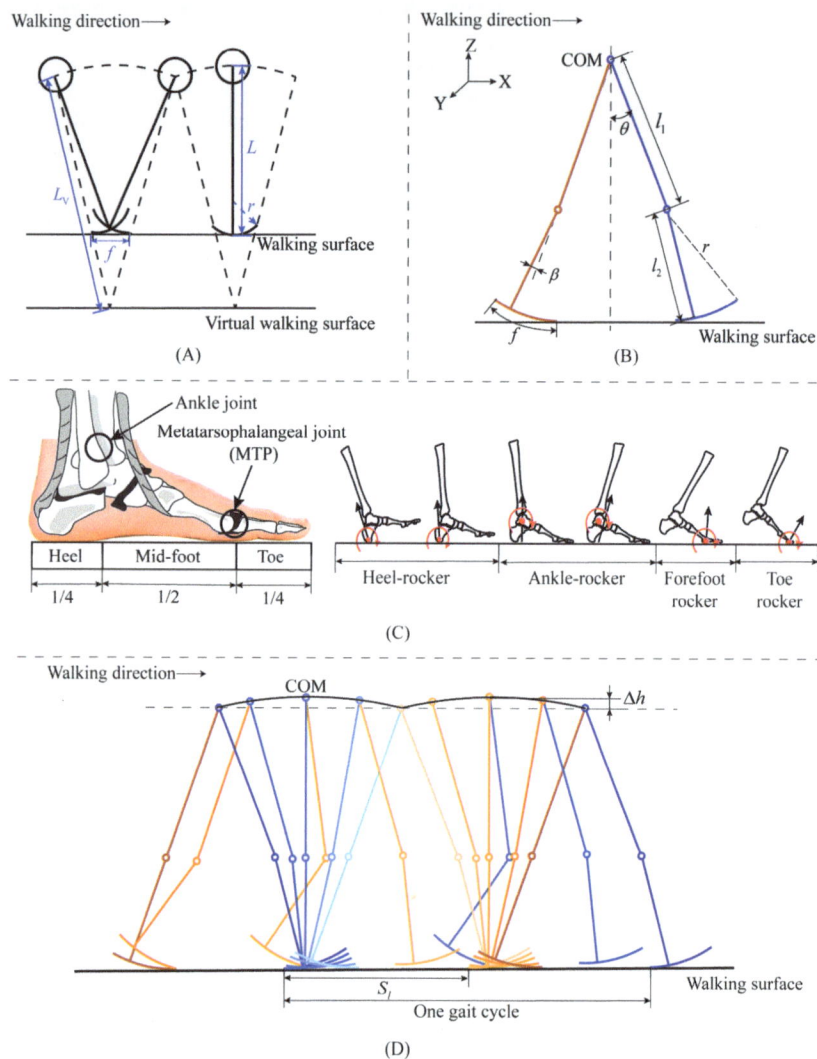

Figure 1. Rocker-based inverted pendulum model of human walk. (**A**): Gard's 1-DOF model, (**B**): the proposed 2-DOF model, (**C**): human foot structure and function, and (**D**): description of step length.

2.2. Gait Parameters

The parameters commonly used in gait analysis include step length, stride length, stride frequency, walking speed, gait cycle, gait phase, as well as the vertical excursion Δh of the COM [28,51]. From Equation (2), the step length can be expressed as

$$S_l = \rho f / (\rho - 1) \tag{3}$$

Considering a single support leg with an arced foot and a massless swing leg as shown in Figure 2, the moment balance centering at the ground contact point (GCP) (indicated by Q in Figure 2) is given with

$$\frac{d\tau}{dt} = r_{com} \times F_{com} \tag{4}$$

where τ represents the rotational momentum around point Q, and r_{com} and F_{com} represent the vector from point Q to the COM and the inertial force acting on the COM, respectively. In a stable gait during the stance phase, since the angular momentum is conserved, Equation (4) equals 0, and the equation of motion can be expressed as

$$m(g + \ddot{y}_{com})(x_{com} - x_a) = m\ddot{x}_{com}(y_{com} - y_a) \tag{5}$$

where x_{com} and y_{com} represent the position of COM in the x and y directions, g is the acceleration of gravity, and m represents the mass of the human body. Geometrically, $x_{com} - x_a$ and $y_{com} - y_a$ can be expressed as

$$x_{com} - x_a \cong -L_{iv}\theta_r' - r(\theta_r - \beta_r) \tag{6}$$

$$y_{com} - y_a = L_{iv}\cos\theta_r' \cong L_{iv} \tag{7}$$

where θ_r' represents the angle of the line of PQ from the vertical direction, L_{iv} represents the distance between point P and point Q, and θ_r and β_r represent the hip angle and the knee angle of the leading leg, respectively. The relationship between θ_r' and θ_r is $\theta_r' \cong \frac{L}{\rho L_{iv}}\theta_r + \frac{l_2-r}{L_{iv}}\beta_r$. Ignoring that β_r as the knee angle in the single leg support phase is small, Equation (5) can be simplified as

$$\ddot{\theta}_r \cong \frac{g}{L}(2-\rho)\theta_r \tag{8}$$

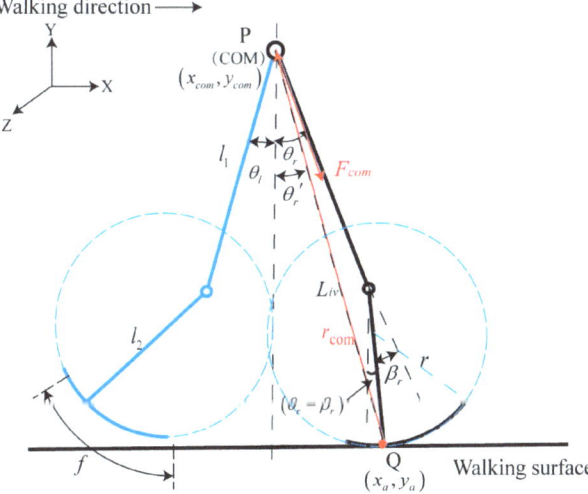

Figure 2. The moment balance centering on the point Q for the 2-DOF model.

The natural frequency of the 2-DOF inverted pendulum model is $\omega = \sqrt{(2-\rho)g/L}$, so the swing period can be expressed as $T = \sqrt{L/g}/\sqrt{2-\rho}$. The cadence (the number of steps per minute) N_C is given with

$$N_C = (1 - 2\xi)\sqrt{2-\rho}/T_0 \tag{9}$$

where ξ represents the percentage of double support in a gait cycle, which is approximately 10% in normal stable walking, and T_0 is the inherent period of the inverted pendulum, where $T_0 = \sqrt{L/g}$.

According to Equations (3) and (9), the gait speed can be expressed as

$$V = \frac{(1-2\zeta)f}{T_0} \frac{\rho\sqrt{2-\rho}}{\rho-1} \tag{10}$$

The vertical excursion of COM (Δh) is given with

$$\Delta h = L - h = L - [l_1 \cos\theta + (l_2 - r)\cos(\theta - \beta) + r] \tag{11}$$

where h represents the vertical height of the COM. According to Equation (2), Equation (11) can be expressed as

$$\Delta h = \rho f^2 / \left[8L(\rho - 1)^2\right] \tag{12}$$

As shown in Equations (3), (9), (10) and (12), the gait kinematics parameters are functions of the leg length L, the foot length f, and the roll factor ρ. Since the leg length and foot length are constant, the gait kinematics parameters are essentially functions of the roll factor ρ.

As shown in Figure 3, a gait cycle can be divided into seven phases: loading response (LR), mid-stance (MSt), terminal stance (TSt), pre-swing (PSw), initial swing (ISw), mid-swing (MSw), and terminal swing (TSw). Hip motion plays an important role when walking forward. In this figure, Hmax represents the highest point of forward flexion of the thigh, and Hmin represents the highest point of backward extension of the thigh. The two points give the thigh span during walking, which is strongly related to the step length. Kmax1 and Kmax2 represent the knee angle to achieve foot clearance at the initial swing phase and the maximum knee flexion angle, respectively. Amax1 represents the dorsiflexion angle at the heel strike, Amin1, the plantar flexion angle at the flat foot, Amax2, the dorsiflexion angle at the heel-off, and Amin2, the plantar flexion angle at the toe-off.

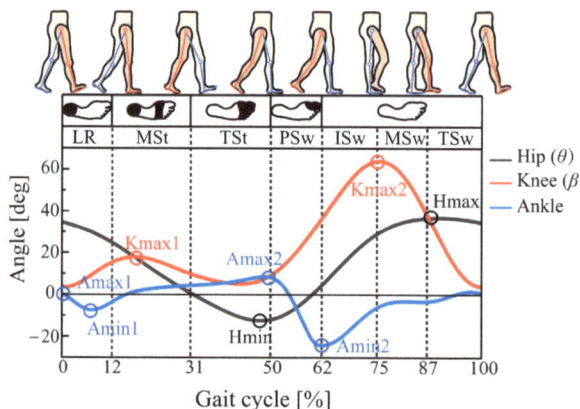

Figure 3. Gait phase division and the important characteristic points of hip, knee, and ankle joint angles.

2.3. Gait Recognition

In normal walking, the step length is always larger than the foot length. Therefore, the minimum value of the roll factor is greater than 1. On the other hand, we understand from Equation (4) that the maximum value of the roll factor is less than 2 for an inverted pendulum motion. This is described in Figure 4. An abnormal gait with a roll factor of less than 1 usually occurs in the elderly with weakened lower limb muscle strength. When the roll factor is larger than 2, the gait is inefficient. Only when the value of the roll factor is between 1 and 2 does the human body walk efficiently and stably as an inverted pendulum. Therefore, we can use the roll factor to judge the walking state of a person.

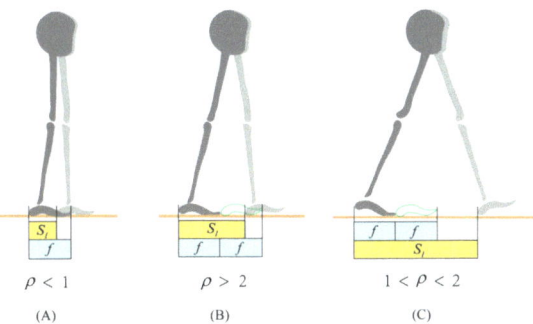

Figure 4. Walking state and roll factor. (**A**): Small broken step walking, (**B**): inefficient walking, and (**C**): inverted pendulum walking.

3. Experiment

3.1. Subjects

Seven healthy adult subjects participated in this study (age = 27.8 ± 1.7 years, height = 169.8 ± 3.4 cm, and weight = 69.9 ± 5.3 kg). Subjects were healthy and regularly participated in moderate activity. They were free of any physical condition or limitation that prevented them from walking on a treadmill.

The test was approved by the ethics committee of Hebei University of Technology, and each subject read and provided written informed consent before the test. (Ethics committee name: the Biomedical Ethics Committee of Hebei University of Technology; approval code: HEBUThMEC2023017.)

3.2. Protocol

Each subject wore specially designed sportswear with reflective markers pasted on it. To perform the motion capture, reflective markers were attached to specific anatomical areas of the lower limbs according to the plug-in gait market set [52,53]. Figure 5A presents the locations of the markers that were pasted symmetrically from left to right, and 39 markers in total were pasted onto each subject. Each subject participated in two experiments, a treadmill test for model verification and a level walk test for gait recognition, under the VICON Motion System (Oxford Metrics Limited, Oxford, UK).

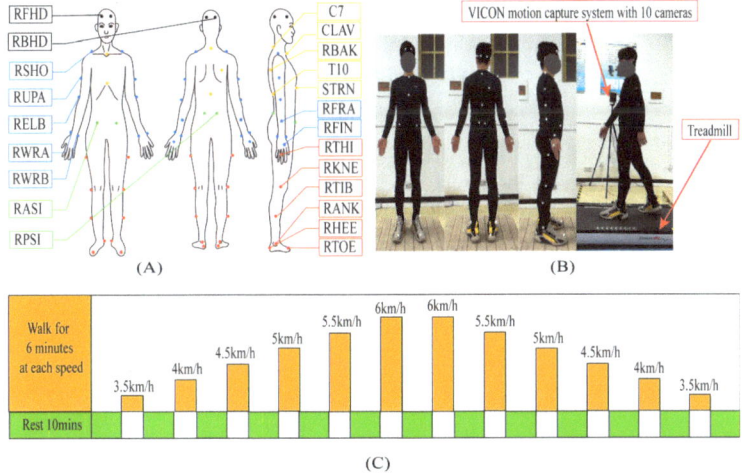

Figure 5. (**A**,**B**): Locations of reflective markers for motion capture, including 4 markers on the head (the black points); 5 markers on the trunk (the yellow points) at the 7th cervical vertebra, the 10th lumbar

vertebra, the upper end of the sternum stem, the lower end of the sternum stem, and the middle of the right scapula; 14 markers on the upper limbs (the blue points, 7 on each side); 4 markers on the pelvis (the green points) at the left and right anterior superior iliac spine and left and right posterior superior iliac spine; and 12 markers on the lower limbs (the red points, 6 on each lower limb). (**C**): Test process.

3.2.1. Treadmill Test for Model Verification

Treadmill tests were conducted at 6 different speeds: 3.5, 4.0, 4.5, 5.0, 5.5, and 6.0 km/h. The test time at each speed was set to be 6 min, and each subject was asked to take a rest of 10 min to ensure physical recovery after the 6 min test at a certain speed (see Figure 5C). The first 3 min of the 6 min test was for warming up to make the subject adapt to the treadmill walk. As shown in Figure 5C, the walking speed in the test was changed from slow to fast and then from fast to slow.

3.2.2. Level Walk Test for Gait Recognition with the 2-DOF Model

Level walk tests were conducted to investigate the usefulness of the proposed 2-DOF model in identifying different gaits. Each subject was asked to walk on the ground in three patterns for 100 steps, without any restriction on walking speed. The three patterns were abnormal small broken steps, inefficient walking, as well as normal walking. Herein inefficient walking means very slow walking with little ankle joint motion.

3.3. Data Collection and Kinematic Parameter Calculation

Data were collected at 100 Hz using the VICON Motion system (Oxford Metrics, Oxford, UK) with 10 cameras (model: VANTAGE-V5-VS-5299). The real marker trajectory data were filtered with a quintic spline filter based on code written by Herman Woltring before the modeling stage [54].

The gait cycle was calculated by taking the time difference between two consecutive heel landings of the left foot. Regarding how to recognize landing, we judged the heel landing of a foot when the marker at the heel of that foot reached its lowest position during walking. The stride was defined as the horizontal distance in the sagittal between the two heel landings, while the step length was half of the stride. The cadence was obtained by counting the number of steps in the test time (three minutes) and dividing the number by three. The vertical position of the COM and the angles of the hip, knee, and ankle joints were obtained by using the plug-in gait model in Vicon Nexus software v1.8.5. The plug-in gait model is a commonly used version of the conventional gait analysis models [55–57]. The output angles for all joints were calculated from the YXZ Cardan angles derived by comparing the relative orientations of the two segments [52].

The roll factor in the proposed 2-DOF inverted pendulum model was calculated using Equation (2), using the information of step length and foot length. The foot length of each subject was measured directly.

Using Vicon Polygon (Oxford Metrics Group, Oxford, UK) [52], kinematic data were extracted to a C3D file or ASCII file, which was then placed in MATLAB software (MATLAB 23.2.0) for post-processing.

The recognition accuracy is the walking state that correctly determines this walking state. And the error rate is other types of walking states mistaken for this walking state. The recognition accuracy and the error rate were calculated using MATLAB software to calculate the roll factor values for each step of each subject in different walking states.

3.4. Statistical Analysis

Statistical analysis was performed using the SPSS statistical software system (SPSS Inc., Chicago, IL, USA; version 22.0). Means and standard deviations for each test condition were calculated. One-way repeated measures analyses of variance with six conditions (six walking speeds) were used to verify the effect of the roll factor on step length, cadence, gait speed, and the vertical excursion of the COM, as well as the angles of the hip, knee, and ankle joints. Pairwise comparisons with Bonferroni post hoc tests were conducted to identify differences between conditions when a statistically significant main effect was identified with the one-way repeated measures analyses of variance. A paired t-test was performed to assess the difference between the roll factor and the kinematic parameters. $p < 0.05$ represented a significant difference. Linear regression and curve-fitting methods were used to fit the measurement curves of the kinematic parameters. Linear regression analyses were performed to calculate the slope of the relationship between the important characteristic points of the hip, knee, and ankle joint angles and the roll factor. The formula for calculating goodness of fit was $R^2 = ESS/TSS = 1 - RSS/TSS$. To determine the correlation strength between the calculation using the proposed 2-DOF model and the measurement, the 2-DOF model calculation and the measurement were compared using Pearson's product-moment correlation coefficients.

4. Results

4.1. Gait Analysis

The kinematic parameters of the seven subjects in the treadmill test are plotted against roll factors in Figure 6 for both measurements and calculations using the proposed 2-DOF model. The black fitting curves of the gait parameter were obtained using the measured values (black points) that were acquired from able-bodied subjects (the goodness-of-fit values were $R^2 = 0.997$, $R^2 = 0.972$, $R^2 = 0.998$, and $R^2 = 0.980$). The red fitting curves of the gait parameter were obtained using the 2-DOF inverted pendulum walk model (the goodness-of-fit values were $R^2 = 0.997$, $R^2 = 0.998$, $R^2 = 0.995$, and $R^2 = 0.998$). The model well agrees with the measurements, demonstrating the validity of the proposed model. The Pearson correlation between the model and the measurements were 0.996, 0.995, 0.998, and 0.994 for step length, cadence, gait speed, and vertical excursion of the COM, respectively ($p < 0.01$).

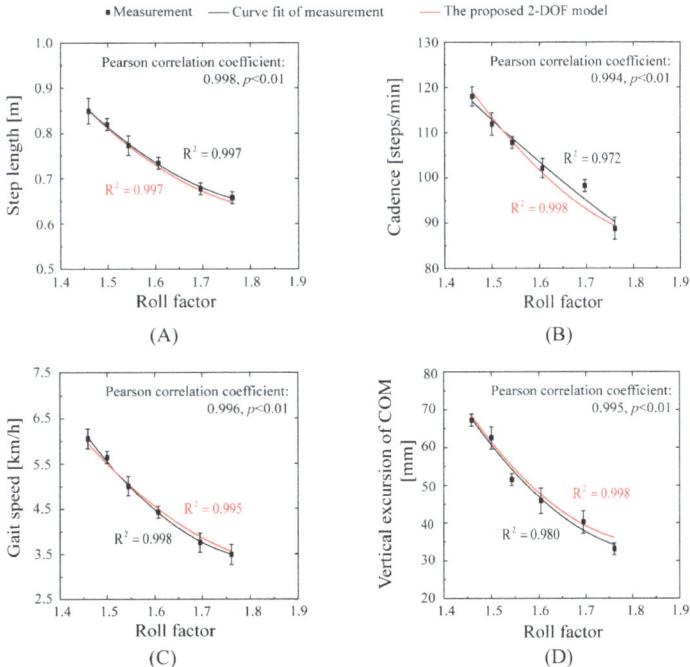

Figure 6. Gait kinematic parameters versus roll factor. (**A**): step length; (**B**): cadence; (**C**): gait speed; (**D**): vertical excursion of COM.

Figure 6 also demonstrates that the roll factor is a comprehensive parameter expressing gait kinematic parameters, including step length, cadence, gait speed, vertical excursion of the COM, etc. During normal walking, the roll factor ranged from 1.4 to 1.8, the vertical excursion of the COM ranged from 3 to 8 cm, and the value was 5 cm at the preferred gait speed.

The hip joint angles at different speeds are shown in Figure 7A. It shows that the Hmax increases with the increase in speed, although there are individual differences between different subjects. From Figure 7B,C, we know that both Hmin and Hmax have a linear relationship with the roll factor (the Hmax goodness-of-fit values are $R^2 = 0.940$, $R^2 = 0.948$, $R^2 = 0.984$, and $R^2 = 0.920$; the Hmin goodness-of-fit values are $R^2 = 0.959$, $R^2 = 0.986$, $R^2 = 0.971$, and $R^2 = 0.975$). As shown in Figure 7D, the difference between Hmax and Hmin also decreases linearly with the roll factor (the goodness-of-fit values are $R^2 = 0.943$, $R^2 = 0.942$, $R^2 = 0.991$, and $R^2 = 0.956$).

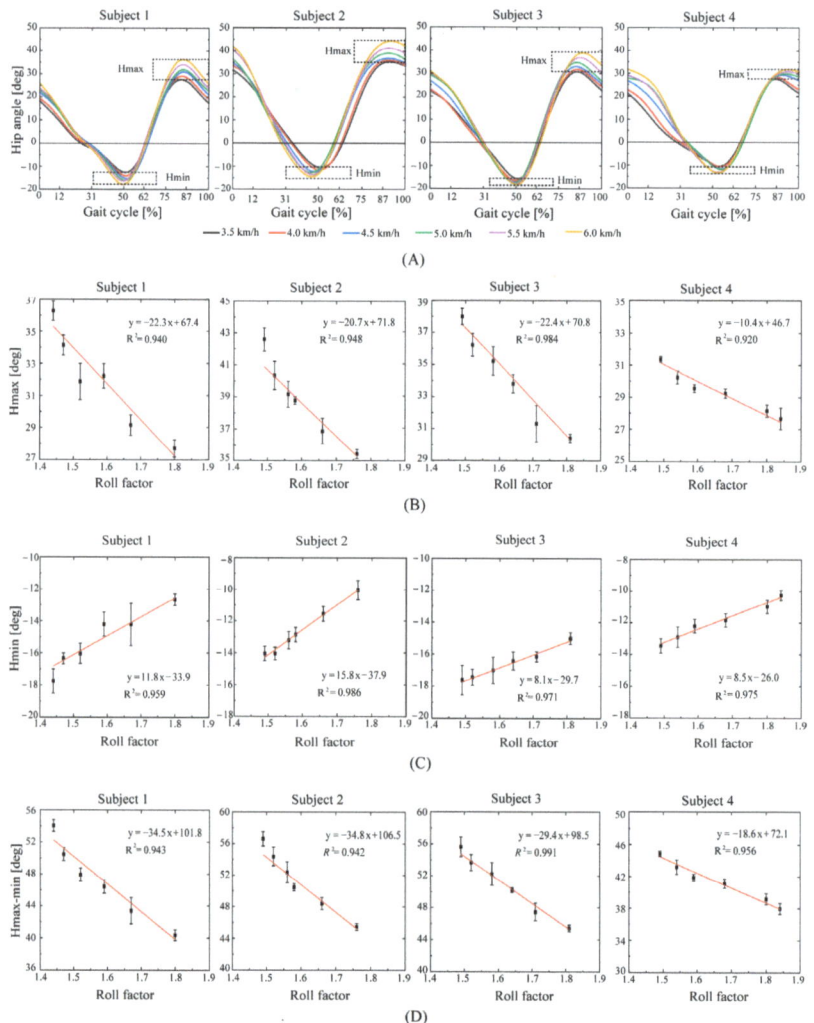

Figure 7. (**A**): The relationship between hip joint angles and roll factor. (**B**): Hmax: the highest point of forward flexion of the thigh; (**C**): Hmin: the highest point of backward extension of the thigh gait; (**D**): the thigh span during walking.

As shown in Figure 8, the knee joint angles increase with the gait speed, but both Kmax1 and Kmax2 decrease linearly with the roll factor (the Kmax1 goodness-of-fit values are $R^2 = 0.973$, $R^2 = 0.952$, $R^2 = 0.939$, and $R^2 = 0.984$; the Kmax2 goodness-of-fit values are $R^2 = 0.944$, $R^2 = 0.987$, $R^2 = 0.982$, and $R^2 = 0.992$). This figure also shows that the roll factor can be used as a factor to express knee motions during walking.

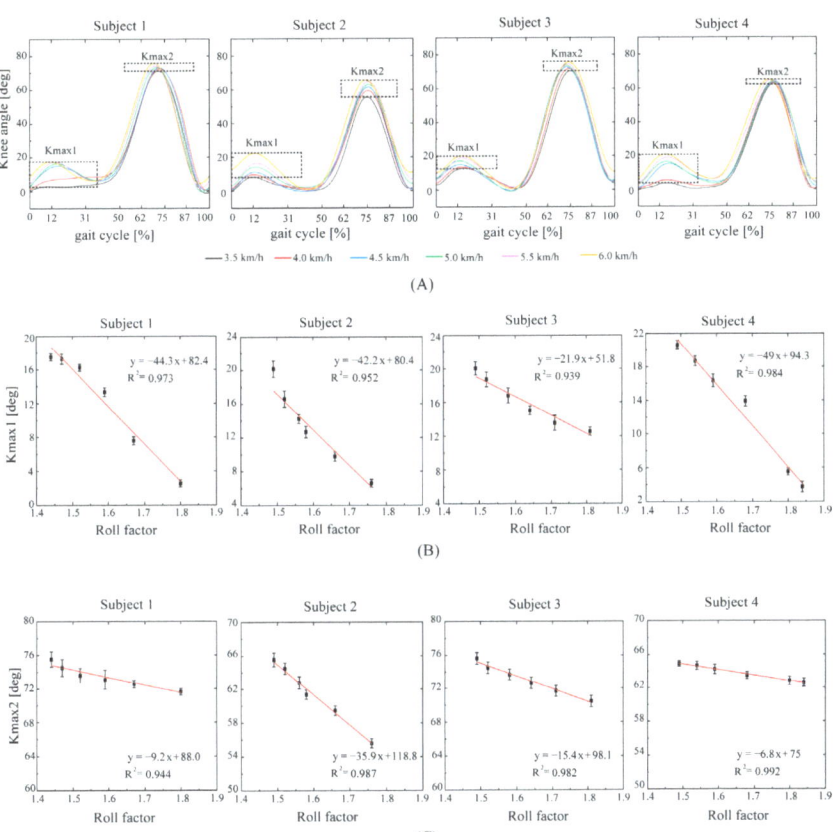

Figure 8. (**A**): The relationship between knee joint angles and the roll factor. (**B**): Kmax1: the maximum knee flexion angle; (**C**): Kmax2: the knee angle to achieve foot clearance at the initial swing phase.

Figure 9 shows that with the decrease in the roll factor, the dorsiflexion angle at heel strike (Amax1) and the plantar flexion angle at flat foot (Amin1) decrease, while the plantar flexion angle at the toe-off (Amin2) increases in the negative direction in a linear way (Figure 9B,C,E), and the dorsiflexion angle at the heel-off (Amax2) increases linearly with the roll factor (Figure 9D). The dorsiflexion angle at the heel strike (the Amax1 goodness-of-fit values are $R^2 = 0.970$, $R^2 = 0.938$, $R^2 = 0.951$, and $R^2 = 0.990$) and the plantar flexion angle at the toe-off (the Amin2 goodness-of-fit values are $R^2 = 0.942$, $R^2 = 0.953$, and $R^2 = 0.967$) have high correlation with the roll factor (Figure 8B,E). In contrast, the Amin1 (Figure 9C) and Amax2 (Figure 9D) show low goodness-of-fit values (the Amin1 goodness-of-fit values are $R^2 = 0.411$, $R^2 = 0.425$, $R^2 = 0.733$, and $R^2 = 0.527$; the Amax2 goodness-of-fit values are $R^2 = 0.006$, $R^2 = 0.112$, $R^2 = 0.668$, and $R^2 = 0.613$). This means the two values have no relationship with the roll factor.

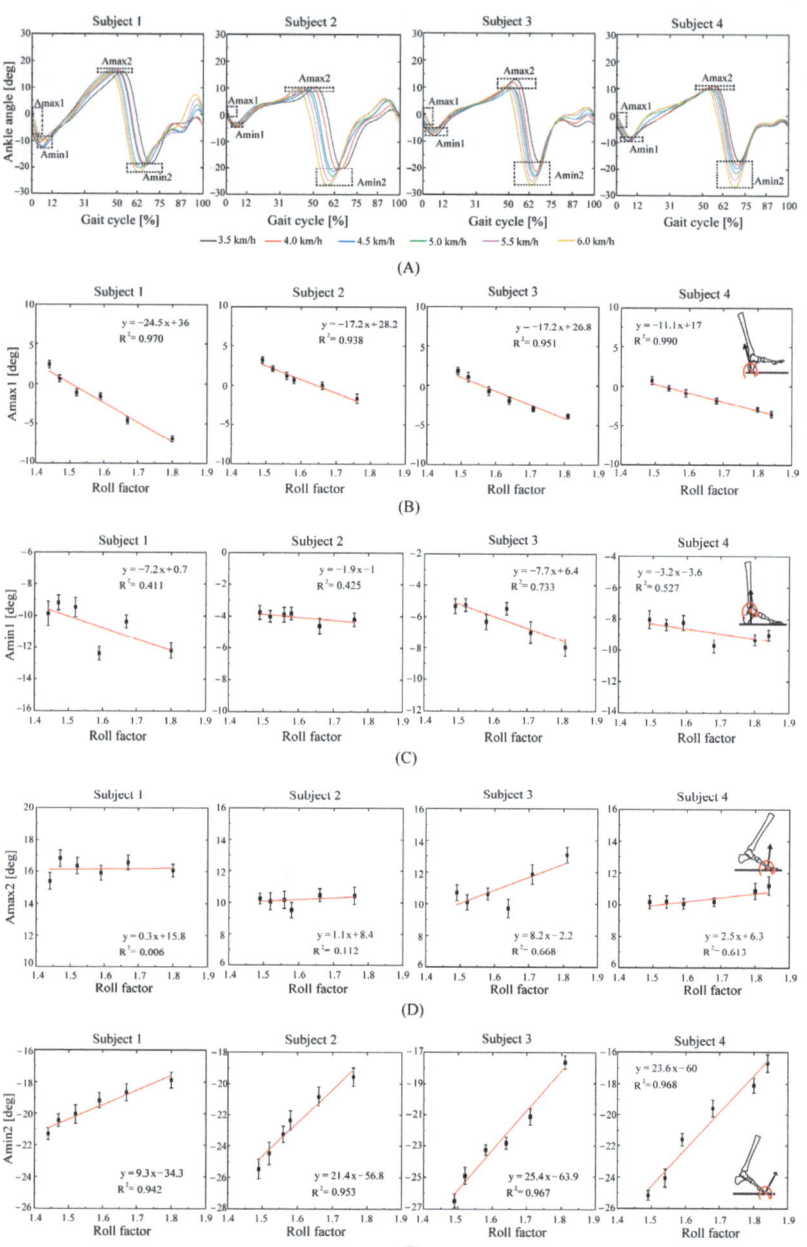

Figure 9. (**A**): The relationship between ankle joint angles and the roll factor. (**B**): Amax1: the dorsiflexion angle at the heel strike; (**C**): Amin1: the plantar flexion angle at the flat foot; (**D**): Amax2: the dorsiflexion angle at the heel-off; (**E**): Amin2: the plantar flexion angle at the toe-off.

In summary, the roll factor of the 2-DOF inverted pendulum model has a similar inverse proportion function to the gait parameters. The 2-DOF model can express the foot rocker function from heel-rocker to toe-rocker via the roll factor.

4.2. Gait Recognition

Since the roll factor has a strong relationship with the kinematics parameters, as shown in the above figures, and that its value is related to the walking style, as shown in Figure 4, we have an idea that uses the roll factor to identify walking styles. The accuracy of recognizing gait according to the value of the roll factor is given in Table 1. The average recognition accuracy for the three typical walking styles of seven subjects is 99.57%, 98.14%, and 99.43%. The results demonstrate that that the roll factor can be used as a parameter to identify walking styles.

Table 1. Recognition accuracy of the three typical walking styles.

Types	Small Broken Step Walking		Inefficient Walking		Inverted Pendulum Walking	
Subject Number	Accuracy [1] (%)	Error Rate [2] (%)	Accuracy (%)	Error Rate (%)	Accuracy (%)	Error Rate (%)
No. 1	100	0	98	0	100	1
No. 2	100	0	100	0	100	0
No. 3	99	0	98	0.5	100	1
No. 4	99	0	100	2.5	96	0
No. 5	100	0	97	0	100	1.5
No. 6	99	0	98	0.5	100	1
No. 7	100	0	96	0	100	2
Average	99.57	-	98.14	-	99.43	-

[1] The accuracy is the walking state correctly determined as this walking state. [2] The error rate is other types of walking states mistaken for this walking state.

5. Discussion

The important characteristic points of hip joint angles are Hmin and Hmax. When the Hmin feature points appear, the extension movement of the thigh reaches its maximum, and the hip flexor muscles are mainly activated, with the peak flexion torque reaching its maximum. When the hip joint rapidly flexes, there is an energy burst in the sagittal plane. At the Hmax feature point, the thigh flexes to its maximum motion, providing assurance for a sufficient step. The flexion and extension of the hip joint help advance the legs forward while maintaining balance in the body. Hmin and Hmax have a linear relationship with the roll factor (Figure 7). The roll factor can be used as an evaluation of thigh extension and flexion. This is consistent with the fact that gait may be improved through the modification of the foot rocker shape proposed by Gard et al. [37].

Knee flexion (Kmax1) provides shock absorption when a human foot follows the ground. The shock absorption is of great significance to the stability of human walking. The larger the Kmax2 flexion angle, the easier to complete the clearance of the foot contour. The effective completion of the flexion angle of the knee joint at the initial swing phase can avoid tripping over obstacles slightly higher than the ground during walking. The roll factor has a linear relationship with the flexion of the knee (Figure 8). The roll factor can be used to judge stable walking.

The four rolling functions of the foot on the ground correspond to the important characteristic points of the ankle joint angles (Amax1: heel-rocker, Amin1: ankle-rocker, Amin2: forefoot-rocker, and Amax2: toe-rocker). The push-off of the trailing leg and the heel collision of the leading leg during the double support phase are important. It can be seen in Figure 9B that the smaller the roll factor, the more obvious the heel-rocker, and the more advantageous the human gait. Human plantigrade gait combined with heel strike appears to be an adaptation for aerobics, long-distance travel, and the effective energetic costs of locomotion. We suggest the continuous use of heel-rocker walking and evaluate it with the roll factor. Figure 9E shows that the toe-rocker becomes more obvious as the roll factor decreases. The ankle joint produces the highest mechanical power with the toe-rocker, with the peak being more than three times the maximum power produced by the other joints [58]. In Figure 8, the 2-DOF model reflects the foot rocker function from heel-rocker to toe-rocker through the roll factor.

The internal factor that causes changes in the kinematic characteristic parameters of the lower limbs is the change in muscle strength. The weakening of lower limb muscle strength greatly reduces the movement of the hip, knee, and ankle joints [59–61]. The roll factor has a high linear correlation with the characteristic points of these angles, indicating that it can reflect the intensity of lower limb muscle strength.

Our study found that the roll factor can not only serve as a criterion for evaluating walking ability, but also as a parameter for adjusting the assist curve of the lower limb assist exoskeleton.

In Equation (2), the step length divided by foot length is a dimensionless ratio. This dimensionless ratio is a directly proportional function of $\rho/(\rho-1)$ (the goodness-of-fit value is $R^2 = 0.998$) (Figure 10A). Therefore, the step length is an amplification of the foot function via the roll factor. In the range of 3.5 to 6.0 km/h of walking speed, the dimensionless ratio is 2.33 to 3.48, and the longer the step length, the better the foot rolling function. Human walking involves an energy exchange between gravitational potential energy (position energy) and forward kinetic energy (motion energy). During stable walking, when the human body is in the highest vertical position, the forward speed is the lowest, and when the human body is in the lowest vertical position, the forward speed is the highest. The total mechanical energy of the human body, i.e., the sum of gravitational potential and kinetic energy, is almost constant. The vertical excursion of the COM reflects the energy conversion in the process of human walking. As shown in Figure 6D, in the range of 1.4–1.7, the smaller the roll factor, the greater the vertical excursion of the COM, and the more gravitational potential energy is converted into kinetic energy. Therefore, the energy conversion during walking can be analyzed with the roll factor, i.e., a longer effective leg length is energetically advantageous [62]. The step length has a trade-off relation with the effective leg length, and the roll factor has an optimal value for low energy consumption during walking (Figure 10B).

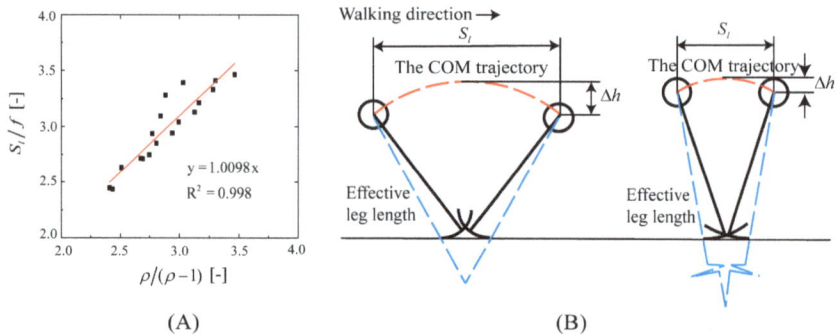

Figure 10. (**A**): The relationship between the dimensionless ratio and $\rho/(\rho-1)$; (**B**): the trade-off relationship between step length and effective leg length.

The optimal value of the roll factor for an efficient walk depends on the walking style. Human walking tends to choose a step length or step frequency that minimizes metabolic energy consumption at a given walking speed [63]. It can be seen in Figures 7–9 that at the same speed, the roll factor value of subject 4 is generally higher than that of the other three subjects. A small step length is a combination of a small hip rotation (Figure 7D), large knee flexion (Figure 8B), small ankle flexion (Figure 9B), and small ankle extension (Figure 9E). This means that as the walking speed increases, subject 4 mainly reduces the energy consumption by increasing the stride frequency.

The roll factor can be used to identify walking styles with high accuracy. Therefore, when wearing the lower-limb-assisted exoskeleton for walking, different assistance plans are carried out in different walking states. When the wearer walks with a small broken step, the exoskeleton does not provide assistance. When the wearer is in an inefficient walking state, the exoskeleton continues to increase assistance until the wearer enters an efficient walking state. After the wearer reaches an efficient walking state, the exoskeleton adjusts the assist function based on the optimal value of the roll factor to provide power that maintains high efficiency and energy conservation. In addition, with the development of rocker sole shoes [64,65], the roll factor can also be used as a method to select rocker shoes that are suitable for efficient and energy-saving walking.

6. Conclusions

This paper proposed a 2-DOF inverted pendulum walk model and defined a new parameter, roll factor, for expressing gait styles. The kinematics of human gait were investigated using this parameter. It was demonstrated that the roll factor has a strong relationship with other gait kinematics parameters, so it can be used as a simple parameter for expressing gait kinematics. In addition, the roll factor can be used to identify walking styles with high accuracy, at 99.57% for small broken step walking, at 98.14% for inefficient walking, and at 99.43% for normal walking. The roll factor can be a criterion for evaluating walking ability. In addition, it can also be a parameter for adjusting the assist function of the lower-limb-assisted exoskeleton. We will try to introduce the proposed 2-DOF inverted pendulum walk model and the defined roll factor into the design of lower limb exoskeletons in future work.

Author Contributions: Q.X.: methodology, software, investigation, formal analysis, validation, data curation, writing—original draft preparation, and writing—review and editing. S.G.: conceptualization, methodology, writing—review and editing, project administration, and funding acquisition. J.W.: writing—review and editing, project administration, and resources. K.H.: investigation and data curation. Y.L. and L.L.: data curation. All authors have read and agreed to the published version of the manuscript.

Funding: This work was supported in part by Hebei Province Key Research Projects No. 22372001D, and in part by the National Natural Science Foundation of China under grant no. 52275018 and no. 62303155.

Institutional Review Board Statement: This study was conducted in accordance with the Declaration of Helsinki and approved by the Biomedical Ethics Committee of the Hebei University of Technology in Tianjin, China. (Ethics committee name: the Biomedical Ethics Committee of Hebei University of Technology; approval code: HEBUThMEC2023017.)

Informed Consent Statement: Informed consent was obtained from all subjects involved in this study.

Data Availability Statement: The original data are available following reasonable request.

Acknowledgments: The authors are grateful to Jiaxin Wang for his technical assistance.

Conflicts of Interest: The authors declare no financial or other relationship that may cause, or are perceived to cause, conflict of interest in relation to this study.

References

1. Alves, F.; Cruz, S.; Ribeiro, A.; Silva, A.B.; Martins, J.; Cunha, I. Walkability Index for Elderly Health: A Proposal. *Sustainability* **2020**, *12*, 7360. [CrossRef]
2. Chan, E.T.H.; Li, T.E.; Schwanen, T. People and Their Walking Environments: An Exploratory Study of Meanings, Place and Times. *Int. J. Sustain. Transp.* **2021**, *15*, 718–729. [CrossRef]
3. Lee, I.M.; Buchner, D.M. The Importance of Walking to Public Health. *Med. Sci. Sport. Exerc.* **2008**, *40*, S512–S518. [CrossRef] [PubMed]
4. McDermott, M.M.; Spring, B.; Tian, L. Effect of Low-Intensity vs High-Intensity Home-Based Walking Exercise on Walk Distance in Patients with Peripheral Artery Disease: The LITE Randomized Clinical Trial. *JAMA* **2021**, *325*, 1266–1276. [CrossRef]
5. Gothe, N.P.; Ehlers, D.K.; Salerno, E.A.; Fanning, J.; Kramer, A.F.; McAuley, E. Physical Activity, Sleep and Quality of Life in Older Adults: Influence of Physical, Mental and Social Well-being. *Behav. Sleep Med.* **2019**, *18*, 797–808. [CrossRef]

6. Xiong, J.; Ye, M.; Wang, L.; Zheng, G. Effects of Physical Exercise on Executive Function in Cognitively Healthy Older Adults: A Systematic Review and Meta-Analysis of Randomized Controlled Trials: Physical Exercise for Executive Function. *Int. J. Nurs. Stud.* **2021**, *114*, 103810. [CrossRef]
7. Kalita, B.; Narayan, J.; Dwivedy, S.K. Development of Active Lower Limb Robotic-Based Orthosis and Exoskeleton Devices: A Systematic Review. *Int. J. Soc. Robot.* **2021**, *13*, 775–793. [CrossRef]
8. Plaza, A.; Hernandez, M.; Puyuelo, G. Lower-Limb Medical and Rehabilitation Exoskeletons: A Review of the Current Designs. *IEEE Rev. Biomed. Eng.* **2021**, *16*, 278–291. [CrossRef] [PubMed]
9. Rodríguez, F.A.; Lobo, P.J.; Font, L.J.M. Systematic Review on Wearable Lower-Limb Exoskeletons for Gait Training in Neuromuscular Impairments. *J. Neuroeng. Rehabil.* **2021**, *18*, 22. [CrossRef] [PubMed]
10. Miller, T.M.; Natividad, R.F.; Lim, D.Y.L. A Wearable Soft Robotic Exoskeleton for Hip Flexion Rehabilitation. *Front. Robot. AI* **2022**, *9*, 835237. [CrossRef]
11. Kapsalyamov, A.; Jamwal, P.K.; Hussain, S.; Ghayesh, M.H. State of the Art Lower Limb Robotic Exoskeletons for Elderly Assistance. *IEEE Access* **2019**, *7*, 95075–95086. [CrossRef]
12. Wang, T.; Zhang, B.; Liu, C.; Liu, T.; Han, Y.; Wang, S.; Ferreira, J.P.; Dong, W.; Zhang, X. A Review on the Rehabilitation Exo-skeletons for the Lower Limbs of the Elderly and the Disabled. *Electronics* **2022**, *11*, 388. [CrossRef]
13. Viteckova, S.; Kutilek, P.; Jirina, M. Wearable Lower Limb Robotics: A review. *Biocybern. Biomed. Eng.* **2013**, *33*, 96–105. [CrossRef]
14. Zhou, J.; Yang, S.; Xue, Q. Lower Limb Rehabilitation Exoskeleton Robot: A review. *Adv. Mech. Eng.* **2021**, *13*, 16878140211011862. [CrossRef]
15. Vidal, A.P.; Morales, J.R.; Torres, G.O.; Vázquez, F.S.; Rojas, A.C.; Mendoza, J.B.; Cerda, J.R. Soft Exoskeletons: Development, Requirements, and Challenges of the Last Decade. *Actuators* **2021**, *10*, 166. [CrossRef]
16. Baud, R.; Manzoori, A.R.; Ijspeert, A.; Bouri, M. Review of Control Strategies for Lower-Limb Exoskeletons to Assist Gait. *J. Neuroeng. Rehabil.* **2021**, *18*, 119. [CrossRef]
17. Chinmilli, P.; Redkar, S.; Zhang, W. A Review on Wearable Inertial Tracking Based Human Gait Analysis and Control Strategies of Lower-Limb Exoskeletons. *Int. Robot. Autom. J.* **2017**, *3*, 398–415.
18. Kolaghassi, R.; Al-Hares, M.K.; Sirlantzis, K. Systematic Review of Intelligent Algorithms in Gait Analysis and Prediction for Lower Limb Robotic systems. *IEEE Access* **2021**, *9*, 113788–113812. [CrossRef]
19. Xiang, Y.J.; Arora, J.S.; Karim, A.M. Physics-Based Modeling and Simulation of Human Walking: A Review of Optimization-Based and Other Approaches. *Struct. Multidisc. Optim.* **2010**, *42*, 1–23. [CrossRef]
20. Rajagopal, A.; Dembia, C.; Demers, M.; Delp, D.; Hicks, J.; Delp, S. Full-Body Musculoskeletal Model for Muscle-Driven Simulation of Human Gait. *IEEE Trans. Biomed. Eng.* **2016**, *63*, 2068–2079. [CrossRef]
21. Sylvester, A.D.; Lautzenheiser, S.G.; Kramer, P.A. A Review of Musculoskeletal Modelling of Human Locomotion. *Interface Focus* **2021**, *11*, 20200060. [CrossRef] [PubMed]
22. Grabke, E.P.; Masani, K.; Andrysek, J. Lower Limb Assistive Device Design Optimization Using Musculoskeletal Modeling: A Review. *J. Med. Devices* **2019**, *13*, 040801. [CrossRef]
23. Yu, J.; Zhang, S.; Wang, A.; Li, W.; Song, L. Musculoskeletal modeling and humanoid control of robots based on human gait data. *PeerJ Comput. Sci.* **2021**, *7*, e657. [CrossRef] [PubMed]
24. Schiehlen, W. Human Walking Dynamics: Modeling, Identification and Control. In Proceedings of the MATEC Web of Conferences, CSNDD 2014-International Conference on Structural Nonlinear Dynamics and Diagnosis, Agadir, Morocco, 19–21 May 2014; Volume 16, p. 05008.
25. Sun, C.; Wu, Q.; Zhang, K.; Li, H. A Simulation Method for Walking Gait of Human Daily Activity Oriented on Intelligent Artificial Limbs and Exoskeleton. In Proceedings of the 5th Annual IEEE International Conference on Cyber Technology in Automation 2015, Control and Intelligent Systems, Shenyang, China, 6–10 June 2015.
26. Cavagna, G.A.; Heglund, N.C.; Taylor, C.R. Mechanical Work in Terrestrial Locomotion: Two Basic Mechanisms for Minimizing Energy Expenditure. *Am. J. Physiol.* **1977**, *235*, R243–R261. [CrossRef]
27. Buczek, F.L.; Cooney, K.M.; Walker, M.R.; Rainbow, M.J.; Concha, M.C.; Sanders, J.O. Performance of an Inverted Pendulum Model Directly Applied to Normal Human Gait. *Clin. Bio.* **2006**, *21*, 288–296. [CrossRef]
28. Kuo, A.D. The Six Determinants of Gait and the Inverted Pendulum Analogy: A Dynamic Walking Perspective. *Hum. Mov. Sci.* **2007**, *26*, 617–656. [CrossRef]
29. Martin, A.E.; Schmiedeler, J.P. Predicting Human Walking Gaits with a Simple Planar Model. *J. Biomech.* **2014**, *47*, 1416–1421. [CrossRef]
30. McGrath, M.; Howard, D.; Baker, R. A Forward Dynamic Modelling Investigation of Cause-and-Effect Relationships in Single Support Phase of Human Walking. *Comput. Math. Methods Med.* **2015**, *2015*, 383705. [CrossRef]
31. Hong, H.; Kim, S.; Kim, C.; Lee, S.; Park, S. Spring-Like Gait Mechanics Observed During Walking in Both Young and Older Adults. *J. Biomech.* **2013**, *46*, 77–82. [CrossRef]
32. Koolen, T.; Boer, T.D.; Rebula, J.; Goswami, A.; Pratt, J. Capturability-Based Analysis and Control of Legged Locomotion, Part 1: Theory and Application to Three Simple Gait Models. *Int. J. Robot. Res.* **2012**, *31*, 1094–1113. [CrossRef]
33. Shahbazi, M.; Babuska, R.; Lopes, G.A.D. Unified Modeling and Control of Walking and Running on the Spring-Loaded Inverted Pendulum. *IEEE Trans. Robot.* **2016**, *32*, 1178–1195. [CrossRef]

34. Srinivasan, M. Fifteen Observations on the Structure of Energy-Minimizing Gaits in Many Simple Biped Models. *J. R. Soc. Interface* **2010**, *8*, 74–98. [CrossRef] [PubMed]
35. Lim, H.; Park, S. Kinematics of Lower Limbs During Walking Are Emulated by Springy Walking Model with a Compliantly Connected, Off-Centered Curvy Foot. *J. Biomech.* **2018**, *71*, 119–126. [CrossRef]
36. Lim, H.; Park, S. A Bipedal Compliant Walking Model Generates Periodic Gait Cycles with Realistic Swing Dynamics. *J. Biomech.* **2019**, *91*, 79–84. [CrossRef]
37. Gard, S.A.; Childress, D.S. What Determines the Vertical Displacement of the Body During Normal Walking. *J. Prosthet. Orthot.* **2001**, *13*, 64–67. [CrossRef]
38. Faraji, S.; Ijspeert, A.J. 3LP: A Linear 3D-Walking Model Including Torso and Swing Dynamics. *Int. J. Robot. Res.* **2017**, *36*, 436–455. [CrossRef]
39. Kuo, A.D.; Donelan, J.M. Dynamic Principles of Gait and Their Clinical Implications. *Phys. Ther.* **2010**, *90*, 157–174. [CrossRef]
40. Lin, B.; Zhang, Q.; Fan, F.; Shen, S. A damped bipedal inverted pendulum for human–structure interaction analysis. *Appl. Math. Model.* **2020**, *87*, 606–624. [CrossRef]
41. Yang, H.; Wu, B.; Li, J.; Bao, Y.; Xu, G. A Spring-Loaded Inverted Pendulum Model for Analysis of Human-Structure Interaction on Vibrating Surfaces. *J. Sound Vib.* **2022**, *522*, 116727. [CrossRef]
42. Lin, B.; Zivanovic, S.; Zhang, Q.; Fan, F. Implementation of Damped Bipedal Inverted Pendulum Model of Pedestrian into FE Environment for Prediction of Vertical Structural Vibration. *Structures* **2023**, *48*, 523–532. [CrossRef]
43. Zhu, A.; Shen, Z.; Shen, H.; Wu, H.; Zhang, X. Design of a Passive Weight-Support Exoskeleton of Human-Machine Multi-Link. In Proceedings of the 2018 15th International Conference on Ubiquitous Robots (UR), Honolulu, HI, USA, 26–30 June 2018; IEEE: Piscatvey, NJ, USA, 2018; pp. 296–301.
44. Hanavan, E.P. *A Mathematical Model of the Human Body*; Technical Report Amrl.; Aerospace Medical Research Laboratories, Aerospace Medical Division, Air Force Systems Command: Dayton, OH, USA, 1964; pp. 64–102.
45. Hurmuzlu, Y.; Genot, F.; Brogliato, B. Modeling, Stability and Control of Biped Robots a General Framework. *Automatica* **2004**, *40*, 1647–1664. [CrossRef]
46. Ishigaki, T.; Yamamoto, K. Dynamics Computation of a Hybrid Multi-Link Humanoid Robot Intergrating Rigid and Soft Bodies. In Proceedings of the 2021 IEEE/RSJ International Conference on Intelligent Robots and Systems (IROS), Prague, Czech Republic, 27 September–1 October 2021; pp. 2816–2821.
47. Borisov, A.V.; Kaspirovich, I.E.; Mukharlyamov, R.G. On Mathematical Modeling of the Dynamics of Multilink Systems and Exoskeletons. *J. Comput. Sys. Sci. Int.* **2021**, *60*, 827–841. [CrossRef]
48. Usherwood, J.R. The Collisional Geometry of Economical Walking Predicts Human Leg and Foot Segment Proportions. *J. R. Soc. Interface* **2023**, *20*, 20220800. [CrossRef] [PubMed]
49. Farris, D.J.; Kelly, L.A.; Cresswell, A.G. The Functional Importance of Human Foot Muscles for Bipedal Locomotion. *Proc. Natl. Acad. Sci. USA* **2019**, *116*, 1645–1650. [CrossRef]
50. Perry, J.; Burnfield, J.M. *Gait Analysis: Normal and Pathological Function*, 2nd ed.; SLACK Incorporated: Thorofare, NJ, USA, 2010.
51. Jeong, B.; Ko, C.Y.; Chang, Y.; Ryu, J.; Kim, G. Comparison of Segmental Analysis and Sacral Marker Methods for Determining the Center of Mass During Level and Slope Walking. *Gait Posture* **2018**, *62*, 333–341. [CrossRef]
52. Vicon Documentation. Available online: https://docs.vicon.com/display/Nexus25/Plug-in+Gait+kinematic+variables (accessed on 20 March 2020).
53. Pfister, A.; West, A.M.; Bronner, S. Comparative Abilities of Microsoft Kinect and Vicon 3D Motion Capture for Gait Analysis. *J. Med. Eng. Technol.* **2014**, *38*, 274–280. [CrossRef]
54. Van, D.B.T. Practical Guide to Data Smoothing and Filtering. 1996, pp. 1–6. Available online: http://isbweb.org/software/sigproc/bogert/filter.pdf (accessed on 31 October 1996).
55. Schwartz, M.H.; Trost, J.P.; Wervey, R.A. Measurement and Management of Errors in Quantitative Gait Data. *Gait Posture* **2004**, *20*, 196–203. [CrossRef]
56. Wright, C.; Seitz, A.L.; Arnold, B.L. Repeatability of Ankle Joint Kinematic Data at Heel Strike Using the Vicon Plug-In Gait model. Available online: https://www.researchgate.net/publication/268380486 (accessed on 16 January 2011).
57. Webber, J.T.; Raichlen, D.A. The Role of Plantigrady and Heel-Strike in the Mechanics and Energetics of Human Walking with Implications for the Evolution of the Human Foot. *J. Exp. Biol.* **2016**, *219*, 3729–3737. [CrossRef]
58. Zhang, J.; Si, Y.; Zhang, Y.; Liu, Y. The Effects of Restricting the Flexion-Extension Motion of the First Metatarsophalangeal Joint on Human Walking Gait. *Bio-Med. Mater. Eng.* **2014**, *24*, 2577–2584. [CrossRef]
59. Khalaj, N.; Vicenzino, B.; Heales, L.J.; Smith, M.D. Is Chronic Ankle Instability Associated with Impaired Muscle Strength? Ankle, Knee and Hip Muscle Strength in Individuals with Chronic Ankle Instability: A Systematic Review with Meta-analysis. *Br. J. Sports Med.* **2020**, *54*, 839–847. [CrossRef] [PubMed]
60. Kim, S.H.; Kwon, O.Y.; Park, K.N.; Jeon, I.C.; Weon, J.H. Lower Extremity Strength and the Range of Motion in Relation to Squat Depth. *J. Hum. Kinet.* **2015**, *45*, 59–69. [CrossRef]
61. Wu, R.; Zhang, Y.; Bai, J.J.; Sun, J.; Bao, Z.J.; Wang, Z. Impact of Lower Limb Muscle Strength on Walking Function Beyond Aging and Diabetes. *J. Int. Med. Res.* **2020**, *48*, 1–9. [CrossRef]
62. Adamczyk, P.G.; Collins, S.H.; Kuo, A.D. The Advantages of a Rolling Foot in Human Walking. *J. Exp. Biol.* **2006**, *209*, 3953–3963. [CrossRef] [PubMed]

63. Kim, J.; Lee, G.; Heimgartner, R.; Revi, D.A.; Karavas, N.; Nathanson, D.; Galiana, I.; Eckert-Erdheim, A.; Murphy, P.; Perry, D.; et al. Reducing the Metabolic Rate of Walking and Running with a Versatile, Portable Exosuit. *Science* **2019**, *365*, 668–672. [CrossRef] [PubMed]
64. Song, Y.; Cen, X.; Zhang, Y. Development and Validation of A Subject-Specific Coupled Model for Foot and Sports Shoe Complex: A Pilot Computational Study. *Bioengineering* **2022**, *9*, 553. [CrossRef] [PubMed]
65. Farzad, M.; Safaeepour, Z.; Nabavi, H. Effect of Different Placement of Heel Rockers on Lower-Limb Joint Biomechanics in Healthy Individuals. *J. Am. Podiatr. Med. Assoc.* **2018**, *108*, 231–235. [CrossRef]

Disclaimer/Publisher's Note: The statements, opinions and data contained in all publications are solely those of the individual author(s) and contributor(s) and not of MDPI and/or the editor(s). MDPI and/or the editor(s) disclaim responsibility for any injury to people or property resulting from any ideas, methods, instructions or products referred to in the content.

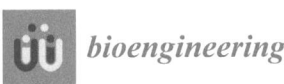

Article

Preliminary Virtual Constraint-Based Control Evaluation on a Pediatric Lower-Limb Exoskeleton

Anthony C. Goo [1], Curt A. Laubscher [2], Douglas A. Wajda [3] and Jerzy T. Sawicki [1,*]

[1] Center for Rotating Machinery Dynamics and Control (RoMaDyC), Washkewicz College of Engineering, Cleveland State University, Cleveland, OH 44115, USA; a.goo@vikes.csuohio.edu

[2] Department of Robotics, Michigan Engineering, University of Michigan Ann Arbor, Ann Arbor, MI 48109, USA; claub@umich.edu

[3] Department of Health Sciences and Human Performance, College of Health, Cleveland State University, Cleveland, OH 44115, USA; d.a.wajda@csuohio.edu

* Correspondence: j.sawicki@csuohio.edu

Abstract: Pediatric gait rehabilitation and guidance strategies using robotic exoskeletons require a controller that encourages user volitional control and participation while guiding the wearer towards a stable gait cycle. Virtual constraint-based controllers have created stable gait cycles in bipedal robotic systems and have seen recent use in assistive exoskeletons. This paper evaluates a virtual constraint-based controller for pediatric gait guidance through comparison with a traditional time-dependent position tracking controller on a newly developed exoskeleton system. Walking experiments were performed with a healthy child subject wearing the exoskeleton under proportional-derivative control, virtual constraint-based control, and while unpowered. The participant questionnaires assessed the perceived exertion and controller usability measures, while sensors provided kinematic, control torque, and muscle activation data. The virtual constraint-based controller resulted in a gait similar to the proportional-derivative controlled gait but reduced the variability in the gait kinematics by 36.72% and 16.28% relative to unassisted gait in the hips and knees, respectively. The virtual constraint-based controller also used 35.89% and 4.44% less rms torque per gait cycle in the hips and knees, respectively. The user feedback indicated that the virtual constraint-based controller was intuitive and easy to utilize relative to the proportional-derivative controller. These results indicate that virtual constraint-based control has favorable characteristics for robot-assisted gait guidance.

Keywords: gait; exoskeletons; virtual constraint control; pediatric

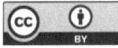

1. Introduction

A lower-limb exoskeleton is a wearable robotic device that provides assistive torque to the joints of the wearer's legs. In medical contexts, exoskeletons can be used to assist or rehabilitate the motion of individuals dealing with gait impairment through robotic-assisted gait training (RAGT). RAGT has been suggested as an alternative or complementary solution to traditional physical therapy options and bodyweight-supported treadmill training. The introduction of a robotic device to guide the gait pattern decreases the physical demands on the physical therapist and offers increased robotic accuracy and controllability to the walking task [1,2]. Previous studies have shown that RAGT can increase the wearer's average walking speed, distance, balance, and other mobility measures [3,4]. Studies have also demonstrated that RAGT can improve the range of motion, increase muscle strength, and decrease spasticity for pediatric subjects with cerebral palsy [5–7].

While children with gait impairments stand to benefit from RAGT, most commercially available exoskeletons are adult-oriented [8,9] and are not designed to serve the pediatric population [10]. Representative pediatric devices currently include the pediatric Lokomat [11], the Trexo robotic walker [12], the very small-sized Hybrid Assistive Limb (2S-HAL) [13], the ATLAS 2020 and 2030 [7,14], the MOTION exoskeleton by

Zhang et al. [15], and the exoskeletons developed by Lerner et al. at the NIH [5]. Of the pediatric devices that do exist, few devices combine the characteristics of a lightweight form factor, community setting mobility, adjustability, and ease of use. Previously, the authors created an anthropometrically parametrized exoskeleton [16], and recently introduced the Cleveland State University (CSU) adjustable pediatric exoskeleton [17,18]. Preliminary human factor testing with the new device demonstrated that the exoskeleton was suitable for preliminary control testing with pediatric subjects [19].

Identifying an appropriate controller for medical exoskeletons remains a challenge, in large part due to the diversity of gait impairment pathologies. The therapeutic objective for those who need walking assistance due to severe neurological injury differs greatly from those seeking gait rehabilitation and guidance, such as individuals recovering from stroke [20]. In this manuscript, the authors wish to investigate controllers suitable for gait guidance and rehabilitation. A common strategy for exoskeleton control includes time-dependent, position tracking controllers such as proportional-derivative (PD) and proportional-integral-derivative (PID) controllers [21–23]. Closely related time-dependent controllers include impedance controllers, which improve human–robot interaction safety by introducing compliant behavior between the wearer and the exoskeleton through model-based control [24,25]. Relevant examples include the LOPES robot by van der Kooij et al. [26], the knee device by Aguirre-Ollinger et al. [27], and the impedance control law used by Tran et al. on the HUALEX [28]. These controllers oftentimes utilize nominal human walking patterns from sources like Winter et al. [29] or Schwartz [30], to define the desired joint motion reference and spatiotemporal gait parameters. However, while time-dependent trajectory tracking controllers are effective at matching a gait pattern and are easy to implement, the strict timing nature can disincentivize user participation in the walking cycle, leading to patient passivity [31,32]. This in turn can lead to less efficient therapy sessions and inconclusive rehabilitation results. Other manuscripts have noted that the strict regulation of gait, especially timing, can lead to gait destabilization [33]. This aligns with the "guidance hypothesis", which predicts that feedback can negatively impact motor learning and rehabilitation when heavily relied upon to complete that learned action [34]. Additionally, these time-dependent trajectory tracking controllers also risk gait desynchronization between the walking cycle of the controller and the intended gait of the wearer. This often results in the user fighting the exoskeleton controller and can lead to gait instability and potential falls. Thus, while these controllers are useful for walking assistance purposes, they are oftentimes not suitable for gait rehabilitation.

The shortcomings of strict time-dependent position controllers for rehabilitation purposes have encouraged the exploration of patient-cooperative and time-independent controllers. A prominent example of these are the "virtual tunnel" controllers utilized by the ALEX [3] and Lokomat [35] exoskeletons. These controllers are designed to provide restorative inputs when a patient deviates from the desired gait pattern by a certain threshold. The ALEX's force-field controller aims to guide the motion of a user's ankle [3], while the Lokomat's path control mode focuses on the overall leg posture through the gait cycle [35]. A continuation of this control methodology can be found in the paper by Martínez et al. [36], which utilizes force-field controllers to guide a lower leg exoskeleton during the swing phase. These controllers enable the wearer's volitional control over the gait cycle and encourage their active participation in the walking activity. They have also been implemented in both time-dependent and -independent formulations. However, while the increased level of volitional control over the gait cycle encourages rehabilitation and user participation in the exercise, it only indirectly encourages a user's dynamic stability during gait.

Recent advances in the control of bipedal robotic systems have yielded a new control methodology in virtual constraint-based controllers, also commonly referred to as hybrid zero dynamic controllers. These controllers enforce relationships between the system's joints such that the biped walker becomes virtually constrained to walk in a certain pattern [37]. The strategic definition and optimization of these virtual constraints, which evolve with respect to the gait phase, can promote a dynamically stable gait for biped systems within their zero dynamics. These controllers can also be implemented in time-invariant formulations by representing the gait phase as a configuration-dependent variable. Extended to exoskeletal systems, these controllers drive the wearer towards the stable gait cycle defined by the virtual constraints, while leaving progression through the gait cycle dependent on the volitional control and effort exerted by the user. While originally implemented in fully robotic bipedal systems in [38–41], virtual constraint-based controllers have begun to see use in both prosthetic and exoskeletal devices [42–44]. Most of these applications, however, are focused on walking assistance for paraplegic patients instead of gait rehabilitation objectives [42,43]. To the author's knowledge, there have been few studies looking to evaluate virtual constraint-based controllers for gait guidance and rehabilitation.

In this manuscript, the authors aim to preliminarily evaluate a virtual constraint-based controller for gait guidance by performing a comparison to time-dependent proportional-derivative control in treadmill walking experiments. Both the virtual constraint and proportional-derivative controllers utilize identical control gains and gait references to increase comparability. The two controllers are evaluated with respect to the kinetic and kinematic effects of the controllers on the subject's gait, the subject's muscle effort quantified through electromyography (EMG), and the subject's perceived effort and controller preferences as indicated through questionnaires. The authors hypothesize the following:

- The two controllers will have comparable kinematics due to their similar error-based architecture and comparable control gains;
- The virtual constraint-based controller will demonstrate less gait pattern variability due to the lower risk of gait desynchronization;
- The virtual constraint-based controller will be preferred over the proportional-derivative controller due to its time-independent nature and lack of step timing restrictions.

This work builds upon the authors' previous work on virtual constraint-based controllers for gait guidance [45,46] by applying a virtual constraint-based controller on a newly developed pediatric exoskeleton system with an able-bodied child subject. This manuscript demonstrates the adjustable pediatric lower-limb exoskeleton's ability to serve as an investigative platform for future gait assistance and rehabilitation control experiments. Thus, the contributions of this manuscript are as follows:

- A preliminary evaluation of virtual constraint-based control for gait guidance by performing a comparison to a more commonly applied time-dependent proportional-derivative controller;
- The demonstration and first application of control on the CSU adjustable pediatric exoskeleton in gait experiments.

The successful implementation of virtual constraint-based control on the exoskeletal system for gait guidance purposes represents an initial motivating step towards larger-scale rehabilitative control studies involving children with gait disabilities. The remainder of the manuscript is split into the following sections. Section 2 details the materials and test facility used in the gait experiments performed in this work. Section 3 details the controller implementations used in this control comparison. Section 4 discusses the experimental procedure. Section 5 presents and discusses the experimental results. Finally, Section 6 consists of the conclusion and points out avenues for future work.

2. Hardware and Facilities

2.1. Adjustable Pediatric Lower-Limb Exoskeleton

The CSU adjustable pediatric exoskeleton provides supplementary torques at the hip and knee joints of the wearer through 144 W brushless DC motors, scaled through a 20.4:1 two-stage belt and chain transmission. The modular actuators can apply up to 5.9 Nm of continuous torque, have been tested to up to 21.1 Nm peak torque, and have a theoretical peak torque of 46.9 Nm. Previous evaluations indicated that the actuators were lightweight, low-friction, and easily backdrivable at the output, making them appropriate for use in a pediatric lower-limb exoskeleton [17]. These actuators were placed into an adjustable pediatric exoskeleton frame designed for children between 6 and 11 years old [18], resulting in the 4.72 kg exoskeleton shown in Figure 1.

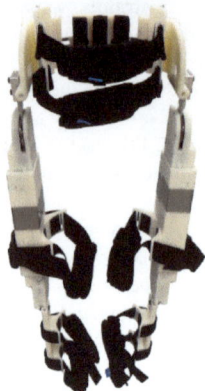

Figure 1. CSU adjustable pediatric exoskeleton.

The ranges of adjustability were determined from estimated limb lengths and widths of children within the target age group, derived from anthropometric averages [47] and census data [48]. For a more detailed discussion of the exoskeleton device and joint actuators, see [17,18]. A preliminary human factor assessment with the unpowered adjustable pediatric exoskeleton and a healthy, 30.8 kg, and 149 cm tall child volunteer subject demonstrated that the hardware was comfortable, easily adjustable, and simple to don and doff [19]. The exoskeleton can provide a measurement of the relative joint angles and velocities for the hips with respect to the torso and the knees with respect to the thigh for both legs through the Hall effect and magnetic angle sensors. A SEN-10736 (Sparkfun Electronics, Boulder, CO, USA) nine-degree-of-freedom inertial measurement unit (IMU) is affixed to the hip cradle to provide angular position and velocity measurements of the torso relative to the gravity vector. The measurement convention for the human–exoskeleton system is shown in Figure 2, with the clockwise rotations in the figure representing positive rotations.

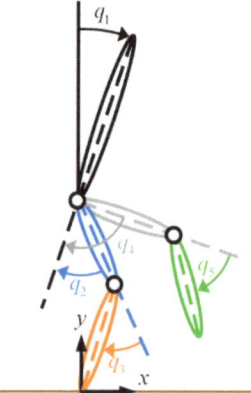

Figure 2. The measurement convention for the exoskeleton system and the controllers discussed. Hip extension and knee flexion correspond to positive values. The horizontal brown line denotes the location of the ground.

2.2. Treadmill, Sensors, and Data Collection

The gait experiments in this manuscript were performed on an R-Mill instrumented split belt treadmill (Motekforce Link, Amsterdam, The Netherlands), shown in Figure 3.

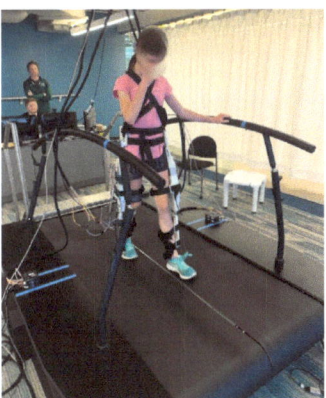

Figure 3. Experimental setup on the instrumented treadmill with the volunteer subject wearing the pediatric exoskeleton.

The system includes parallel bar structures and an overhead harness suspension system to assist with the subject's lateral balance and provide a safety precaution in case of a fall. The instrumented treadmill provides ground reaction force (GRF) signals as analog outputs from the force plates for both the left and right sides.

The subject's muscle activations were measured through a Trigno wireless EMG system (Delsys Incorporated, Natirck, MA, USA). The authors measured activations in the Vastus Medialis (VM), the Rectus Femoris (RF), the Biceps Femoris (BF), the Tibialis Anterior (TA), the Gastrocnemius Medialis (GM), and the Gastrocnemius Lateralis (GL). The Vastus Lateralis was originally measured but the associated EMG sensor fell off mid-experiment, so the analysis on this muscle was excluded. Only the dominant leg of the subject was equipped with EMG sensors. The outputs of the EMG sensors were filtered through a second-order Butterworth bandpass filter between 30 and 300 Hz, full-wave rectified, and then low-pass filtered with a second-order Butterworth filter with a cutoff frequency of 20 Hz to yield the linear envelope of the signal.

The control and partial data acquisition for this experiment were facilitated through a dSPACE MicroLabBox DS1202 (dSPACE, Wixom, MI, USA). The dSPACE system collected the joint angle and velocity measurements from the exoskeleton, and GRF data from the instrumented treadmill. Separately, the wireless EMG sensors and GRF measurements were also recorded through D-Flow (version 3.34.3) and CORTEX (64-bit, version 8.1.0.2017) software to yield data files sampled at 10 kHz. These data sets were then unified in time by aligning both sets' measurements of the GRF data.

3. Control Overview

This manuscript compares the performance of a time-dependent proportional-derivative (PD) trajectory tracking controller and a virtual constraint-based (VC) controller. An unassisted (UA) condition, with the subject walking in the unpowered exoskeleton, was also tested to serve as a baseline condition for comparison.

In the PD controller, the input torque is defined proportionally to the position and velocity error of the system relative to a reference gait pattern. The reference gait profiles for each joint were derived from the unassisted walking pattern of the wearer using the unpowered exoskeleton, taken on a previous testing day. This was chosen over nominal gait to represent the gait closest to the subject's natural walking cycle while constrained by the movements allowed by the exoskeleton. This gait pattern served as the desired gait profile across all the controlled conditions. The proportional and derivative control gains applied to the system were chosen by the subject. For ease of implementation and for the sake of comparison, the same set of control gains were used across all the hip and knee joints and were used for both the PD and VC controllers. The time-dependent nature of the PD controller necessitated a method to align the controller step timing with the user. This was achieved by synchronizing a metronome to the gait period such that an audial cue was given to the subject on when to time their heel strike.

For a more in-depth review and stability analysis of VC-based controllers, the authors point the reader to the seminal works of Grizzle and Westervelt et al. [37,49]. In general, the virtual constraint-based control method generates a set of constraint functions $h(s(q))$ for the hip and knee joints that are dependent on a monotonically increasing phase variable $s(q)$. This phase variable represents the progression of gait and is dependent on the configuration variable vector q. In prior experiments, the authors found that some phase variable definitions were sensitive to natural human gait variability, which led to unnatural human–exoskeleton behavior during control implementation [45]. Thus, the authors utilized a phase definition determined via optimization as performed in previous works, using the gait data from the UA condition [46]. This optimization identifies a phase variable definition of the form shown in Equation (1):

$$s(q) = cq + s_0 \tag{1}$$

The row vector c and the constant s_0 reflect the set of constants identified through the optimization. The optimization of the phase definition was subject to the following constraints:

$$\begin{aligned} s(q^-) &= 0 \\ s(q^+) &= 1 \\ s'(q_i) &> 0 \end{aligned} \tag{2}$$

and minimizes the cost function shown in Equation (3):

$$J_s = \sum_{i=1}^{N} (s'(q_i) - 1)^2 \tag{3}$$

The expression of q^- and q^+ represents the joint configuration vector of the human–exoskeleton model at the beginning and ending of a step, respectively, while q_i represents the system configuration at a single datapoint $1 \leq i \leq N$. The expression for the phase rate with respect to normalized time $\hat{t}$ is denoted as $s' = \Delta s / \Delta \hat{t}$. The result is an optimal phase definition that evenly distributes the phase's sensitivity to natural human gait variability over the entire gait step and is roughly equivalent to normalized time.

This phase definition is then utilized in a second offline optimization that generates constraint functions $h(s(q))$. The optimization aligns the gait cycle described by the constraint functions with the gait cycle recorded from the UA baseline. The optimization is carried out via the Trajectory Optimization in CasADi (TROPIC 1.18.2021) toolbox [50], utilizing the cost function shown in Equation (4).

$$J_{TROPIC} = \sum_{i=1}^{N} \|h(s(q)) - r_i\| \tag{4}$$

In the above equation, r_i is the desired reference gait cycle recorded from the UA condition, where the subscripts denote the percent of step phase. Additional optimization constraints ensure that the walking speed of the optimized gait cycle matches the walking speed of the UA baseline, and that the step period was within two standard deviations of the baseline.

A time-invariant feedback controller then enforces the constraint functions. While theoretical implementations of virtual constraint-based controllers utilize feedback linearization controllers to demonstrate controller stability and convergence, practical implementations in simulation and hardware applications have demonstrated that phase-based PD works to drive the system towards the desired cyclical gait [38,49,51]. The control law used in this virtual constraint-based controller is shown below.

$$Pe + D\dot{e} = u \quad (5)$$

$$e = h(s(q)) - Hq \quad (6)$$

$$\dot{e} = \frac{\partial h(s(q))}{\partial s}\dot{s} - H\dot{q} \quad (7)$$

The error vectors e and $\dot{e}$ represent the position and velocity errors of the system with respect to the virtual constraint functions. The matrix H consists of ones and zeros and maps the controlled joints of q and $\dot{q}$ to their appropriate constraint functions. Specifically, $H = [0_{4\times1}\ I_{4\times4}]$, where $I_{4\times4}$ is a 4-by-4 identity matrix. P and D are positive diagonal gain matrices.

The VC controller relies on a pinned model of the human–exoskeleton system. However, human gait exhibits periods of double support and the swapping of stance and swing legs. In traditional virtual constraint-based controllers, the double support phase is modeled as an instantaneous impact event with a transformation of the system states and the swapping of the swing and stance leg definitions. In this paper, the bilateral mixing strategy from [45,46] is used. It defines two symmetric full-body controllers, u_l and u_r, which assume that either the left or right leg are in the stance phase, respectively. The total control inputs to the system u_{tot} are then defined as a convex combination of the two controllers, where the weights of the two controllers, w_l and w_r, are based on GRF measurements. The bilateral mixing strategy is shown in Equation (8), and the definition of the weighting coefficients are defined in Equation (9), with respect to the left and right vertical GRF f_r and f_l.

$$u_{tot} = w_l u_l + w_r u_r \quad (8)$$

$$w_{l/r} = \begin{cases} \frac{f_{l/r}}{f_l+f_r}, & f_l + f_r \neq 0 \\ 0, & f_l + f_r \approx 0 \end{cases} \quad (9)$$

This bilateral mixing strategy enables transitions across double stance phases without discontinuous control inputs. Additionally, it allows for automatic control switching between the two controllers when either the left or right leg is serving as the stance leg.

4. Experimental Procedure

An 11-year-old female volunteer subject participated in this study along with their adult caretaker. The subject weighed 30.8 kg and measured 149 cm in height. They had been exposed to the exoskeletal device through the previous human factor assessment [19]. The exoskeleton was comfortably compatible with the subject and was adjusted to their anthropometrics at the start of the experiment. The anthropometric parameters of the subject's limbs were estimated from census data using their overall height and weight. The parameters of the exoskeleton system were manually measured or derived from CAD models of the system. The two models were combined to generate an approximate human–exoskeleton rigid body model, with parameters listed in Table 1 for the torso, thigh, and shank.

The volunteer participant was informed of the experiment's motivations and purpose, and written assent and informed consent was given by both the subject and their parent/guardian prior to the start of the study in accordance with the Institutional Review Board at Cleveland State University. The procedure consisted of three sessions. The first session was to familiarize the subject with the placement of the EMG sensors, and to perform preliminary sensor and control calibrations. A research assistant modeled the placement of the EMG sensors on their own leg so that the parent/guardian could accurately place the sensors on the child's limbs. Torque saturation limits were identified for each joint of the exoskeleton by having the subject maintain a neutral single stance standing position while a slowly ramping torque was applied to the joints of the non-stance leg. The subject indicated the upper limit of torque that they were able to overpower or resist from the exoskeleton. These torque limits were implemented as a safety precaution so that the wearer could forcibly exercise control over the gait cycle in case of controller desynchronization. Torque ranges from -5 to 8 Nm and from -4 to 4 Nm were identified for the subject's hips and knees, respectively. Next, the subject walked on the treadmill while wearing the exoskeleton in an unpowered condition. After the subject became accustomed to walking with the exoskeleton, a set of gait data for unassisted walking was taken to serve as the baseline reference for the PD and VC control conditions.

Table 1. Parameters of the human–exoskeleton system.

Link	Mass (kg)	Length (m)	CoM (m)	Inertia (kg·m^2)
Torso	21.89	0.70	0.42	2.63
Thigh	4.51	0.36	0.16	0.06
Shank	2.12	0.42	0.25	0.06

Center of mass locations (CoM) are reported as distances along the body segments' axial length with respect to the proximal joint. Inertia is reported with respect to the link center of mass.

The next session served as a practice day. The subject practiced walking with the exoskeleton in the unassisted, PD-, and VC-controlled conditions for 6 min each. This training day allowed the subject to learn how to walk with the exoskeleton under each control condition before data were recorded. This practice day was conducted to mitigate the temporary effects of the patient's learning period during final data acquisition. During these early gait sessions, preliminary subject-selected control gains were identified as a starting point for the later gait experiments.

The third experimental session consisted of the final set of gait experiments and the collection of data and subject questionnaires. Each of the tested walking conditions started with a gait synchronization event. This allowed the researchers to synchronize the D-Flow and dSPACE data sets in time by aligning the GRF measurements during data processing. The treadmill system was sped up to a user-selected walking speed of 0.8 m/s. The controller inputs were then incrementally increased until the subject-selected gains for the control condition were reached. The subject walked for 3 min under the controlled condition. Afterwards, the control inputs and treadmill speed were ramped back down. Following each test condition, the subject was given a 3-min rest period, during which a questionnaire was completed to allow the subject to give feedback and rate their perceived physical effort using the Borg Rating of Perceived Effort scale [52]. On the day of the experiment, the control conditions were applied in the following order: PD, VC, and finally, UA. After all the tested conditions were completed, the subject was asked to rank the applied controllers based on their exertion and subjective personal preference from least to greatest.

5. Results and Discussion

The subject made no notes regarding discomfort while wearing the exoskeleton and did not indicate excessive levels of fatigue. There were no recorded trips or falls during testing. On the day of the experiments, the subject chose control gains that produced conservative control inputs. The proportional and derivative gains for both the PD and VC conditions were left at 7.8 Nm·rad^{-1} and 0.12 Nm·s·rad^{-1} across both the hip and knee joints.

The gait information was partitioned into step cycles based on the GRF information such that the beginning and end of each gait cycle corresponded with the heel strike event. The left and right leg gait cycles were combined for the kinematic analysis. Only the right leg information was used for the EMG sensors analysis, as only the patient's dominant leg was equipped with sensors.

5.1. Kinematics and Kinetics

To compare hip and knee angles across the conditions, a one-way analysis of variance (ANOVA) statistical test was performed. This was performed by comparing the hip and knee joint angles in each tested condition (PD, VC) to that of the UA baseline and taking the average root mean square (rms) difference. Each comparison was performed using a *t*-test (significance level of 0.050) with a Tukey–Kramer multiple-comparisons correction. Figure 4 illustrates the ensemble-averaged gait cycle accomplished under the different controlled conditions, plotted with respect to the UA condition performance.

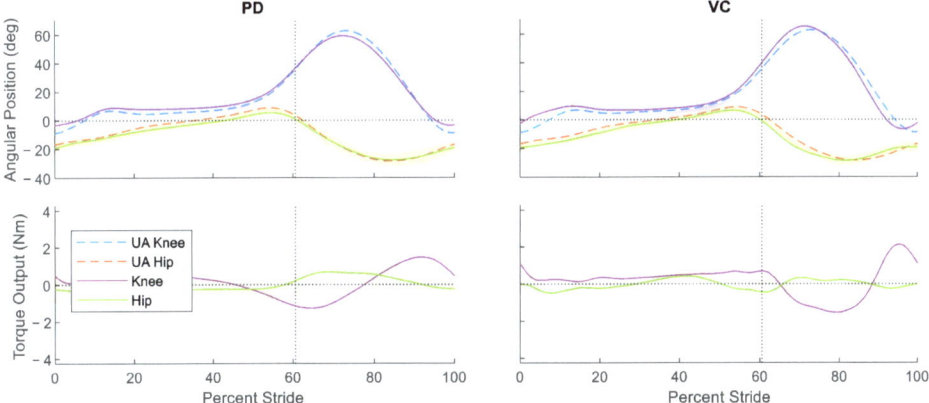

Figure 4. Ensemble-averaged position performance and torque input of the hip and knee joints for the proportional-derivative (PD) and virtual constraint-based (VC) control. They are plotted with respect to the joint performance of the unassisted (UA) baseline condition. The shaded regions show ±1 standard deviation for both position performance and control inputs. The vertical dotted line denotes the approximate location of toe-off.

Table 2 lists the quantified performance metrics averaged over the gait cycle such as the mean rms difference with respect to the UA baseline, their mean standard deviations, and the mean rms torque output.

Table 2. Performance and torque outputs of the control conditions.

Condition	Kinematic Difference *		Kinetics	
	Hip (deg)	Knee (deg)	Hip (Nm)	Knee (Nm)
UA	– ± 4.88	– ± 6.33	–	–
PD	2.50 ± 3.70	3.75 ± 6.78	0.39	0.90
VC	3.06 ± 3.04	4.59 ± 5.30	0.25	0.86

* Mean ± standard deviation. UA only reports standard deviation. – Represents a null entry.

Low angular differences were recorded across the controlled conditions for both the hips and knees. The PD-controlled condition reported an rms difference of 2.50 and 3.75 degrees in the hips and knees, respectively, while the VC-controlled condition reported slightly higher differences of 3.06 and 4.59 degrees for the hips and knees. The rms differences for both the hip and knee positions relative to the UA baseline were sufficiently similar such that statistically significant ($p < 0.05$) differences were not identified between the PD vs. VC conditions in the 275 gait cycles compared. This indicates that the gait cycles in the PD- and VC-controlled conditions were comparable despite the difference in the controller used. This is further corroborated when looking at the effect size between the conditions, which are listed in Table 3.

Table 3. Effect size from control comparisons.

Comparison	Hip (Mean + Std)	Knee (Mean + Std)
UA-PD	0.4833 ± 0.3016	0.4766 ± 0.2302
UA-VC	0.6616 ± 0.2877	0.5769 ± 0.3535
PD-VC	0.5488 ± 0.2893	0.4765 ± 0.3070

UA, PD, and VC represent the unassisted, proportional-derivative, and virtual constraint-based controlled conditions respectively. Hyphens denotes the pairwise comparisons between conditions.

For all the comparisons (UA-PD, UA-VC, and PD-VC), the differences in the kinematics were moderate with an average absolute effect size within 0.48–0.67 for the hip and 0.47–0.58 for the knee. This suggests the gait patterns are largely similar, often within a standard deviation of one another across all the pairs of conditions. In the context of the experiment performed, this is unsurprising, as the subject was a healthy individual and the control gains were tuned such that the subject could manually exert control over the gait cycle. However, while the average gait profiles in each condition were similar, a point-wise calculation of the standard deviation was obtained and then averaged to quantify the gait variability. The mean standard deviation of the hip and knee angles decreased in the VC condition relative to the UA and PD conditions. The VC controller decreased the wearer's gait variability from 4.88 to 3.04 degrees in the hip and 6.33 to 5.30 degrees in the knee between the UA and VC conditions. This represents a relative reduction in the mean standard deviation at the hip and knee joints of 36.72% and 16.28%, respectively. In the PD controller, the mean standard deviation of the hip joints decreased to 3.70, or only 27.03%, and for the knee, increased to 6.78 degrees, representing a 7.10% increase. These changes in the standard deviation indicate that the VC controller increased the wearer's gait regularity and consistency more than the PD controller.

An additional ANOVA and multiple comparisons t-test was performed on the rms torque profiles of each controlled condition to quantify the changes in the amount of applied intervention. There was a statistically significant ($p < 0.050$) reduction in the rms torques applied by the VC controller relative to the PD controller in the hip and knee joints. With regard to the ensemble-averaged torque profiles applied, the VC controller reduced the rms torques applied from 0.39 to 0.25 Nm and 0.90 Nm to 0.86 Nm for the hip and knee joints relative to the PD controller, representing a 35.89% and a 4.44% reduction in the overall robotic intervention, respectively. The kinematic and kinetic data indicate that the mean gait cycles of the VC- and PD-controlled conditions were similar, but the VC controller demonstrated a greater degree of gait regularity in the subject's walking pattern while using less robotic intervention.

5.2. EMG Sensors and Perceived Exertion

Only the right leg of the subject was equipped with EMG sensors, which means the total number of gait cycles available for analysis was around half of those used in the kinematic data analysis. A total of 136 gait cycles were compared between the UA, PD, and VC conditions for the EMG analysis. Before the analysis, the EMG signals of each muscle were normalized with respect to the mean output of the muscle during the UA condition. Figure 5 plots the normalized mean and standard deviation of the EMG readings for each muscle group measured across all the tested conditions, while Figure 6 plots their normalized value over the gait cycle. These values are also listed in Table 4, along with Borg scale ratings and the post-experiment exertion rankings provided by the child subject.

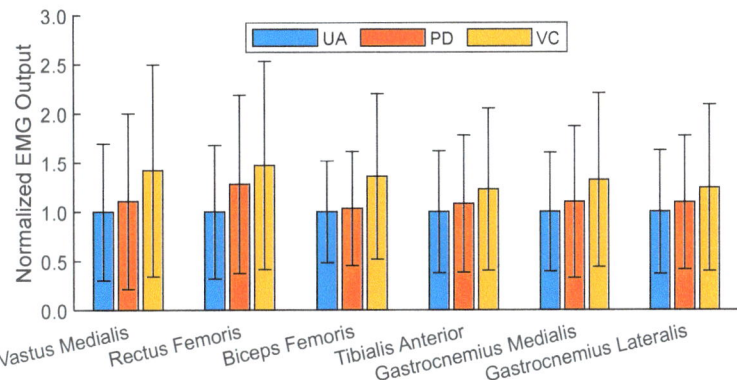

Figure 5. The normalized mean EMG outputs for each muscle and condition tested. The normalized standard deviations for the EMG outputs are represented as error bars.

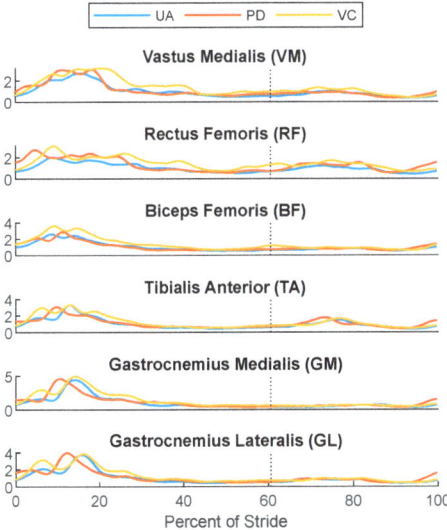

Figure 6. The normalized ensemble-averaged EMG outputs over the gait cycle, starting and ending with heel strike. The vertical dotted line denotes the approximate location of toe-off.

Table 4. Ratings of perceived exertion and normalized EMG outputs.

Condition	Borg	Rank	VM	RF	BF	TA	GM	GL
UA	7	1	1.00	1.00	1.00	1.00	1.00	1.00
PD	8	3	1.10	1.28	1.06	1.09	1.10	1.10
VC	9	2	1.43	1.46	1.36	1.24	1.32	1.25

Vastus Medialis (VM), Rectus Femoris (RF), Biceps Femoris (BF), Tibialis Anterior (TA), Gastrocnemius Medialis (GM), Gastrocnemius Lateralis (GL).

To quantify the differences in the muscle activation levels, a similar statistical analysis was performed on the normalized EMG outputs for each muscle. Statistically significant differences in the muscle activation levels were found in the VC vs. PD and the VC vs. UA comparison, but not in the UA vs. PD comparison. The general trends demonstrate that the UA condition required the least amount of physical exertion based on the EMG measurements. The second lowest average EMG outputs were measured for PD, at about 11.8% higher than those of UA, followed by VC, at 34.4%.

The analysis of the child subject's ratings of perceived exertion show some inconsistencies, and a discrepancy between the muscle activation levels and controller preference. The Borg scale ratings given after each tested condition indicates that the extent of perceived exertion between the PD- and VC-controlled conditions were similar. The PD-controlled condition was initially listed as a slightly lower effort controller than the VC condition, though this perception may have been affected by the order in which the controlled conditions were applied. The PD controller was applied before any other control conditions, and thus, there is likely some recency bias associated with the Borg scale rankings. The post experiment user rankings given at the end of all the gait experiments indicate that the user found the VC controller preferable to PD. These results stand in opposition to the fact that the muscle activations in the VC controller are higher than those in the PD-controlled condition. While more effort was expended by the user to walk under the VC-controlled condition, the controller was still seen as preferable to the PD controller. A potential explanation for this discrepancy is that the final rankings of preference in these experiments might serve more as a measure of ease of use, or how intrusive the controller was with respect to the wearer's gait. For instance, the time dependency of the PD controller dictates a certain rate of gait progression and step timing. If the subject's intended gait is lagging or leading the PD controller's reference, this could result in the controller pushing or resisting the motion of the user. Gait desynchronization could lead to the user fighting the controller at certain points in the gait profile even if the PD controller is working cooperatively with the wearer for most of the motion. There were a few instances of gait desynchronization between the user and PD controller during the experiment, including a few gait cycles where the user and controller were completely desynched. Additionally, the standard deviation of the torque curve in Figure 4 is noticeably larger than that of the VC-controlled condition, suggesting a greater degree of variance in the control inputs, which themselves stem from how well the user's gait is synchronized to the controller. In contrast, the VC-controlled condition leaves the gait timing entirely up to the wearer's volition. While these controllers may not push the user through the gait cycle at any point, they never actively resist the intention of the wearer.

Across all the controlled conditions, the EMG outputs for each muscle increased relative to the UA case. Similarly, the Borg scale ratings and the finalized rankings of the tested conditions indicated that the subject found it more difficult to walk with external controllers than without. This suggests that for able-bodied subjects, the introduction of control inputs in this experiment acted more as a system disturbance as opposed to a restorative or assistive force.

5.3. Study Limitations

There are a few limitations to the conducted study. This study utilized only a single volunteer pediatric subject, which limits the generalizability of these results to other individuals. Additionally, the control inputs applied by the exoskeleton remained low. The average peak torque input was in the VC condition at merely 2.91 ± 0.63 Nm at the knee. This represents around 15.36% of the 18.94 Nm peak knee torque expected based on Winter gait data for a 30.8 kg subject [29]. The low control input can be attributed to the fact that the subject did not have any form of gait impairment, and so the amount of control input exerted by the exoskeleton remained low throughout the walking cycle. Additionally, the control gains applied in the experiment were tuned based on user comfort, resulting in gains that minimally affected the already well-performing gait cycle. However, repeated exposure to the exoskeleton and controllers may encourage the user to adopt a more cooperative walking strategy, or increase the subject's confidence in the device, leading to the use of higher control gains and inputs. Additionally, a user with gait impairment may be more amenable to increased robotic intervention.

For similar reasons, the interpretation of the EMG-measured outputs should be taken with caution. While statistically significant differences in EMG activations were found between the controlled conditions, it is unclear whether the comparisons and relationships discussed in this paper will hold true when greater control inputs are allowed by a healthy individual or a user with gait impairment.

6. Conclusions

This paper presented a comparison of a virtual constraint-based controller with a traditional proportional-derivative controller to evaluate their suitability for gait guidance. Control was applied on a newly developed adjustable pediatric exoskeleton, marking the device's first use in a control study. During the experiment, the subject gave no indication of discomfort due to the applied controller or the physical hardware. The authors successfully conducted multiple gait experiments using the exoskeleton under different controllers. The successful control implementation demonstrates that the adjustable pediatric lower-limb exoskeleton may serve as a platform in future experiments on rehabilitative and assistive controllers for children.

The virtual constraint-based controller achieved similar levels of gait performance relative to the proportional-derivative controller, as evidenced by the moderate effect size values. However, the VC controller was able to decrease the level of gait variability by 36.72% and 16.28% for the hips and knees, respectively. Conversely, the PD controller decreased variability in the hip joint by only 27.03% and increased the gait variability in the knee joint by 7.10%. Additionally, the VC controller utilized 35.89% and 4.44% less torque in the hip and knee joints relative to the PD controller. A comparison of the EMG outputs between the two controllers indicated that the virtual constraint-based controller required more effort to utilize. However, the user's post-experiment controller rankings indicated that the VC-based controller was easier to utilize. This could be attributed to the difference in time dependence between the PD and VC controllers, which is evidenced by both the large standard deviation in the control torque inputs and the observations of gait desynchronization made by both the wearer and authors during the PD-controlled experiment.

The results of this study's comparison suggest that virtual constraint-based controllers have favorable characteristics relative to standard PD control due to their perceived ease of use, decreased gait variability, and ability to reduce the control torque required to achieve good performance all while maintaining a time-invariant control implementation. The VC controller also allows the user to retain volitional control over the step timing and removes the risk of gait desynchronization during walking. Thus, virtual constraint-based controllers merit further investigation in larger multi-subject rehabilitation-oriented studies. The efficacy of virtual constraint-based controllers for rehabilitation should also be evaluated through the application of control on a pediatric subject dealing with gait impairment. The authors also propose a multi-subject study utilizing the newly validated exoskeleton platform to better demonstrate the exoskeleton's ability to adjust to several pediatric subjects.

Author Contributions: Conceptualization, A.C.G., C.A.L. and J.T.S.; methodology, A.C.G., C.A.L. and D.A.W.; software, A.C.G. and C.A.L.; validation, A.C.G. and C.A.L.; formal analysis, A.C.G. and C.A.L.; investigation, A.C.G., C.A.L. and D.A.W.; resources, J.T.S.; data curation, A.C.G. and C.A.L.; writing—original draft preparation, A.C.G. and C.A.L.; writing—review and editing, A.C.G., C.A.L., D.A.W. and J.T.S.; visualization, A.C.G. and C.A.L.; supervision, J.T.S.; project administration, J.T.S.; funding acquisition, J.T.S. All authors have read and agreed to the published version of the manuscript.

Funding: This research received no external funding.

Institutional Review Board Statement: This study was conducted according to the guidelines of the Declaration of Helsinki, and approved by the Institutional Review Board (or Ethics Committee) of Cleveland State University (IRB-FY2022-90, Approved on 18 April 2022).

Informed Consent Statement: Informed consent was obtained from all subjects involved in the study.

Data Availability Statement: The data presented in this study are available on request from the corresponding author.

Acknowledgments: The authors would like to thank Jason J. Wiebrecht and Jacob A. Strick for their assistance in supporting the conducted experiments.

Conflicts of Interest: The authors declare no conflicts of interest.

References

1. Viteckova, S.; Kutilek, P.; Jirina, M. Wearable Lower Limb Robotics: A Review. *Biocybern. Biomed. Eng.* **2013**, *33*, 96–105. [CrossRef]
2. Westlake, K.P.; Patten, C. Pilot Study of Lokomat versus Manual-Assisted Treadmill Training for Locomotor Recovery Post-Stroke. *J. NeuroEng. Rehabil.* **2009**, *6*, 18. [CrossRef] [PubMed]
3. Banala, S.K.; Kim, S.H.; Agrawal, S.K.; Scholz, J.P. Robot Assisted Gait Training with Active Leg Exoskeleton (ALEX). *IEEE Trans. Neural Syst. Rehabil. Eng.* **2009**, *17*, 2–8. [CrossRef] [PubMed]
4. Nam, K.Y.; Kim, H.J.; Kwon, B.S.; Park, J.-W.; Lee, H.J.; Yoo, A. Robot-assisted gait training (Lokomat) improves walking function and activity in people with spinal cord injury: A systematic review. *J. NeuroEng. Rehabil.* **2017**, *14*, 24. [CrossRef] [PubMed]
5. Lerner, Z.F.; Damiano, D.L.; Bulea, T.C. A Lower-Extremity Exoskeleton Improves Knee Extension in Children with Crouch Gait from Cerebral Palsy. *Sci. Transl. Med.* **2017**, *9*, eaam9145. [CrossRef] [PubMed]
6. Wallard, L.; Dietrich, G.; Kerlirzin, Y.; Bredin, J. Robotic-assisted gait training improves walking abilities in diplegic children with cerebral palsy. *Eur. J. Paediatr. Neurol.* **2017**, *21*, 557–564. [CrossRef] [PubMed]
7. Cumplido-Trasmonte, C.; Ramos-Rojas, J.; Delgado-Castillejo, E.; Garcés-Castellote, E.; Puyuelo-Quintana, G.; Destarac-Eguizabal, M.A.; Barquín-Santos, E.; Plaza-Flores, A.; Hernández-Melero, M.; Gutiérrez-Ayala, A.; et al. Effects of ATLAS 2030 gait exoskeleton on strength and range of motion in children with spinal muscular atrophy II: A case series. *J. NeuroEng. Rehabil.* **2022**, *19*, 75. [CrossRef] [PubMed]
8. Rodríguez-Fernández, A.; Lobo-Prat, J.; Font-Llagunes, J.M. Systematic Review on Wearable Lower-Limb Exoskeletons for Gait Training in Neuromuscular Impairments. *J. NeuroEng. Rehabil.* **2021**, *18*, 22. [CrossRef] [PubMed]
9. Gardner, A.D.; Potgieter, J.; Noble, F.K. A Review of Commercially Available Exoskeletons' Capabilities. In Proceedings of the 2017 24th International Conference on Mechatronics and Machine Vision in Practice (M2VIP), Auckland, New Zealand, 21–23 November 2017; pp. 1–5. [CrossRef]
10. Fosch-Villaronga, E.; Čartolovni, A.; Pierce, R.L. Promoting Inclusiveness in Exoskeleton Robotics: Addressing Challenges for Pediatric Access. *Paladyn J. Behav. Robot.* **2020**, *11*, 327–339. [CrossRef]
11. Koenig, A.; Wellner, M.; Köneke, S.; Meyer-Heim, A.; Lünenburger, L.; Riener, R. Virtual Gait Training for Children with Cerebral Palsy Using the Lokomat Gait Orthosis. *Stud. Health Technol. Inform.* **2008**, *132*, 204–209. Available online: https://europepmc.org/article/med/18391287 (accessed on 7 May 2020).
12. Diot, C.M.; Thomas, R.L.; Raess, L.; Wrightson, J.G.; Condliffe, E.G. *Robotic Lower Extremity Exoskeleton Use in a Non-Ambulatory Child with Cerebral Palsy: A Case Study*; Taylor & Francis: Abingdon, UK, 2021; Volume 18, pp. 1–5. [CrossRef]
13. Kuroda, M.; Nakagawa, S.; Mutsuzaki, H.; Mataki, Y.; Yoshikawa, K.; Takahashi, K.; Nakayama, T.; Iwasaki, N. Robot-assisted gait training using a very small-sized Hybrid Assistive Limb® for pediatric cerebral palsy: A case report. *Brain Dev.* **2020**, *42*, 468–472. [CrossRef] [PubMed]
14. Sanz-Merodio, D.; Pereze, M.; Prieto, M.; Sancho, J.; Garcia, E. Result of Clinical Trials with Children with Spinal Muscular Atrophy Using the ATLAS 2020 Lower-Limb Active Orthosis. In *Human-Centric Robotics, Proceedings of the CLAWAR 2017: 20th International Conference on Climbing and Walking Robots and the Support Technologies of Mobile Machines, Porto, Portugal, 11–13 September 2017*; World Scientific: Singapore, 2017; pp. 48–55. [CrossRef]
15. Zhang, Y.; Bressel, M.; De Groof, S.; Dominć, F.; Labey, L.; Peyrodie, L. Design and Control of a Size-Adjustable Pediatric Lower-Limb Exoskeleton Based on Weight Shift. *IEEE Access* **2023**, *11*, 6372–6384. [CrossRef]
16. Laubscher, C.A.; Farris, R.J.; van den Bogert, A.J.; Sawicki, J.T. An Anthropometrically Parameterized Assistive Lower-Limb Exoskeleton. *ASME J. Biomech. Eng.* **2021**, *143*, 105001. [CrossRef] [PubMed]
17. Goo, A.; Laubscher, C.A.; Farris, R.J.; Sawicki, J.T. Design and Evaluation of a Pediatric Lower-Limb Exoskeleton Joint Actuator. *Actuators* **2020**, *9*, 138. [CrossRef]
18. Goo, A.; Laubscher, C.A.; Wiebrecht, J.J.; Farris, R.J.; Sawicki, J.T. Hybrid Zero Dynamics Control for Gait Guidance of a Novel Adjustable Pediatric Lower-Limb Exoskeleton. *Bioengineering* **2022**, *9*, 208. [CrossRef] [PubMed]
19. Goo, A.; Wiebrecht, J.J.; Wajda, D.A.; Sawicki, J.T. Preliminary Human Factors Assessment of a Novel Pediatric Lower Limb Exoskeleton. *MDPI Robot.* **2023**, *12*, 26. [CrossRef]
20. Baud, R.; Manzoori, A.R.; Ijspeert, A.; Bouri, M. Review of control strategies for lower-limb exoskeletons to assist gait. *J. NeuroEng. Rehabil.* **2021**, *18*, 119. [CrossRef] [PubMed]
21. Yan, T.; Cempini, M.; Oddo, C.M.; Vitiello, N. Review of Assistive Strategies in Powered Lower-Limb Orthoses and Exoskeletons. *Robot. Auton. Syst.* **2015**, *64*, 120–136. [CrossRef]
22. Kalita, B.; Narayan, J.; Dwivedy, S.K. Development of Active Lower Limb Robotic-Based Orthosis and Exoskeleton Devices: A Systematic Review. *Int. J. Soc. Robot.* **2021**, *13*, 775–793. [CrossRef]
23. Anam, K.; Al-Jumaily, A.A. Active Exoskeleton Control Systems: State of the Art. *Procedia Eng.* **2012**, *41*, 988–994. [CrossRef]

24. Marchal-Crespo, L.; Reinkensmeyer, D.J. Review of Control Strategies for Robotic Movement Training after Neurologic Injury. *J. NeuroEng. Rehabil.* **2009**, *6*, 20. [CrossRef] [PubMed]
25. Perez Ibarra, J.C.; Siqueira, A.A.G. Impedance Control of Rehabilitation Robots for Lower Limbs, Review. In Proceedings of the 2014 Joint Conference on Robotics: SBR-LARS Robotics Symposium and Robocontrol, Sao Carlos, Brazil, 18–23 October 2014. [CrossRef]
26. Veneman, J.F.; Kruidhof, R.; Hekman, E.E.G.; Ekkelenkamp, R.; Van Asseldonk, E.H.F.; van der Kooij, H. Design and Evaluation of the LOPES Exoskeleton Robot for Interactive Gait Rehabilitation. *IEEE Trans. Neural Syst. Rehabil. Eng.* **2007**, *15*, 379–386. [CrossRef] [PubMed]
27. Aguirre-Ollinger, G.; Colgate, J.E.; Peshkin, M.A.; Goswami, A. Active-Impedance Control of a Lower-Limb Assistive Exoskeleton. In *Rehabilitation Robotics, 2007. ICORR 2007, Proceedings of the 2007 IEEE 10th International Conference on Rehabilitation Robotics, Noordwijk, The Netherlands, 13–15 June 2007*; IEEE: Piscataway, NJ, USA, 2007; pp. 188–195.
28. Tran, H.T.; Cheng, H.; Rui, H.; Lin, X.; Duong, M.K.; Chen, Q. Evaluation of a Fuzzy-Based Impedance Control Strategy on a Powered Lower Exoskeleton. *Int. J. Soc. Robot.* **2016**, *8*, 103–123. [CrossRef]
29. Winter, D.A. *The Biomechanics and Motor Control of Human Gait: Normal, Elderly and Pathological*; University of Waterloo Press: Waterloo, ON, Canada, 1991.
30. Schwartz, M.H.; Rozumalski, A.; Trost, J.P. The Effect of Walking Speed on the Gait of Typically Developing Children. *J. Biomech.* **2008**, *41*, 1639–1650. [CrossRef] [PubMed]
31. Hidler, J.M.; Wall, A.E. Alterations in Muscle Activation Patterns during Robotic-Assisted Walking. *Clin. Biomech.* **2005**, *20*, 184–193. [CrossRef] [PubMed]
32. Israel, J.F.; Campbell, D.D.; Kahn, J.H.; Hornby, T.G. Metabolic Costs and Muscle Activity Patterns during Robotic- and Therapist-Assisted Treadmill Walking in Individuals with Incomplete Spinal Cord Injury. *Phys. Ther.* **2006**, *86*, 1466–1478. [CrossRef] [PubMed]
33. Murray, S.A.; Ha, K.H.; Hartigan, C.; Goldfarb, M. An Assistive Control Approach for a Lower-Limb Exoskeleton to Facilitate Recovery of Walking Following Stroke. *IEEE Trans. Neural Syst. Rehabil. Eng.* **2015**, *23*, 441–449. [CrossRef]
34. Winstein, C.J.; Pohl, P.S.; Lewthwaite, R. Effects of Physical Guidance and Knowledge of Results on Motor Learning: Support for the Guidance Hypothesis. *Res. Q. Exerc. Sport* **1994**, *65*, 316–323. [CrossRef]
35. Duschau-Wicke, A.; von Zitzewitz, J.; Caprez, A.; Lunenburger, L.; Riener, R. Path Control: A Method for Patient-Cooperative Robot-Aided Gait Rehabilitation. *IEEE Trans. Neural Syst. Rehabil. Eng.* **2010**, *18*, 38–48. [CrossRef]
36. Martínez, A.; Lawson, B.; Goldfarb, M. A Controller for Guiding Leg Movement during Overground Walking with a Lower Limb Exoskeleton. *IEEE Trans. Robot.* **2018**, *34*, 183–193. [CrossRef]
37. Westervelt, E.R.; Grizzle, J.W.; Koditschek, D.E. Hybrid Zero Dynamics of Planar Biped Walkers. *IEEE Trans. Automat. Contr.* **2003**, *48*, 42–56. [CrossRef]
38. Chevallereau, C.; ABBA, G.; Aoustin, Y.; Plestan, F.; Westervelt, E.; Canudas de Wit, C.; Grizzle, J. RABBIT: A Testbed for Advanced Control Theory. *IEEE Control Syst. Mag.* **2003**, *23*, 57–79.
39. Sreenath, K.; Park, H.-W.; Poulakakis, I.; Grizzle, J.W. A Compliant Hybrid Zero Dynamics Controller for Stable, Efficient and Fast Bipedal Walking on MABEL. *Int. J. Robot. Res.* **2011**, *30*, 1170–1193. [CrossRef]
40. Yang, T.; Westervelt, E.R.; Schmiedeler, J.P.; Bockbrader, R.A. Design and Control of a Planar Bipedal Robot ERNIE with Parallel Knee Compliance. *Auton. Robot.* **2008**, *25*, 317–330. [CrossRef]
41. Reher, J.; Cousineau, E.A.; Hereid, A.; Hubicki, C.M.; Ames, A.D. Realizing Dynamic and Efficient Bipedal Locomotion on the Humanoid Robot DURUS. In Proceedings of the 2016 IEEE International Conference on Robotics and Automation (ICRA), Stockholm, Sweden, 16–21 May 2016; pp. 1794–1801. [CrossRef]
42. Agrawal, A.; Harib, O.; Hereid, A.; Finet, S.; Masselin, M.; Praly, L.; Ames, A.D.; Sreenath, K.; Grizzle, J.W. First Steps towards Translating HZD Control of Bipedal Robots to Decentralized Control of Exoskeletons. *IEEE Access* **2017**, *5*, 9919–9934. [CrossRef]
43. Gurriet, T.; Finet, S.; Boeris, G.; Duburcq, A.; Hereid, A.; Harib, O.; Masselin, M.; Grizzle, J.; Ames, A.D. Towards Restoring Locomotion for Paraplegics: Realizing Dynamically Stable Walking on Exoskeletons. In Proceedings of the 2018 IEEE International Conference on Robotics and Automation (ICRA), Brisbane, Australia, 21–25 May 2018; IEEE: Brisbane, QLD, Australia, 2018; pp. 2804–2811. [CrossRef]
44. Gregg, R.D.; Lenzi, T.; Hargrove, L.J.; Sensinger, J.W. Virtual Constraint Control of a Powered Prosthetic Leg: From Simulation to Experiments with Transfemoral Amputees. *IEEE Trans. Robot.* **2014**, *30*, 1455–1471. [CrossRef]
45. Goo, A.; Laubscher, C.A.; Sawicki, J.T. Hybrid Zero Dynamics-Based Control of an Underactuated Lower-Limb Exoskeleton for Gait Guidance. *ASME J. Dyn. Syst. Meas. Control* **2022**, *144*, 061008. [CrossRef]
46. Laubscher, C.A.; Goo, A.; Sawicki, J.T. Optimal phase-based gait guidance control on a lower-limb exoskeleton. *Control Eng. Pract.* **2023**, *139*, 105651. [CrossRef]
47. Winter, D.A. *Biomechanics and Motor Control of Human Movement*, 4th ed.; John Wiley & Sons: Hoboken, NJ, USA, 2009.
48. Fryar, C.D.; Carroll, M.D.; Qiuping, G.; Afful, J.; Ogden, C.L. *Anthropometric Reference Data for Children and Adults: United States, 2015–2018*; Vital Health Statistics 46; National Center for Health Statistics: Hyattsville, MD, USA, 2021; pp. 1–44.
49. Westervelt, E.R.; Grizzle, J.W.; Chevallereau, C.; Choi, J.H.; Morris, B. *Feedback Control of Dynamic Bipedal Robot Locomotion*, 1st ed.; CRC Press: Boca Raton, FL, USA, 2018. [CrossRef]

50. Fevre, M.; Wensing, P.M.; Schmiedeler, J.P. Rapid Bipedal Gait Optimization in CasADi. In Proceedings of the 2020 IEEE/RSJ International Conference on Intelligent Robots and Systems (IROS), Las Vegas, NV, USA, 24 October 2020–24 January 2021; IEEE: Las Vegas, NV, USA, 2020; pp. 3672–3678. [CrossRef]
51. Harib, O.; Hereid, A.; Agrawal, A.; Gurriet, T.; Finet, S.; Boeris, G.; Duburcq, A.; Mungai, M.E.; Masselin, M.; Ames, A.D.; et al. Feedback Control of an Exoskeleton for Paraplegics: Toward Robustly Stable Hands-free Dynamic Walking. *IEEE Control Syst. Mag.* **2018**, *38*, 61–87. Available online: http://arxiv.org/abs/1802.08322 (accessed on 28 May 2020). [CrossRef]
52. Williams, N. The Borg Rating of Perceived Exertion (RPE) Scale. *Occup. Med.* **2017**, *67*, 404–405. [CrossRef]

Disclaimer/Publisher's Note: The statements, opinions and data contained in all publications are solely those of the individual author(s) and contributor(s) and not of MDPI and/or the editor(s). MDPI and/or the editor(s) disclaim responsibility for any injury to people or property resulting from any ideas, methods, instructions or products referred to in the content.

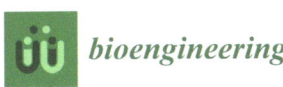 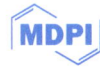

Article

Compensation Method for Missing and Misidentified Skeletons in Nursing Care Action Assessment by Improving Spatial Temporal Graph Convolutional Networks

Xin Han [1], Norihiro Nishida [2], Minoru Morita [1], Takashi Sakai [2] and Zhongwei Jiang [1,*]

1. Faculty of Engineering, Yamaguchi University Graduate School of Sciences and Technology for Innovation, 2-16-1 Tokiwadai, Ube City 755-0097, Yamaguchi Prefecture, Japan; hxyamaguchiu@163.com (X.H.); mmorita@yamaguchi-u.ac.jp (M.M.)
2. Department of Orthopedic Surgery, Yamaguchi University Graduate School of Medicine, 1-1-1 Minamikogushi, Ube City 755-8505, Yamaguchi Prefecture, Japan; nishida3@yamaguchi-u.ac.jp (N.N.); cozy@yamaguchi-u.ac.jp (T.S.)
* Correspondence: jiang@yamaguchi-u.ac.jp

Abstract: With the increasing aging population, nursing care providers have been facing a substantial risk of work-related musculoskeletal disorders (WMSDs). Visual-based pose estimation methods, like OpenPose, are commonly used for ergonomic posture risk assessment. However, these methods face difficulty when identifying overlapping and interactive nursing tasks, resulting in missing and misidentified skeletons. To address this, we propose a skeleton compensation method using improved spatial temporal graph convolutional networks (ST-GCN), which integrates kinematic chain and action features to assess skeleton integrity and compensate for it. The results verified the effectiveness of our approach in optimizing skeletal loss and misidentification in nursing care tasks, leading to improved accuracy in calculating both skeleton joint angles and REBA scores. Moreover, comparative analysis against other skeleton compensation methods demonstrated the superior performance of our approach, achieving an 87.34% REBA accuracy score. Collectively, our method might hold promising potential for optimizing the skeleton loss and misidentification in nursing care tasks.

Keywords: work-related musculoskeletal disorders; ergonomic posture risk assessment; REBA; skeleton compensation; ST-GCN

1. Introduction

The nursing industry has consistently exhibited a high prevalence of work-related musculoskeletal disorders (WMSDs) [1]. Among nursing professionals, the incidence of work-related musculoskeletal disorders is even more pronounced, particularly in rehabilitation and geriatric care settings, reaching a staggering 92% [2,3]. The most effective preventive approach lies in conducting ergonomic posture risk assessments for nursing personnel and promptly addressing high-risk postures through corrective measures [4,5].

The predominant methods for assessing ergonomic posture typically rely on field observation or video monitoring to measure joint angles. These joint angles are then utilized in scoring tools, such as the Rapid Upper Limb Assessment (RULA) [6] and Rapid Entire Body Assessment (REBA) [7], to determine the level of postural risk and guide the implementation of suitable intervention measures. Nevertheless, limitations exist when conducting posture assessments through field observation. Firstly, subjective judgments made by assessors are prone to biases influenced by viewing angles and fatigue [8,9]. Secondly, manual observation is time-consuming and inefficient. As a result, researchers have sought to develop machine-based automated assessment methods as a replacement for manual evaluation. Initially, some researchers employed contact-based sensors to capture human posture movements. While this method provides high accuracy and frequently serves as a validation benchmark for emerging recognition techniques [10,11], it requires a significant number of sensors, resulting in increased equipment costs and requiring extensive sensor calibration. Moreover, the use of sensors may impede the normal work of healthcare personnel [12,13]. In contrast, vision-based posture motion capture methods offer a non-contact approach that does not disrupt the tasks of healthcare providers [14]. Currently, this approach primarily relies on machine learning algorithms to recognize motion pose keypoints from images or videos [15,16], enabling the automatic calculation of the REBA posture score using these keypoints. Compared to the Microsoft Kinect camera [17] and various pose estimation networks (e.g., PoseNet [18], DensePose [19], HRNet [20]), OpenPose [21] is presently recognized as a widely utilized and reliable algorithm for human pose estimation, demonstrating stable skeletal tracking capabilities even in non-frontal views and video sequences.

We endeavored to incorporate OpenPose into the automatic REBA assessment of caregiver postures. However, our findings revealed significant discrepancies in the REBA scores and substantial fluctuations in joint angles. To explore the underlying reasons for this issue, we conducted an analysis of caregiver postures. The results revealed that when healthcare professionals were involved in posture estimation, the overlapping of limbs between nurses and patients not only led to the loss of skeletal information but also introduced complexities in distinguishing the skeletal structures of both parties. Consequently, this significantly compromised the accuracy of OpenPose in estimating caregiver postures, resulting in considerable fluctuations and errors in both REBA scores and joint angles. The simultaneous estimation of poses for multiple individuals presents inherent challenges that may compromise the accuracy of joint angle calculations and lead to inaccurate REBA scores, particularly in scenarios involving overlapping, occlusion, and intricate interactions among various body parts.

To improve the pose estimation deficiencies caused by body occlusion in nursing interactions, researchers have utilized the principle of left–right symmetry to compensate for missing skeleton keypoints [22]. However, this approach is applicable to pose captured from a frontal camera perspective, and deviations in camera angles result in corrected skeletal keypoints being positioned outside the body. To overcome this limitation, the Mask RCNN method has been utilized to detect human boundaries, thereby constraining the skeletal keypoints within the body's boundaries [23]. Nonetheless, compensating for skeletal keypoints using the symmetry principle often encounters challenges when dealing with complex movements. To restore occluded keypoints, researchers have explored the utilization of unoccluded skeletal keypoints in a Euclidean distance matrix [24]. This skeleton compensation method has proven successful in mitigating skeletal occlusion issues. However, ignoring temporal attributes and their association with skeletal motion trends leads to disparities between the compensated skeleton and the action dynamics. Furthermore, certain approaches have introduced the concept of "Human Dynamics" [25], which predicts future body poses based on multiple frames in the current video, even in the absence of subsequent frames. This method has demonstrated remarkable effectiveness in compensating for missing skeletal keypoints. However, limitations still persist regarding skeletal misidentification.

To tackle the challenges of skeleton loss and misidentification caused by body contact in nursing tasks, we proposed an enhanced spatial temporal graph convolutional network (ST-GCN) method that incorporated action feature weighting for skeleton time series. Additionally, we introduced a skeleton discrimination method based on kinematic chains, which identified skeletal loss and misidentification by combining skeleton and action features. This information was then utilized to provide feedback to the skeleton interpolation compensation network and skeleton correction network, enabling the reconstruction of missing and misidentified skeletal structures. The following are the main contributions of this study:

(1) An improved ST-GCN framework is proposed for skeleton action prediction.

(2) A kinematic-chain-based method for missing and misidentified skeletons is proposed for skeleton compensation in scenes with limb overlapping.

(3) Our results illustrate that the skeleton compensation and correction methods can effectively improve the calculation accuracy of skeleton joint angles and REBA score.

2. Methods

2.1. Overview

In our study, we introduced a novel kinematic chain skeleton discrimination method to assess the integrity of the pose skeleton, distinguishing loss and misidentification. By analyzing the heterogeneity of action features obtained from the ST-GCN network and their corresponding skeleton mappings within a predefined temporal threshold, we identified instances of skeleton misidentification from a pose-based kinematic chain perspective. To optimize skeletal loss, we proposed a temporal-based skeleton interpolation compensation method. This involved utilizing temporal features, traversing complete skeletons preceding and subsequent to the temporal sequence, and employing interpolation algorithms to rectify missing skeleton data. In cases of skeleton misidentification, we presented a method to optimize action feature heterogeneity. This technique involved optimizing action features with lower weights within the predefined temporal range, compensating for gaps by utilizing consistent action features from previous and subsequent temporal sequences, and updating the corresponding skeletons mapped with the action features to rectify misidentification of the pose skeleton. The overview of our skeleton compensation method is shown in Figure 1. The following supporting information can be downloaded at: https://github.com/Nicxhan/Skeleton-compensation-and-correction (accessed on 1 January 2024).

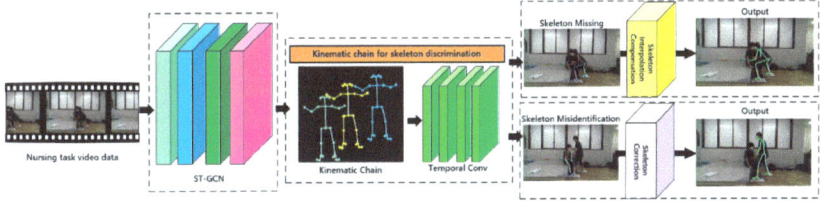

Figure 1. Overview of our skeleton compensation method.

2.2. ST-GCN

The ST-GCN has demonstrated its extraordinary ability to extract dynamic skeletal features from both spatial and temporal dimensions by capitalizing on a sequence of skeletal graphs [26]. Our adjusted ST-GCN structure comprises the spatial and spatial temporal feature layer (Figure 2a). Through the fusion of spatial temporal features of the skeleton, it enables the allocation of distinct action labels and weights to the temporal variations of skeletal features, redefining posture with actions.

The construction of the Spatial Feature layer entailed the integration of multiple Spatial Conv layers through residual structures. Each Spatial Conv layer was complemented by batch normalization (BN) and ReLU modules (Figure 2b), thereby bolstering the stability and facilitating the capture of intricate non-linear linkages among joints. The Spatial Feature layer aimed to discern the interconnected features that manifested between skeletal nodes and their neighboring counterparts, originating from the spatial information encapsulated within the pivotal nodes of the skeletal graph. Consequently, it exerted a discernible influence on the estimation of human poses by representing localized attributes of individual skeletal joints alongside the distinctive characteristics exhibited by adjacent nodes [27]. The Spatial–Temporal Feature layer, constructed by intricately interweaving multiple spatial temporal feature extraction units, manifested as a dense connection structure [28]. Encompassing a stack of Temporal Conv and Spatial Conv (Figure 2c), each Spatial–Temporal Conv aimed to extract motion trend features from skeletal joint nodes that exhibited correspondence across frames in the skeletal graph. This extraction process facilitated the depiction of motion trends between matched joint nodes in consecutive frames. By acquiring a comprehensive understanding of these features, the prediction of pose actions within the skeletal structure was enhanced.

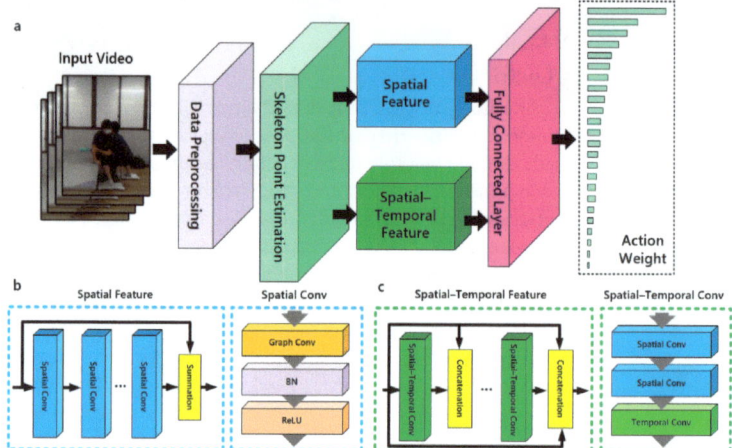

Figure 2. (**a**) Spatial temporal graph convolutional network structure. (**b**) Spatial Feature layer and Spatial Conv structure. (**c**) Spatial Temporal Feature layer and Spatial–Temporal Conv structure.

2.3. Kinematic Chain for Skeleton Discrimination

The integration of spatial and temporal features within the label mapping framework enables the determination of action weights for postures, with the highest-weighted action label signifying each unique posture. To address challenges related to missing or misidentified skeletons in complex scenarios, we introduced a Kinematic Chain Skeleton Discrimination Network in the extra layer of the ST-GCN. This novel approach evaluated both skeletal pose completeness and the comparison of fused action weight features, distinct from prior research [29]. Anomalous action weights within a defined temporal sequence were identified as misidentified actions and skeletons, and corrective feedback was provided for both. Skeletal connections, denoting the links between adjacent keypoints in the human skeletal structure, form a $2 \times M$ matrix K, where M represents the predefined number of skeletal keypoints. Matrix $\Psi = K^T K$ acts as a feature for discriminating skeletal integrity, with diagonal elements in Ψ representing squared joint lengths, while the remaining elements signify weighted angles between pairs of skeletal keypoints, serving as internal indicators. Inspired by kinematic chains, we introduced a temporal kinematic chain, defined as Equation (1)

$$\Phi = K_{t+i}^T K_{t+i} - K_t^T K_t \quad (1)$$

where i represents the temporal interval between successive frames within the temporal kinematic chain. The diagonal elements within matrix Φ depict alterations in skeletal joint lengths, while the remaining elements signify changes in angles between pairs of skeletal keypoints.

We established the prediction of temporal kinematic chains by connecting the coordinates of skeletal keypoints, which were subsequently input into a Temporal Convolutional Network (TCN) to construct a posture discrimination network. This methodology not only accounted for the integrity of posture skeletons across frames but also ensured the coherence of weight variations in action feature changes across frames. It optimized abnormal action weights and provides feedback for skeleton compensation or correction. Building upon the framework of a Generative Adversarial Network [30], we constructed the posture discrimination network and employed this framework to generate regularization loss for pose estimation.

2.4. Skeleton Interpolation Compensation

In the case of missing skeleton states detected in the pose estimation results, the skeleton interpolation compensation network initiated the process by considering the current time sequence of the missing skeleton as the starting point. Subsequently, it traversed through the skeletal information of the preceding and succeeding time sequences to identify complete skeletons. In terms of temporal proximity to the missing skeleton, the nearest preceding and succeeding complete skeletons were chosen as references for interpolating the missing skeleton. Based on the spatial and temporal features offered by the complete skeletons, the linear interpolation algorithm was employed to fill in the missing skeletal keypoints. Simultaneously, the motion characteristics of the temporal sequence were taken into account to ensure alignment between the generated skeleton and the actual kinematic features, the process of skeleton compensation is depicted in Figure 3. To determine the temporal features within the interpolation compensation process, the traversal range for the preceding and succeeding temporal skeletons was set to 10 frames. This selection of a 10-frame range, sampled at a frequency of 50 Hz, provided the optimal interpolated data for motion skeleton interpolation [31].

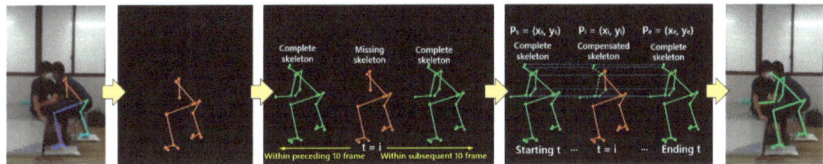

Figure 3. Skeleton compensation for missing frames (left to right: skeleton loss in OpenPose, missing skeleton frame, complete skeleton traverse, skeleton interpolation compensation, compensated skeleton).

Assuming that the motion velocity of skeletal keypoints remained independent and constant within the missing region, when there were n missing skeletal keypoints between the temporal sequences $P_s(x_s, y_s)$, $P_e(x_e, y_e)$, P_s and P_e represented the starting and ending points of the complete skeletal information with a temporal distance of 10 frames, respectively. The missing point was denoted as $P_1(x_1, y_1)$, $P_2(x_2, y_2)$, ..., $P_n(x_n, y_n)$. The equation for computing the interpolated compensatory coordinates of the missing skeleton keypoints was determined by Equations (2)–(4).

$$x_i = (1-t)x_s + tx_e \qquad (2)$$

$$y_i = (1-t)y_s + ty_e \qquad (3)$$

$$t = i/(n+1) \ (i = 1, 2, \ldots, n) \qquad (4)$$

2.5. Skeleton Correction

In the case of pose estimation results indicating skeletal misidentification states, we proposed a novel approach termed heterogeneous action feature optimization. By leveraging the inherent action features associated with each stage of the skeleton, we could rectify the misidentified skeleton by focusing on the correction of action features. The process of skeleton correction is depicted in Figure 4. The skeleton correction network commenced the process using the current time sequence of the misidentification skeleton as the starting point. It subsequently traversed the action features of the preceding and succeeding 10 frames within the temporal sequence. Following this, the weight proportions of the action features were calculated in the predefined time thresholds. For example, if the skeleton action features were denoted as A and B, within the specified time threshold, a comparison was made between the weights of action features A and B. Dominant action features were identified as those with a weight proportion exceeding 60%, while the remaining action features were considered heterogeneous. Consequently, the heterogeneous features were replaced with the dominant features, and the skeleton was accordingly updated. This approach effectively rectified the misidentified skeleton, demonstrating its efficacy in practice.

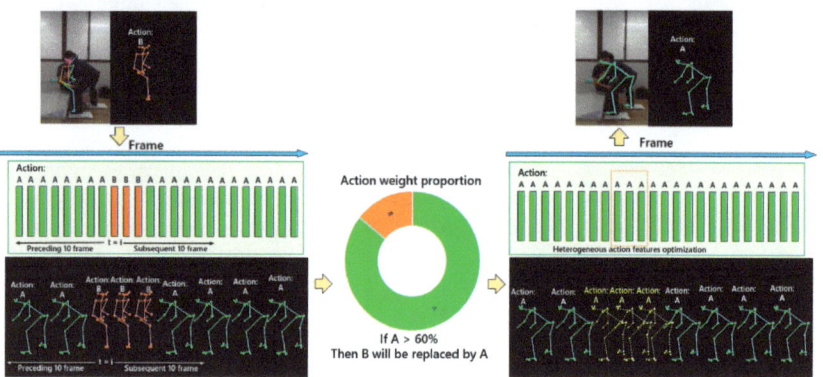

Figure 4. Skeleton correction for misidentified frames. It was accomplished by employing action features and weights when skeleton misidentification was detected, A and B represented the skeleton action features.

To prevent the disregard of preceding and succeeding frames due to estimation errors in the current frame, we incorporated the Kalman filtering algorithm to perform noise smoothing on the time series of coordinates for each skeletal point [32]. This procedure enhanced the congruity between the corrected skeleton and the actual movement. Assuming the independent calculation of each skeletal point, without considering skeletal constraints, we observed a natural correlation between the horizontal and vertical actions of the skeleton. Additionally, when disregarding action trends, the preceding and subsequent temporal states exhibited the same characteristics. Hence, Equations (5)–(9) were met.

$$\hat{x}_k^- = A\hat{x}_{k-1} + Bu_k \tag{5}$$

$$\hat{P}_k^- = AP_{k-1}A^T + Q \tag{6}$$

$$K_k = \left(P_k^- C^T\right) / \left(CP_k^- C^T + R\right) \tag{7}$$

$$\hat{x}_k = \hat{x}_k^- + K_k\left(y_k - C\hat{x}_k^-\right) \tag{8}$$

$$P_k = (I - K_kC)P_k^- \tag{9}$$

where $\hat{x}_k$ and $\hat{x}_{k-1}$ represent the posterior state estimates of the skeleton points at time series $k-1$ and k, respectively. $\hat{x}_k^-$ represents the prior state estimate of the skeleton point at time series k. P_{k-1} and P_k represent the posterior estimated covariance values at time series $k-1$ and k, respectively. $\hat{P}_k^-$ represents the a priori estimated covariance value at time series k. C represents the transformation matrix from state variables to measured values. y_k represents the input value. K_k represents the Kalman coefficient. A represents the state transition matrix. B represents the control input matrix. Q represents the process excitation noise covariance value. R represents the measurement noise covariance value.

2.6. Study Design

The data used in this study was acquired by recruiting volunteers to simulate the task of patient transfer. The recruited volunteers had no history of musculoskeletal disorders in the past year. Volunteers were tasked with transferring the standard patient from the bed to the wheelchair.

A single monocular RGB camera was employed for recording the nursing care task videos. A motion capture system comprising multiple inertial sensors was utilized to measure the angles of various joints in the body [33], with a high correlation observed between the results obtained from this system and those obtained from optical motion capture systems, making it suitable for joint angle measurement research. Additionally, inertial sensors possess strong occlusion resistance and find extensive application in fields like rehabilitation medicine and ergonomic analysis [34,35]. Hence, the joint angle measurements obtained from the inertial sensors can be employed as a ground truth value to assess the precision of visually based angle measurements [36].

Statistical analysis was conducted using SPSS v27 software (SPSS Inc., Chicago, IL, USA) and GraphPad Prism 9 (GraphPad Inc., San Diego, CA, USA). Paired *t*-tests were employed for paired continuous data, mean values and standard deviations were reported for all statistical tests. A *p*-value less than 0.05 was considered statistically significant.

2.7. Joint Angle and Scoring Tool

The nursing task videos were processed by OpenPose and our method to predict the human body skeleton and compute the skeleton joint angles. A total of 25 skeletal keypoints were identified for each participant (Figure 5), and based on the scoring criteria of the REBA, a total of eight joint angles were calculated. The computation of joint angles and their corresponding skeletal keypoints were summarized in Table 1. Due to the wrist being in a nearly fixed position during the nursing tasks, the wrist angle was considered constant for the purpose of angle measurement and posture risk assessment in this study.

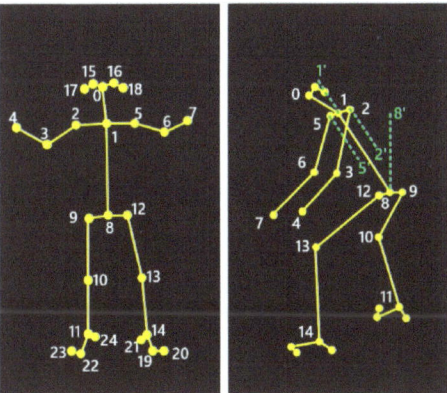

Figure 5. Pose estimation skeleton key points numbers. OpenPose detects 25 key skeletal points on the human body for joint construction and skeleton analysis. Numbers 0 to 24 represent different bone points.

Table 1. Joint angles list.

Joint Angle	Involved Skeletal Points
Trunk flexion angle	∠1, 8, 8′
Neck flexion angle	∠0, 1, 1′
Left leg flexion angle	∠12, 13, 14
Right leg flexion angle	∠9, 10, 11
Left upper arm flexion angle	∠5′, 5, 6
Right upper arm flexion angle	∠2′, 2, 3
Left lower arm flexion angle	∠5, 6, 7
Right lower arm flexion angle	∠2, 3, 4

The REBA method was chosen as a tool for evaluating ergonomic risks in the workplace. Its objective was to swiftly assess the WMSD risk of postures to determine which work positions require additional attention and improvement, thereby reducing the risk of bodily discomfort and injury associated with work. The REBA algorithm involved evaluating the angle changes of key joints (trunk, neck, legs, upper arms, lower arms, wrists), external loads, and hand coupling capability. REBA scores range from 1 to 12, with higher scores indicating greater WMSD risk (Table 2).

Table 2. REBA risk level list.

Action Level	REBA Score	Risk Level	Correction Suggestion
0	1	Negligible	None necessary
1	2–3	Low	Maybe necessary
2	4–7	Medium	Necessary
3	8–10	High	Necessary soon
4	11–15	Very high	Necessary now

2.8. Accuracy Verification

To validate the accuracy of our approach in posture risk assessment, a comparison was conducted among OpenPose, inertial sensors, and our method in terms of joint angles and REBA scores. The nursing task videos were separated into individual frames, and for each frame, the joint angles and REBA scores were calculated independently, as shown in Table 3. The mean absolute error (MAE) of the joint angles and the precision of the REBA scores were used to assess the performance of our method. The MAE measured the absolute difference between the joint angles computed by different methods. Although it did not distinguish between positive and negative errors, this value represented the actual magnitude of the error. The mathematical equation for MAE was determined by the Equations (10) and (11).

$$MAE_1 = \left(\sum_{i=1}^{n}|A_i - A_{si}|\right)/n \qquad (10)$$

$$MAE_2 = \left(\sum_{i=1}^{n}|A_{oi} - A_{si}|\right)/n \qquad (11)$$

where MAE_1 was measured by our method and the inertial sensors; MAE_2 was measured by OpenPose and the inertial sensors. Assuming the number of frames with consistent REBA scores between the inertial sensors and our method was denoted as F_m, and the total number of frames was denoted as F, the REBA precision calculation was determined by Equation (12).

$$Acc = F_m/F \times 100\% \qquad (12)$$

Table 3. Accuracy calculation parameters.

	Nursing Task Video	Frame 1	Frame 2	Frame i	Frame n
OpenPose	Joint angle	A_{o1}	A_{o2}	A_{oi}	A_{on}
	REBA	R_{o1}	R_{o2}	R_{oi}	R_{on}
Inertial sensors	Joint angle	A_{s1}	A_{s2}	A_{si}	A_{sn}
	REBA	R_{s1}	R_{s2}	R_{si}	R_{sn}
Ours	Joint angle	A_1	A_2	A_i	A_n
	REBA	R_1	R_2	R_i	R_n
Accuracy	Joint angle error	$[A_{o1}, A_{s1}, A_1]$	$[A_{o2}, A_{s2}, A_2]$	$[A_{oi}, A_{si}, A_i]$	$[A_{on}, A_{sn}, A_n]$
	REBA score error	$[R_{o1}, R_{s1}, R_1]$	$[R_{o2}, R_{s2}, R_2]$	$[R_{oi}, R_{si}, R_i]$	$[R_{on}, R_{sn}, R_n]$

3. Results

3.1. Missing and Misidentified Skeletons

During the application of OpenPose for posture risk assessment in nursing tasks, notable challenges arise from complex interactions and overlapping body configurations between nurses and patients. These challenges often lead to incomplete or erroneous skeletal estimations, resulting in deviations and fluctuations in joint angles (Figure 6a). For instance, as depicted in Figure 6b, when a skeleton corresponding to the upper arm was misidentified, substantial fluctuations in the upper arm angle occurred, resulting in discontinuous states. In contrast, our method optimized the misidentification problem (Figure 6c), maintaining a stable and continuous state for the joint angles of the upper arm. Likewise, in scenarios where the skeleton was missing, such as the legs, there might be deviations or even a complete absence of leg angles. However, our method optimized the identification of the skeleton, achieving the continuity of leg angle measurements.

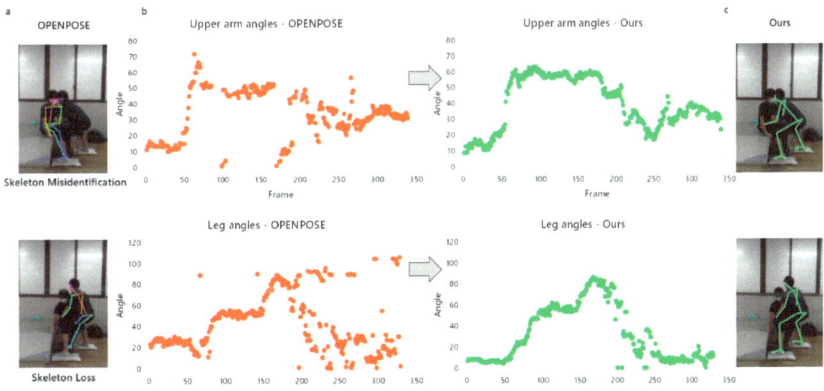

Figure 6. (a) The utilization of OpenPose for pose estimation in the nursing task gave rise to issues concerning missing and misidentified skeletons. (b) The variations in the angles of the upper arm and leg in the presence of skeleton loss and misidentification (Orange represents the angle data obtained by OpenPose) and subsequent skeleton compensation (Green represents the angle data obtained by our method). (c) The effect of our skeleton compensation method.

We compared the overall skeleton missing rate and misidentification rate for all frames (Table 4). The results revealed that our approach achieved a skeletal misidentification rate of 2.18%. Regarding the skeleton missing rate, except for the right lower arm (Lower arm-R) caused by limb occlusion, significant skeleton compensation effects were observed for all other missing skeletons. These outcomes highlighted the efficacy and potential of our approach in optimizing missing skeletons and misidentification the field of skeletal analysis.

Table 4. Overall skeleton missing rate and misidentification rate for all frames.

Joints	Skeleton Missing Rate		Skeleton Misidentification Rate	
	OpenPose	Ours	OpenPose	Ours
Trunk	0.18%	0.07%		
Leg-R	16.79%	5.96%		
Upper arm-R	22.42%	10.36%		
Lower arm-R	64.68%	51.67%	20.60%	2.18%
Neck	22.06%	7.01%		
Leg-L	8.47%	1.78%		
Upper arm-L	11.19%	0.29%		
Lower arm-L	12.75%	0.58%		

3.2. Joint Angles Error

To assess the accuracy of our approach in measuring joint angles, we conducted a comparative analysis of angle errors among various methods. The analysis involved three distinct groups, each focused on evaluating the errors within a specific context. $E_{angle1} = A_{oi} - A_{si}$ represented the error between the joint angles obtained from OpenPose and the ground truth values; $E_{angle2} = A_i - A_{si}$ represented the error between our method and the ground truth values; $E_{angle3} = A_i - A_{oi}$ represented the error in joint angle errors between our method and OpenPose (Table 5).

Table 5. Errors between different joint angles.

Joints	E_{angle1} (N = 8)	p-Value $p1$	E_{angle2} (N = 8)	p-Value $p2$	E_{angle3} (N = 8)	p-Value $p3$
Trunk	−0.166 ± 18.526	p = 0.628	−0.019 ± 2.345	p = 0.659	−0.017 ± 18.800	p = 0.961
Leg-R	3.880 ± 18.591	p < 0.001	−0.060 ± 2.324	p = 0.160	0.882 ± 6.090	p < 0.001
Upper arm-R	3.145 ± 10.742	p < 0.001	−0.186 ± 4.475	p = 0.025	0.755 ± 10.136	p < 0.001
Lower arm-R	3.969 ± 30.840	p < 0.001	−0.226 ± 4.427	p = 0.006	−0.108 ± 18.481	p = 0.752
Neck	−1.956 ± 14.891	p < 0.001	−0.072 ± 2.281	p = 0.087	1.963 ± 14.436	p < 0.001
Leg-L	−1.069 ± 7.174	p < 0.001	−0.125 ± 4.512	p = 0.134	−4.098 ± 30.771	p < 0.001
Upper arm-L	−1.014 ± 10.605	p < 0.001	−0.059 ± 2.292	p = 0.165	0.773 ± 9.903	P < 0.001
Lower arm-L	2.473 ± 27.971	p < 0.001	0.006 ± 4.586	p = 0.942	−3.001 ± 27.793	p < 0.001

We presented a detailed analysis of joint angle errors based on comprehensive experimental results (Table 5). When comparing joint angle errors between OpenPose and ground truth values (E_{angle1}), all angles, except Trunk angles ($p1$ = 0.628), displayed significant statistical differences ($p1$ < 0.001), indicating substantial joint angle deviations. Conversely, our method exhibited minimal errors compared to ground truth values (E_{angle2}), with significant statistical differences observed only in Upper arm-R ($p2$ = 0.025) and Lower arm-R ($p2$ = 0.006) joint angles. This highlighted the reliability of our method in calculating skeletal joint angles. Additionally, significant differences were found in joint angle errors ($p3$ < 0.001) between our method and OpenPose (E_{angle3}), except for Trunk ($p3$ = 0.961) and Lower arm-R angles ($p3$ = 0.752), demonstrating the effectiveness of our approach in enhancing pose estimation accuracy and improving the precision of skeletal joint angle calculation.

MAE was employed to evaluate the stability and accuracy of measuring joint angles. A smaller MAE value indicated better measurement accuracy. Our method consistently achieved an overall MAE (MAE1) below 10°, demonstrating superior accuracy in measuring joint angles (Figure 7). In contrast, OpenPose exhibited an MAE exceeding 10° for all joints, except the trunk, indicating significant error fluctuations. Both MAE1 and

MAE2 showed statistically significant differences across all joint angles ($p < 0.05$). These discrepancies could be attributed to the skeleton loss and misidentification issues encountered in OpenPose during estimation of nursing care poses, resulting in frequent variations in angle differences and increased error fluctuation. In contrast, our proposed method addressed these challenges by optimizing skeleton loss and misidentification and reducing error fluctuations. This significantly enhanced the accuracy of joint angle calculations, as evidenced by the lower MAE values and reduced error fluctuations observed in Figure 7.

3.3. REBA Score Error

To verify the performance of our method in REBA scoring, we conducted a comparative analysis of the error in REBA scores among different skeletal joints. $E_{REBA1} = R_{oi} - R_{si}$ denoted the error between OpenPose and the ground truth values, while $E_{REBA2} = R_i - R_{si}$ signified the error between our method and the ground truth values. The results, in accordance with the REBA scoring rules, are presented in Table 6.

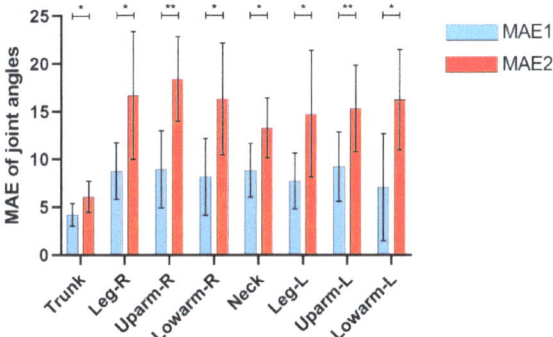

Figure 7. MAE of different joint angles. * $p < 0.05$, ** $p < 0.01$.

Table 6. Errors between joint angle score and REBA score.

Joints	EREBA1 (N = 8)	p-Value	EREBA2 (N = 8)	p-Value
Trunk	−0.001 ± 0.207	$p = 0.788$	0 ± 0.159	$p = 1$
Leg-R	0.255 ± 0.568	$p < 0.001$	0.015 ± 0.465	$p = 0.066$
Upper arm-R	−0.176 ± 0.644	$p < 0.001$	−0.005 ± 0.302	$p = 0.296$
Lower arm-R	−0.154 ± 0.635	$p < 0.001$	0.235 ± 0.448	$p < 0.001$
Neck	0.003 ± 0.132	$p = 0.124$	−0.003 ± 0.395	$p = 0.638$
Leg-L	−0.027 ± 0.282	$p < 0.001$	0.012 ± 0.506	$p = 0.186$
Upper arm-L	0.013 ± 0.282	$p = 0.013$	0.001 ± 0.186	$p = 0.619$
Lower arm-L	0.098 ± 0.309	$p < 0.001$	0.234 ± 0.508	$p = 0.325$
REBA	0.116 ± 1.128	$p < 0.001$	−0.003 ± 0.208	$p = 0.373$

Based on the comprehensive results presented in Table 6, notable differences ($p < 0.001$) were observed in the joints scores and REBA scores between the OpenPose and the ground truth values (E_{REBA1}), except for Trunk ($p = 0.788$) and Neck ($p = 0.124$). These observations indicated that the reliability of REBA scores derived from the OpenPose method for assessing nursing care task postures was suboptimal, with considerable deviations. Conversely, when considering the REBA scores obtained through our proposed method (E_{REBA2}), a significant difference was only observed for the Lower arm-R score ($p < 0.001$) compared to the ground truth values, while no significant differences were detected for other joint scores. Moreover, the final REBA scores showed no significant discrepancy compared to the ground truth values ($p = 0.373$). These outcomes demonstrated that the REBA scores computed using our method closely aligned with the ground truth values, highlighting the substantial feasibility and reliability of our approach for assessing nursing task posture.

Moreover, to evaluate the effectiveness of our method in tackling the issues of skeleton loss and misidentification within nursing care task scenarios, we conducted a comprehensive performance comparison against several existing methods, including that of Tsai et al. [23], a left–right skeletal symmetry skeleton compensation method; Guo et al. [24], a Euclidean distance matrix skeleton compensation method; and Kanazawa et al. [25], a Human-Dynamics-based temporal skeleton compensation method. The evaluation metric employed for this analysis was the precision of REBA scores. To uphold the scientific integrity of the comparative results, all assessments of the methods were conducted using standardized hardware configurations and nursing care posture datasets. Nonetheless, it was vital to exercise caution when interpreting these findings, as discrepancies in algorithmic parameters and model metrics might introduce variations that require careful consideration [37]. The summarized results of this comparative evaluation can be found in Table 7.

Table 7. Accuracy of REBA score by different methods in nursing care tasks.

Joints	Acc				
	OpenPose	Tsai et al. [23]	Guo et al. [24]	Kanazawa et al. [25]	Ours
Trunk	91.92%	90.34%	92.36%	95.32%	95.65%
Leg-R	81.43%	86.61%	86.42%	88.33%	87.47%
Upper arm-R	71.61%	72.41%	72.98%	75.79%	76.95%
Lower arm-R	47.76%	59.87%	60.14%	62.87%	64.31%
Neck	76.96%	82.86%	87.95%	86.97%	87.96%
Leg-L	82.94%	83.14%	89.76%	91.61%	90.81%
Upper arm-L	80.25%	85.27%	92.31%	91.89%	92.13%
Lower arm-L	84.26%	87.35%	91.14%	95.57%	91.68%
REBA	58.33%	63.29%	76.63%	80.46%	87.34%

The findings in Table 7 indicated that OpenPose achieved an accuracy exceeding 90% for specific skeletal joints, yet its final accuracy in REBA scoring remains at 58.33%. This was associated with the issues of skeleton loss and misidentification, which caused low accuracy of REBA. In contrast, our approach attained an accuracy of 87.34%, outperforming alternative methods and improving the skeleton loss and misidentification in nursing care tasks. Importantly, our method exhibited promising potential for pose assessment in interaction-based nursing tasks.

4. Discussion

4.1. Main Findings and Contributions

In this study, we identified concerning accuracy issues in the integration of OpenPose with the REBA assessment for nursing postures. This inadequacy stemmed from the inherent challenges posed by motion interactions and limb occlusions in nursing tasks, resulting in skeleton missing and misidentification in the OpenPose pose estimation. Consequently, these deviations and fluctuations in skeletal joint angles had a direct impact on the accuracy of REBA scoring. To address this problem, we have devised an innovative method that built upon the ST-GCN framework by incorporating action feature inverse skeleton compensation and correction. Hence, we enhanced the tracking of pose skeletons in scenarios involving overlapping bodies and interactive movements during nursing tasks. This improvement ensured the continuity and stability of skeletal joint angle calculations, ultimately resulting in an enhanced accuracy of REBA scoring.

To validate the reliability and feasibility of our proposed method, we conducted a comprehensive comparison of skeleton missing rate, skeleton misidentification rate, joint angles, REBA score, and REBA scoring accuracy. We have identified significant differences between the joint angles and scores obtained from OpenPose and the inertial sensors, primarily due to the influence of skeleton loss and misidentification. In contrast, our method yielded joint angles and scores that did not differ from the ground truth values, demonstrating the effectiveness of our approach in mitigating skeleton loss and misidentification challenges (Tables 5 and 6). Furthermore, it was important to highlight that substantial angle errors were observed in the right upper and lower arm joints (Table 5, Upper arm-R ($p2 = 0.025$), Lower arm-R ($p2 = 0.006$)). This discrepancy could be attributed to the interaction between the arms and patients during the caregiving process, resulting in the loss of arm joint tracking features. It is important to note that such limitations are commonly encountered in vision-based pose estimation algorithms. It could be overcome by employing marker-based wearable sensor measurement methods, but the use of sensors itself may impede the normal work of healthcare personnel [12]. It seems that improving the performance of pose estimation algorithms is more convenient and effective [10]. While our method showed smaller error fluctuation (Figure 7), improvements could be made in the future studies, particularly in addressing errors related to the Leg, Upper arm, and Lower arm joints on the side that is occluded by the limb. These joints experience significant challenged in terms of skeleton loss during the pose estimation process within multi-person interaction nursing care tasks. Therefore, future research efforts should prioritize enhancing the recognition accuracy of these specific joints.

While numerous studies have demonstrated the reliability of OpenPose in calculating joint angles for simple poses [38,39], its performance in complex scenarios involving overlapping bodies and interactions among multiple individuals remains suboptimal. Skeletal compensation methods that rely on left–right skeletal symmetry are often proved to be highly dependent on camera perspective settings [22]. Additionally, when employing Mask RCNN to confine the boundaries of compensated skeletal points in scenes with multiple individuals, the accuracy of pose skeleton estimation is not ideal enough [23]. Existing methods that compensate for occluded skeletons based on a Euclidean distance matrix [24] or that predict future pose skeletons using Human Dynamics [25] share a common limitation: they fail to address the problem of skeletal misidentification, leading to a uniform compensation approach for both correctly identified and misidentified skeletons. Consequently, the compensated skeletons fail to match the target pose skeleton, exacerbating differences in pose skeleton angles and REBA scores. Taking inspiration from skeleton kinematics, we proposed a novel skeleton discrimination method based on skeleton kinematic chains, which effectively distinguished different states of skeletal misidentification. Furthermore, we introduced a heterogeneous action feature optimization method that updated heterogeneous action features at the temporal sequences level. Leveraging the ST-GCN network's ability to assign action labels to different temporal skeletons, we could focus on updating the action features to correct misidentified skeletons. Comparative analysis of the accuracy of REBA scores demonstrated the distinct advantages of our method compared to alternative approaches (Table 7).

Furthermore, the primary objective of this study was to conduct a comparative analysis between our method and the OpenPose in terms of the predictive accuracy of skeletal joint angles at the algorithmic level of 2D pose estimation. It is important to note that the REBA scoring criteria encompasses not only joint angle assessment but also incorporates additional scores for joint rotation and extra points. To ensure consistency across all methods, we manually defined the parameters for rotation and extra point interventions. While previous research has explored posture risk assessment based on monocular camera 3D pose estimation [40,41], achieving good recognition accuracy, it is essential to recognize the inherent limitations of 3D pose evaluation. The computational demands associated with 3D pose estimation make it less suitable for real-time pose estimation, and the reliance on depth cameras or specialized sensors to capture depth data introduces complexities in terms of hardware and data collection. In contrast, 2D pose estimation algorithms exhibit greater resilience to challenging conditions such as lighting variations and occlusions in comparison to their 3D counterparts. Significantly, most existing monocular camera 3D pose estimation techniques primarily focus on simple pose estimation scenarios, while the complexities arising from multi-person interactions and limb occlusions present more substantial obstacles for accurate 3D pose estimation.

Collectively, our approach initially explored solutions for multi-person pose estimation from a 2D perspective before transitioning to 3D pose estimation research. The current research findings underscored the feasibility of our method, which might hold wide-ranging applicability in popular mobile devices or surveillance cameras through the utilization of lightweight models. Moreover, our method could be integrated into Internet of Things (IoT) devices equipped with RGB cameras, including smartphones and surveillance systems. Leveraging neural network models and image processing techniques, our method enables the inference of posture information, facilitating risk assessment and visual guidance for WMSDs associated with nursing postures. Looking ahead, the realization of an integrated intelligent nursing posture assessment system becomes a tangible possibility, driven by the advancements achieved through our method.

4.2. Limitations

It is important to acknowledge that our skeletal compensation and correction mechanisms rely on traversing temporal features over a span of 10 frames. Any instances of skeleton loss beyond this range might increase the skeleton miss rate of our method, resulting in our method's REBA score accuracy being limited to 87.34%. As such, future investigations should focus on mitigating these limitations and exploring a suitable traversing temporal scope for improving accuracy. Furthermore, exploring the application of monocular camera 3D caregiving pose evaluation would be merited to improve the performance in the limb occlusion scenario, as investigating the effectiveness of 3D compared to 2D approaches would carry significant implications and contribute to the advancement of the field.

4.3. Directions for Further Research

In light of the demonstrable benefits associated with the capture of temporal features over a 10-frame interval in nursing care action interaction actions, the accuracy of skeleton compensation within this temporal range is influenced by the speed and complexity of these actions across diverse application scenarios. Consequently, it is imperative for future research to prioritize the investigation of pose actions' intricacy and subsequently determine the optimal time span required to match these actions accurately. The development of a model that establishes the relationship between action complexity and time span would significantly enhance the efficiency and effectiveness of skeleton compensation, thereby unlocking the substantial potential for intelligent selection of time intervals in various pose estimation scenarios. Furthermore, augmenting the precision of monocular-camera-based 3D techniques in multi-person pose skeleton estimation is pivotal for improving the accuracy of caregiving posture assessment, particularly in scenarios involving rotational movements and changes in perspective. Exploring the integration of skeleton compensation and correction techniques derived from 2D approaches into 3D scenes represents a promising avenue for future research, as it addresses the challenge of compensating for skeleton occlusion during rotational maneuvers and visual alterations. Additionally, proactive exploration of the integration of our approach into Internet of Things (IoT) devices equipped with RGB cameras, such as smartphones and monitoring systems, holds substantial potential. Leveraging neural network models and image processing techniques to infer pose information can facilitate risk assessment and visual guidance pertaining to work-related musculoskeletal disorders (WMSDs), offering significant opportunities for the implementation of integrated intelligent pose assessment systems.

5. Conclusions

This study introduced an enhanced ST-GCN-based skeletal compensation method that effectively optimized skeletal occlusion and misidentification in nursing care tasks. Our approach integrated distinct action features and weights for posture skeletons, utilizing a skeletal discrimination network to evaluate skeleton integrity. To mitigate occlusion, we employed a skeletal interpolation compensation network that utilized adjacent temporal contexts. In instances of misidentification, a skeletal correction network optimized abnormal action features and updated skeletons accordingly. Our method improved joint angle calculations and enhanced the accuracy of REBA scores, which exhibited higher accuracy compared to the traditional OpenPose, achieving high precision in REBA scores for nursing task postures. Such improvements are crucial in mitigating the risk of WMSDs in the nursing profession.

Supplementary Materials: A demo could be found at https://github.com/Nicxhan/Skeleton-compensation-and-correction, accessed on 1 January 2024.

Author Contributions: Conceptualization, X.H., N.N. and Z.J.; methodology, X.H., N.N. and Z.J.; software, X.H.; validation, X.H., M.M. and T.S.; formal analysis, X.H., M.M. and T.S.; investigation, X.H., M.M. and T.S.; writing—original draft preparation, X.H.; writing—review and editing, N.N. and Z.J.; visualization, X.H.; supervision, N.N. and Z.J. All authors have read and agreed to the published version of the manuscript.

Funding: This research received no external funding.

Institutional Review Board Statement: The study was conducted in accordance with the Declaration of Helsinki and approved by the ethics committee at the Center for Clinical Research of the co-authors' hospital (H2019−182).

Informed Consent Statement: Informed consent was obtained from all subjects involved in the study.

Data Availability Statement: The data presented in this study are available on request from the corresponding author.

Acknowledgments: The authors would like to thank the motion capture system and related supporting equipment provided by the Micro Mechatronics Laboratory of Yamaguchi University Graduate School of Sciences and Technology for Innovation. The authors would also like to thank the professional medical staff of the Department of Orthopedic Surgery, Yamaguchi University Graduate School of Medicine, for their enthusiastic assistance and guidance.

Conflicts of Interest: The authors declare no conflicts of interest.

References

1. Jacquier-Bret, J.; Gorce, P. Prevalence of Body Area Work-Related Musculoskeletal Disorders among Healthcare Professionals: A Systematic Review. *Int. J. Environ. Res. Public Health* **2023**, *20*, 841. [CrossRef]
2. Heuel, L.; Lübstorf, S.; Otto, A.-K.; Wollesen, B. Chronic stress, behavioral tendencies, and determinants of health behaviors in nurses: A mixed-methods approach. *BMC Public Health* **2022**, *22*, 624. [CrossRef]
3. Naidoo, R.N.; Haq, S.A. Occupational use syndromes. *Best Pract. Res. Clin. Rheumatol.* **2008**, *22*, 677–691. [CrossRef]
4. Asuquo, E.G.; Tighe, S.M.; Bradshaw, C. Interventions to reduce work-related musculoskeletal disorders among healthcare staff in nursing homes; An integrative literature review. *Int. J. Nurs. Stud. Adv.* **2021**, *3*, 100033. [CrossRef]
5. Xu, D.; Zhou, H.; Quan, W.; Gusztav, F.; Wang, M.; Baker, J.S.; Gu, Y. Accurately and effectively predict the ACL force: Utilizing biomechanical landing pattern before and after-fatigue. *Comput. Meth. Programs Biomed.* **2023**, *241*, 107761. [CrossRef] [PubMed]
6. McAtamney, L.; Corlett, E.N. RULA: A survey method for the investigation of work-related upper limb disorders. *Appl. Ergon.* **1993**, *24*, 91–99. [CrossRef] [PubMed]
7. Hignett, S.; McAtamney, L. Rapid entire body assessment (REBA). *Appl. Ergon.* **2000**, *31*, 201–205. [CrossRef] [PubMed]
8. Graben, P.R.; Schall, M.C., Jr.; Gallagher, S.; Sesek, R.; Acosta-Sojo, Y. Reliability Analysis of Observation-Based Exposure Assessment Tools for the Upper Extremities: A Systematic Review. *Int. J. Environ. Res. Public Health* **2022**, *19*, 10595. [CrossRef] [PubMed]
9. Kee, D. Comparison of OWAS, RULA and REBA for assessing potential work-related musculoskeletal disorders. *Int. J. Ind. Ergon.* **2021**, *83*, 103140. [CrossRef]
10. Kim, W.; Sung, J.; Saakes, D.; Huang, C.; Xiong, S. Ergonomic postural assessment using a new open-source human pose estimation technology (OpenPose). *Int. J. Ind. Ergon.* **2021**, *84*, 103164. [CrossRef]
11. Xu, D.; Zhou, H.; Quan, W.; Jiang, X.; Liang, M.; Li, S.; Ugbolue, U.C.; Baker, J.S.; Gusztav, F.; Ma, X.; et al. A new method proposed for realizing human gait pattern recognition: Inspirations for the application of sports and clinical gait analysis. *Gait Posture* **2024**, *107*, 293–305. [CrossRef]
12. Lind, C.M.; Abtahi, F.; Forsman, M. Wearable Motion Capture Devices for the Prevention of Work-Related Musculoskeletal Disorders in Ergonomics—An Overview of Current Applications, Challenges, and Future Opportunities. *Sensors* **2023**, *23*, 4259. [CrossRef]

13. Kalasin, S.; Surareungchai, W. Challenges of Emerging Wearable Sensors for Remote Monitoring toward Telemedicine Healthcare. *Anal. Chem.* **2023**, *95*, 1773–1784. [CrossRef] [PubMed]
14. Han, X.; Nishida, N.; Morita, M.; Mitsuda, M.; Jiang, Z. Visualization of Caregiving Posture and Risk Evaluation of Discomfort and Injury. *Appl. Sci.* **2023**, *13*, 12699. [CrossRef]
15. Yu, Y.; Umer, W.; Yang, X.; Antwi-Afari, M.F. Posture-related data collection methods for construction workers: A review. *Autom. Constr.* **2021**, *124*, 103538. [CrossRef]
16. Xu, D.; Quan, W.; Zhou, H.; Sun, D.; Baker, J.S.; Gu, Y. Explaining the differences of gait patterns between high and low-mileage runners with machine learning. *Sci. Rep.* **2022**, *12*, 2981. [CrossRef] [PubMed]
17. Clark, R.A.; Mentiplay, B.F.; Hough, E.; Pua, Y.H. Three-dimensional cameras and skeleton pose tracking for physical function assessment: A review of uses, validity, current developments and Kinect alternatives. *Gait Posture* **2019**, *68*, 193–200. [CrossRef] [PubMed]
18. Kendall, A.; Grimes, M.; Cipolla, R. Posenet: A convolutional network for real-time 6-dof camera relocalization. In Proceedings of the IEEE International Conference on Computer Vision, Santiago, Chile, 7–13 December 2015; pp. 2938–2946.
19. Güler, R.A.; Neverova, N.; Kokkinos, I. Densepose: Dense human pose estimation in the wild. In Proceedings of the IEEE Conference on Computer Vision and Pattern Recognition, Salt Lake City, UT, USA, 18–22 June 2018; pp. 7297–7306.
20. Huang, J.; Zhu, Z.; Huang, G. Multi-stage HRNet: Multiple stage high-resolution network for human pose estimation. In Proceedings of the IEEE/CVF Conference on Computer Vision and Pattern Recognition (CVPR), Long Beach, CA, USA, 15–20 June 2019.
21. Cao, Z.; Simon, T.; Wei, S.E.; Sheikh, Y. Realtime multi-person 2d pose estimation using part affinity fields. In Proceedings of the IEEE Conference on Computer Vision and Pattern Recognition, Honolulu, HI, USA, 21–26 July 2017; pp. 7291–7299.
22. Huang, C.C.; Nguyen, M.H. Robust 3D skeleton tracking based on openpose and a probabilistic tracking framework. In Proceedings of the 2019 IEEE International Conference on Systems, Man and Cybernetics (SMC), Bari, Italy, 6–9 October 2019; pp. 4107–4112.
23. Tsai, M.F.; Huang, S.H. Enhancing accuracy of human action Recognition System using Skeleton Point correction method. *Multimed. Tools Appl.* **2022**, *81*, 7439–7459. [CrossRef]
24. Guo, X.; Dai, Y. Occluded joints recovery in 3d human pose estimation based on distance matrix. In Proceedings of the 2018 24th International Conference on Pattern Recognition (ICPR), Beijing, China, 20–24 August 2018; pp. 1325–1330.
25. Kanazawa, A.; Zhang, J.Y.; Felsen, P.; Malik, J. Learning 3d human dynamics from video. In Proceedings of the IEEE/CVF Conference on Computer Vision and Pattern Recognition, Long Beach, CA, USA, 15–20 June 2019; pp. 5614–5623.
26. Yan, S.; Xiong, Y.; Lin, D. Spatial temporal graph convolutional networks for skeleton-based action recognition. In Proceedings of the AAAI Conference on Artificial Intelligence, New Orleans, LA, USA, 2–7 February 2018; p. 32.
27. Chen, Y.; Zhang, Z.; Yuan, C.; Li, B.; Deng, Y.; Hu, W. Channel-wise topology refinement graph convolution for skeleton-based action recognition. In Proceedings of the IEEE/CVF International Conference on Computer Vision, Montreal, BC, Canada, 11–17 October 2021; pp. 13359–13368.
28. Li, G.; Zhang, M.; Li, J.; Lv, F.; Tong, G. Efficient densely connected convolutional neural networks. *Pattern Recognit.* **2021**, *109*, 107610. [CrossRef]
29. Wandt, B.; Ackermann, H.; Rosenhahn, B. A kinematic chain space for monocular motion capture. In Proceedings of the European Conference on Computer Vision (ECCV) Workshops, Munich, Germany, 8–14 September 2018.
30. Natarajan, B.; Elakkiya, R. Dynamic GAN for high-quality sign language video generation from skeletal poses using generative adversarial networks. *Soft Comput.* **2022**, *26*, 13153–13175. [CrossRef]
31. Howarth, S.J.; Callaghan, J.P. Quantitative assessment of the accuracy for three interpolation techniques in kinematic analysis of human movement. *Comput. Methods Biomech. Biomed. Eng.* **2010**, *13*, 847–855. [CrossRef] [PubMed]
32. Gauss, J.F.; Brandin, C.; Heberle, A.; Löwe, W. Smoothing skeleton avatar visualizations using signal processing technology. *SN Comput. Sci.* **2021**, *2*, 429. [CrossRef]
33. Miyajima, S.; Tanaka, T.; Imamura, Y.; Kusaka, T. Lumbar joint torque estimation based on simplified motion measurement using multiple inertial sensors. In Proceedings of the 2015 37th Annual International Conference of the IEEE Engineering in Medicine and Biology Society (EMBC), Milan, Italy, 25–29 August 2015; pp. 6716–6719.
34. Liang, F.Y.; Gao, F.; Liao, W.H. Synergy-based knee angle estimation using kinematics of thigh. *Gait Posture* **2021**, *89*, 25–30. [CrossRef]
35. Figueiredo, L.C.; Gratão, A.C.M.; Barbosa, G.C.; Monteiro, D.Q.; Pelegrini, L.N.d.C.; Sato, T.d.O. Musculoskeletal symptoms in formal and informal caregivers of elderly people. *Rev. Bras. Enferm.* **2021**, *75*, e20210249. [CrossRef]
36. Yu, Y.; Li, H.; Yang, X.; Kong, L.; Luo, X.; Wong, A.Y.L. An automatic and non-invasive physical fatigue assessment method for construction workers. *Autom. Constr.* **2019**, *103*, 1–12. [CrossRef]
37. Li, L.; Martin, T.; Xu, X. A novel vision-based real-time method for evaluating postural risk factors associated with musculoskeletal disorders. *Appl. Ergon.* **2020**, *87*, 103138. [CrossRef] [PubMed]
38. Li, Z.; Zhang, R.; Lee, C.-H.; Lee, Y.-C. An evaluation of posture recognition based on intelligent rapid entire body assessment system for determining musculoskeletal disorders. *Sensors* **2020**, *20*, 4414. [CrossRef]
39. Xu, D.; Zhou, H.; Quan, W.; Gusztav, F.; Baker, J.S.; Gu, Y. Adaptive neuro-fuzzy inference system model driven by the non-negative matrix factorization-extracted muscle synergy patterns to estimate lower limb joint movements. *Comput. Meth. Programs Biomed.* **2023**, *242*, 107848. [CrossRef]

40. Yuan, H.; Zhou, Y. Ergonomic assessment based on monocular RGB camera in elderly care by a new multi-person 3D pose estimation technique (ROMP). *Int. J. Ind. Ergon.* **2023**, *95*, 103440. [CrossRef]
41. Liu, P.L.; Chang, C.C. Simple method integrating OpenPose and RGB-D camera for identifying 3D body landmark locations in various postures. *Int. J. Ind. Ergon.* **2022**, *91*, 103354. [CrossRef]

Disclaimer/Publisher's Note: The statements, opinions and data contained in all publications are solely those of the individual author(s) and contributor(s) and not of MDPI and/or the editor(s). MDPI and/or the editor(s) disclaim responsibility for any injury to people or property resulting from any ideas, methods, instructions or products referred to in the content.

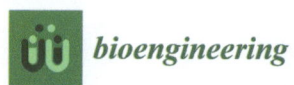

Article

Musculoskeletal Disorder Risk Assessment during the Tennis Serve: Performance and Prevention

Philippe Gorce [1,2] and Julien Jacquier-Bret [1,2,*]

1. International Institute of Biomechanics and Occupational Ergonomics, 83418 Hyères, France; gorce@univ-tln.fr
2. University of Toulon, CS60584, 83041 Toulon, France
* Correspondence: jacquier@univ-tln.fr

Abstract: Addressing the risk of musculoskeletal disorders (MSDs) during a tennis serve is a challenge for both protecting athletes and maintaining performance. The aim of this study was to investigate the risk of MSD occurrence using the rapid whole-body assessment (REBA) ergonomic tool at each time step, using 3D kinematic analysis of joint angles for slow and fast serves. Two force platforms (750 Hz) and an optoelectronic system including 10 infrared cameras (150 Hz, 82 markers located on the whole body and on the racket) were used to capture the kinematics of the six REBA joint areas over five services in two young male and two young female ranked players. The mean REBA score was 9.66 ± 1.11 (ranging from 7.75 to 11.85) with the maximum value observed for the loading and cocking stage (REBA score > 11). The intermediate scores for each of the six joint areas ranged between 2 and 3 and the maximum value of their respective scales. The lowest scores were observed for the shoulder. Neck rotation and shoulder flexion are parameters that could be taken into account when analyzing performance in the context of MSD prevention.

Keywords: biomechanics; optoelectronic system; 3D motion analysis; ergonomic assessment; REBA; tennis serve; performance; coaching

Citation: Gorce, P.; Jacquier-Bret, J. Musculoskeletal Disorder Risk Assessment during the Tennis Serve: Performance and Prevention. *Bioengineering* **2024**, *11*, 974. https://doi.org/10.3390/bioengineering11100974

Academic Editors: Guang Yue and Ravinder Reddy Regatte

Received: 3 September 2024
Accepted: 20 September 2024
Published: 27 September 2024

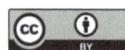

Copyright: © 2024 by the authors. Licensee MDPI, Basel, Switzerland. This article is an open access article distributed under the terms and conditions of the Creative Commons Attribution (CC BY) license (https://creativecommons.org/licenses/by/4.0/).

1. Introduction

The tennis serve is a complex movement that must be mastered to gain an advantage over the opponent. Control of ball velocity and trajectory is conditioned by racket control, which is linked to the kinematics of the player's body. In order to study the execution of a serve, many authors have divided it into phases based on key postures. Kovacs and Ellenbecker [1] proposed a three-phase decomposition with eight stages as follows: the preparation phase with four stages (start, release, loading, and cocking), the acceleration phase with two stages (acceleration and ball contact), and the follow-up phase with two stages (deceleration and finishing). Five key points of interest have been classically identified in the literature [1,2]. These are (1) the initial position with the racket at rest (start); (2) the ball release (BR) when the ball leaves the non-serving hand; (3) the trophy position (TP) with minimal vertical elbow position and maximum knee flexion; (4) the racket low point (RLP) when lateral shoulder rotation is maximal and the racket head is pointing downwards; and (5) the ball impact (BI).

To master this technique, a detailed knowledge of kinematics is needed to improve performance, often considered in terms of ball or racket velocity. These parameters are affected by several factors, such as service side, service type, or stance style, as many studies have demonstrated. For example, Reid et al. reported a difference in knee extension velocity as a function of stance style [3]. The foot-up technique (placing the back foot next to the foot before the jump) generates a greater knee extension velocity than the foot-back technique (keeping the feet offset, one forward and the other backward, until the jump [4]). Hornestam et al. [5] also reported that knee flexion had an impact on racket velocity. Comparing two groups with different flexions, the authors showed that the group with the lowest knee flexion generated a lower racket velocity than the group with the highest knee flexion. Reid et al. also showed that a kick serve led to a lower racket velocity than a flat serve in high-level players [6].

Kinematic analyses were also carried out at different key points, especially TP, RLP, and BI [7]. For TP, the authors mainly studied trunk position as well as knee and ankle flexions (front and back) as a function of several parameters. Trunk inclination and rotation, respectively, assessed from $17.0 \pm 11.0°$ to $34.3 \pm 7.6°$ and from $4.0 \pm 10.0°$ to $27.3 \pm 25.5°$, were affected by age (children, teenagers, and adults [8]), level (expert vs. non-expert [9]), and stance style (foot-up vs. foot-back [3]). Knee and ankle flexions were analyzed as a function of sex [10,11], age [12], type of serve (flat, slice, and topspin serve [13]), and racket size [14] with values ranging between $47.0 \pm 21.0°$ and $82.8 \pm 12.8°$ for the knees and between $0.3 \pm 22.3°$ and $19.8 \pm 3.4°$ for the ankles. For these two joint angles, some authors compared the values obtained for the front and rear lower limbs [13–15]. A few studies reported values for the upper limb, notably, on shoulder axial rotation (from $60.0°$ to $76°$ [16,17]), elbow flexion ($77.8 \pm 35.1°$ to $107.0 \pm 30.0°$), and wrist flexion ($2.0 \pm 10.0°$ to $16.0 \pm 11.0°$) [9,12].

For RLP, the joint angle most studied in the literature has been shoulder lateral rotation, which is the parameter that defines this key point [1]. The value of shoulder lateral rotation has been measured as a function of multiple parameters such as the type of serve (flat: $89.8°$ [18]; kick: $119.0 \pm 18.3°$ [6]), the side of serve (deuce: $136.7 \pm 10.6°$; ad: $138.1 \pm 11.4°$ [19]), fatigue condition ($125.0°$ with and without fatigue [16]), and age (children: $152.0 \pm 32°$ [2]; adults: $141.0 \pm 7.0°$ [8]).

The player's posture at the moment of ball impact has also been the subject of numerous studies under a variety of conditions. Shoulder abduction and elbow flexion were the two most commonly reported parameters in these studies. The results showed a slight elbow flexion at BI for the following conditions: sex (male $10.7 \pm 6.6°$; female: $34.7 \pm 4.0°$ [10]), age (children: $44.0 \pm 13.0°$ [2]; adults: $27.0 \pm 8.0°$ [8]), level (expert: $5.4 \pm 7.8°$; non-expert: $79.9 \pm 4.9°$ [9]), and side of serve (deuce: $18.0 \pm 7.8°$; ad: $18.0 \pm 8.5°$ [19]). Shoulder abduction was assessed at nearly $100°$ under the following conditions: sex (male $150.3 \pm 4.9°$; female: $161.1 \pm 1.3°$ [10], age (children: $92.0 \pm 9.0°$ [2]; adults: $104.0 \pm 13.0°$ [8]), and side of serve (deuce: $114.0 \pm 6.4°$; ad: $114.5 \pm 6.4°$ [19]). Trunk inclination (>$25°$ [2,20]), wrist flexion (20 to $30°$ [11,19]), knee flexion (20 to $30°$ [19,21]), and ankle extension (approx. $40°$ [8,11]) have also been reported in some studies.

In conjunction with the kinematic analysis of the serve, the question of preventing musculoskeletal disorders (MSDs) and their consequences in tennis players has been addressed in the literature in a descriptive way. MSDs are defined by the World Health Organization as health problems of the locomotor apparatus, i.e., muscles, tendons, bone skeleton, cartilage, ligaments, and nerves. This includes any type of complaint, from slight transitory discomforts to irreversible and incapacitating injuries [22]. They can be caused by acute trauma (e.g., fractures, sports injuries), tissue degeneration (e.g., osteoarthritis, spinal stenosis), genetic aberrancies (e.g., muscular dystrophy), and autoimmunity (e.g., rheumatoid arthritis) [23]. Martin et al. compared differences in the onset time of several biomechanical events between a group of healthy and a group of injured players [24]. However, to our knowledge, no study has objectively quantified and qualified the level of risk when serving in tennis. There are many tools available to assess MSD risk. Gómez-Galán et al. proposed an exhaustive list of these tools and classified them into three groups as follows: direct, indirect, and semi-direct methods [25]. Semi-direct methods use posture evaluation grids and additional activity-related criteria to assess MSD risk. Among the 18 methods listed, the REBA—Rapid Entire Body Assessment [26] method enables the whole body to be taken into account in posture assessment, using angular value thresholds, unlike other methods such as RULA—Rapid Upper Limb Assessment [27], LUBA—postural loading on the upper body assessment [28], OWAS—Ovako Working Posture Analyzing System [29], and RAMP—Risk Assessment and Management tool for manual handling Proactively [30].

The aim of the present study was to evaluate tennis serve performance by integrating an MSD risk assessment using the REBA in order to prevent and better understand the onset of MSDs. Perkins and Davis proposed a list of musculoskeletal injuries most commonly encountered in tennis players by joint area [31]. Thus, a detailed analysis of MSD risk by region using REBA intermediate scores was proposed to identify the areas most at risk during a slow and fast serve. The ergonomic scores were computed at each moment of the shift by quantified posture analysis using an optoelectronic system.

2. Materials and Methods

2.1. Participants

Four right-handed young tennis players (17.8 ± 2.2 years, 56.5 ± 4.6 kg, and 1.66 ± 0.08 m) ranked in the first series in the French national ranking voluntarily participated in the experiment. The sample included 2 young males and 2 young females. Detailed characteristics are presented in Table 1. None of them suffered from any joint or muscle injury that might affect serve performance. After a detailed and comprehensive presentation of the entire protocol, each player gave written informed consent before taking part in the experiment. The protocol conformed to the Declaration of Helsinki. The Ethics Committee of the International Institute of Biomechanics and Occupational Ergonomics approved the experiment (IIBOE23-E53).

Table 1. Detailed characteristics of the measured players.

	Player 1	Player 2	Player 3	Player 4	Mean ± Std
Sex	Male	Male	Female	Female	
Age (year)	21	17	17	16	17.8 ± 2.2
Height (m)	1.75	1.74	1.63	1.59	1.66 ± 0.08
Weight (kg)	58.1	61.0	58.8	50.4	56.5 ± 4.6
BMI	19.0	20.2	22.1	19.9	20.3 ± 1.3
Training by week (h)	15.0	15.0	15.0	15.0	15.0 ± 0.0
Level	National	National	National	National	

2.2. Experimental Task

Each subject faced a wall 11.88 m away, onto which a tennis net of the required dimensions was projected to reproduce the conditions of a tennis court. The net was surmounted by a target zone to be reached corresponding to a theoretically successful serve. Each player began with a 15 min warm-up session to prevent injury during the experiment. Next, the task was to perform a series of flat serves until five attempts were usable. Each serve was followed by a one-minute rest.

2.3. Equipment

After the warm-up session, the players were fitted with 74 markers (14 mm in diameter) positioned all over the body. Fifty-six were anatomical markers positioned on anatomical landmarks identified by palpation in accordance with the recommendations of the International Society of Biomechanics (ISB) [32,33]. Eighteen technical markers were added in clusters of 3 on both arms, forearms, and thighs in order to reconstruct the trajectories of the anatomical markers in the case of occultation. Eight markers were placed around the sieve and on the racket handle to record its position throughout the serve. The markers were carefully positioned so as not to interfere with the racket's grip [34].

The 3D marker trajectories were recorded using an optoelectronic system comprising ten M5 infrared cameras (Qualisys AB, Göteborg, Sweden) sampled at 150 Hz. A digital camera (Samsung galaxy S20 FE, Samsung Electronics, Seoul, Republic of Korea) was added in the sagittal plane of the player (left) to record each serve entirely and detect the serve key points of interest and the ball's position.

Two force platforms (600×400 mm Kistler 5695A DAQ, Winterthur, Eulachstrasse, Switzerland, 750 Hz) were used to record 3D ground reaction forces (anteroposterior, mediolateral, and vertical axes) throughout the serve. Each subject was asked to start with one foot on each platform and then execute the serve.

2.4. Data Processing

Qualisys Track Manager Software (v2020.3 build 6020—Qualisys AB, Gothenburg, Sweden) was used for body tracking and automatic marker labeling. The cubic spline gap-filling function was used to reconstruct anatomical markers in the case of occultation [34,35]. A trial was considered usable if occultations were less than 10 frames. The 20 selected trials (5 trials × 4 subjects) were exported to Matlab (R2023a Update 5, v9.14.0.2237262, The Mathworks, Natick, MA, USA). A Butterworth anti-aliasing low-pass filter (order 2, with a cut-off frequency of 8 Hz) was applied to the data set. The body was modeled in 15 segments as follows: neck, truck, pelvis, left and right arms, forearms, hands, thighs, legs, and feet. An anatomical landmark was defined for each segment at each moment of the serve, based on anatomical markers and in accordance with ISB recommendations. The pelvis was considered the origin of the model, and its 3D position was analyzed in the global reference frame associated with the laboratory with X corresponding to the anteroposterior axis pointing forward, Y corresponding to the vertical axis pointing upwards, and Z corresponding to the mediolateral axis pointing to the right. From this segment, the joint angles of the hips, knees, and ankles, for the lower limbs, and of the neck, trunk, shoulders, elbows, and wrists, for the upper body, were derived from the rotation matrices obtained from the coordinate system of two consecutive segments. The ZXY rotation sequence recommended by ISB was used to compute lower limb joint angles, as well as trunk, neck, elbow, and wrist angles. Only the shoulder sequence was different. Based on recent work, the XZY rotation sequence is preferred to the ISB sequence (YXY), as it is better suited to the analysis of the tennis serve [36].

Twenty-three joint angles were computed at every instant of the serve as follows: neck and trunk flexion (−)/extension (+), left (−)/right (+) inclination and left (+)/right (−) rotation, pelvis anteversion (−)/retroversion (+), left (−)/right (+) inclination and left (+)/right (−) rotation, shoulder and hip flexion (+)/extension (−), abduction (−)/adduction (+) and medial (+)/lateral (−) rotation, elbow flexion (+) and knee flexion (−), forearm pronation (+)/supination (−) wrist flexion (+)/extension (−) and radio (−)/ulnar (+) deviation, and ankle flexion (+)/extension (−).

MSD risk assessment was carried out using the REBA [26]. The proposed grid detailed by Raman et al. was used to compute the REBA score between 1 and 12 [37] (see Appendix A). REBA has the following 5 risk levels: 1 = negligible risk, no action required; 2–3 = low risk, change may be needed; 4–7 = medium risk, further investigation, change soon; 8–10 = high risk, investigate and implement change; 11–12 = very high risk, implement change. A specific script was developed with Matlab to compute the intermediate scores and the final REBA score at each instant of the serve.

Six intermediate scores were successively considered as follows: neck, trunk, leg, upper arm, lower arm, and wrist scores. Joint angle values and specific parameters were used to obtain these six scores. Vertical reaction forces were used to identify take-off and landing instants and thus, the number of ground supports. This information was used to compute the leg score. The force/load score was set to 0, as the weight of a tennis racket is well under 5 kg. The coupling score was also set to 0 because the racket is handled with a power grip. Finally, the activity score was set to 1 because the serve is a fast action with a wide range of changes in posture. All this information was then used to read the intermediate scores needed to determine the final REBA score.

The temporal evolution of the REBA score and each intermediate score was analyzed to determine which joint areas were most at risk and, therefore, which pathologies were likely to appear as a result of repeated service. These data were coupled with the time course of the corresponding kinematic variables for slow and fast services.

Seven key points were selected to analyze the serve. Five of them, i.e., start, BR, TP, RLP, and BI, were defined as presented in the literature [1,2] and characterized using 3D anatomical marker data. Only BI was identified using the camera previously synchronized with the optoelectronic system. The following key points were added: (1) finish, which corresponds to the end of racket displacement that follows BI before the preparation movement for the next stroke, as presented by Kovacs et al. [1], and (2) backward, which corresponds to the moment when the player's center of gravity reaches its greatest backward position (smallest value along the X axis of the laboratory global reference frame). The different stages of the serve were defined based on the following 7 key points: release backward between start and backward, release forward between backward and BR, loading between BR and TP, cocking between TP and RLP, acceleration between RLP and BI, and follow through between BI and finish. This division enabled us to study the temporal course of the tennis serve. Figure 1 illustrates the position of the 82 markers for each key point and their trajectory during the serve. Figure 2 shows the entire process of data analysis and ergonomic evaluation using REBA.

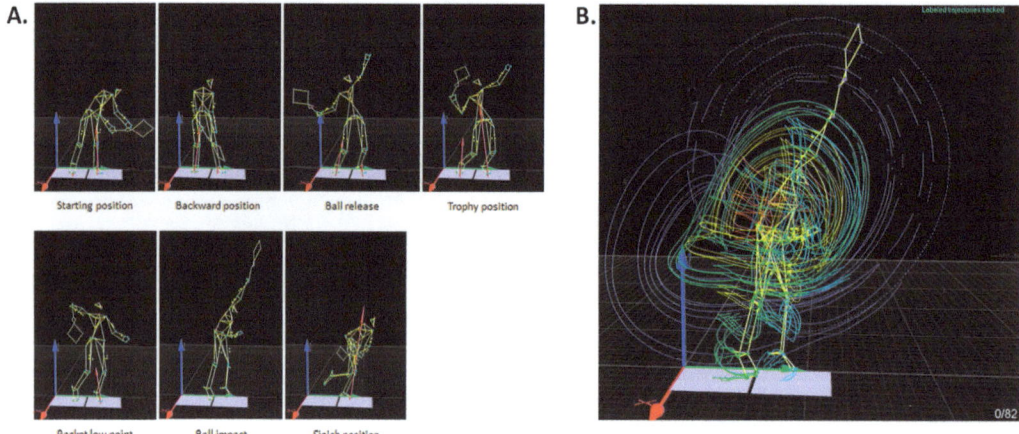

Figure 1. Three-dimensional visualization of markers positioned on players. (**A**) Position of markers at each key point of interest. (**B**) Marker trajectories during the serve. The illustration shows the first attempt by the first male player. The green and blue markers represent anatomical points on the right and left sides respectively. Yellow markers represent technical markers. The purple markers relate to the racket. The two blue squares represent the two force plates. The red vertical arrows represent ground reaction forces.

2.5. Statistical Analysis

A descriptive analysis (mean ± standard deviation) of intermediate and total REBA scores and the corresponding temporal assessment of joint angle was performed for the entire tennis serve. A repeated-measures ANOVA was performed to compare total REBA scores at each key point, taking into account all 20 serves (Statistica 7.1, Statsoft, Tulsa, OK, USA). The significance level was set at 5%.

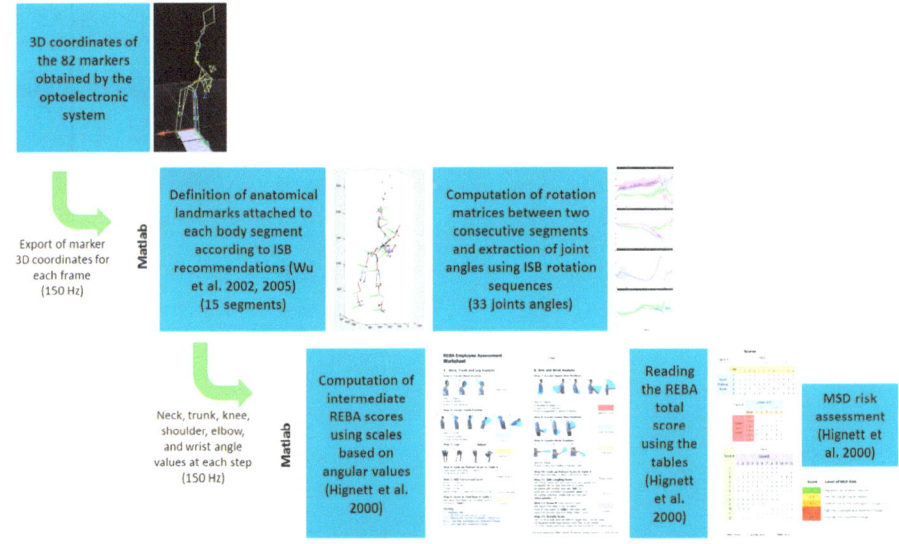

Figure 2. Presentation of the experimental data processing used to carry out an ergonomic assessment of MSD risks during the tennis serve using REBA.

3. Results

3.1. MSD Assessment: REBA Analysis

The mean REBA score was 9.7 ± 1.1. Figure 3 shows the evolution of this score during the serve. The average REBA score ranged from 7.7 to 11.8. The lowest scores were observed during the release backward phase. From the second half of the release forward phase, the score increased beyond 11 and was maintained during the loading and cocking phases. A decrease was observed just after BI, followed by an increase to a value close to 11 during the follow-through phase. These scores indicate that the tennis serve presents a high or very high risk with the need to implement changes from an ergonomic point of view. Table 2 presents the REBA score for each serve of each player as well as the mean score for each of the seven key points considered. The highest scores were recorded for TP, RLP, and finish (11.5 ± 0.6, 11.2 ± 0.9, and 11.0 ± 0.3, respectively, $p < 0.05$), while the lowest scores were observed for start, backward, and BI (8.6 ± 1.8, 8.9 ± 0.9, 9.6 ± 1.0, respectively, $p < 0.05$).

The following section presents the REBA results by joint area, according to the REBA evaluation grid: neck, trunk, leg, shoulder, elbow, and wrist.

The neck score ranges from 1 to 4. The mean value obtained during the serve was 3.6 ± 0.2, with values ranging from 3 to 4 throughout the cycle (Figure 4). Peak values were observed during the loading and the follow-through phases. The lowest values were found around BI. Kinematic evaluation showed that neck extension increased throughout the serve (0° to 60°). Contralateral axial rotation (on the left for right-handed players) increased from 20° to 45° during release and loading phases, with a maximum at the start of the cocking phase, then became zero at RLP and increased again in homolateral rotation (on the right for right-handed players) to 30° at the end of the follow-through phase. Neck inclination averaged between −10° and 10°.

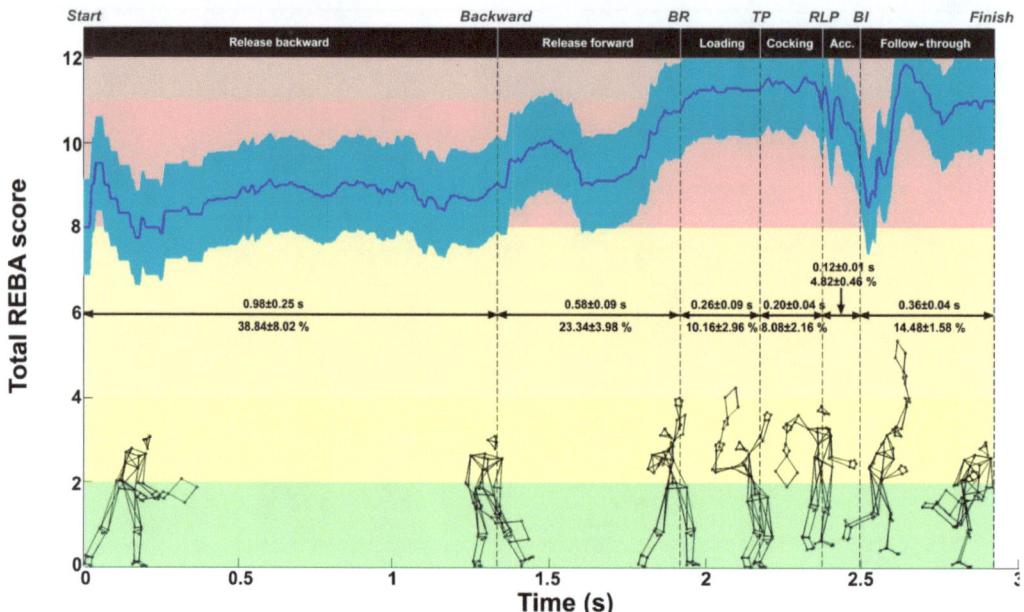

Figure 3. Evolution of the REBA score (mean ± standard deviation) during the tennis serve. The background colors represent the REBA risk level (see last part of Figure 2).

Table 2. REBA score for each serve and each player computed for the 7 key points of interest.

		Start	Backward	BR	TP	RLP	BI	Finish
	Serve 1	9	9	11	11	10	9	11
	Serve 2	10	9	11	11	11	9	12
	Serve 3	9	9	11	11	11	9	11
	Serve 4	9	9	11	11	11	9	11
	Serve 5	10	9	11	11	11	9	11
	Serve 1	7	10	11	12	12	7	11
	Serve 2	7	10	7	12	12	10	11
Player 2	Serve 3	7	8	8	11	10	10	10
	Serve 4	8	8	7	12	10	10	11
	Serve 5	7	8	7	12	10	10	11
	Serve 1	11	10	12	12	12	12	11
	Serve 2	12	10	12	11	12	11	11
	Serve 3	11	10	12	10	12	10	11
	Serve 4	8	8	12	12	12	9	11
	Serve 5	10	9	11	11	12	9	11
	Serve 1	7	8	11	12	11	10	11
	Serve 2	7	10	11	12	11	9	11
Player 4	Serve 3	5	8	10	12	9	10	11
	Serve 4	10	8	11	12	12	9	11
	Serve 5	7	8	10	12	12	10	11
	Mean	8.6 ± 1.8 [3457]	8.9 ± 0.9 [3457]	10.4 ± 1.7 [124]	11.5 ± 0.6 [1236]	11.2 ± 0.9 [126]	9.6 ± 1.0 [457]	11.0 ± 0.3 [126]

[1] different from start; [2] different from backward; [3] different from BR; [4] different from TP; [5] different from RLP; [6] different from BI; [7] different from finish.

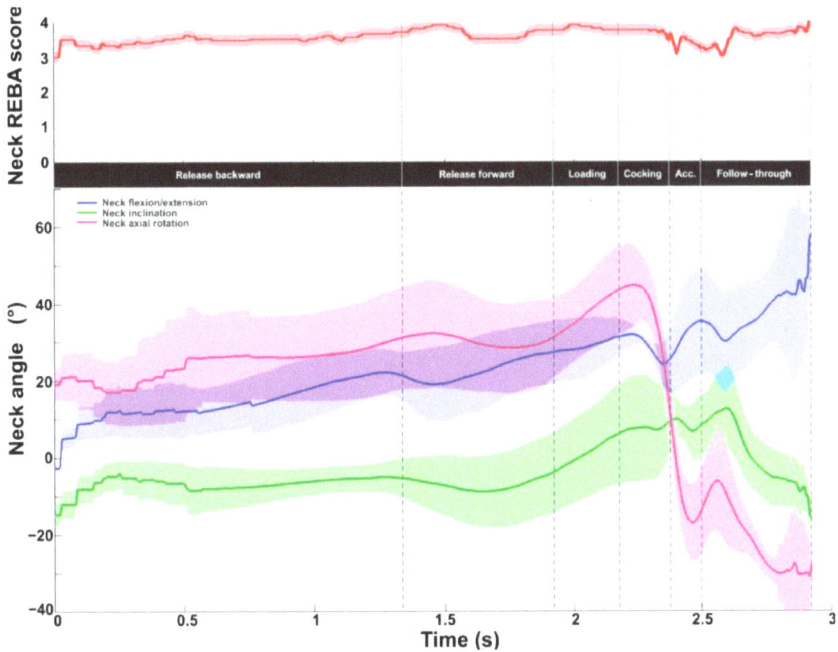

Figure 4. Neck kinematic and ergonomic evaluations during the tennis serve. **Top panel**: Mean (±standard deviation) intermediate neck REBA score. **Bottom panel**: Mean (±standard deviation) neck flexion/extension, inclination, and axial rotation.

Figure 5 depicts the intermediate trunk REBA score evaluated between 1 and 6. The mean value was 3.5 ± 0.7, with values ranging from 2.4 to 5.0. The lowest values were found during the release backward phase. The values then increased to a peak value of 5 during the cocking phase. The values dropped to 3 at BI, then increased to around 4 during the follow-through phase. Trunk extension increased from the beginning to its peak value at RLP ($38.4 \pm 5.9°$) and then decreased to zero. Axial rotation increased on the homo-lateral side (right for right-handed players) to reach a peak value in the middle of the cocking phase ($-21.6 \pm 7.0°$). A rapid rotation to the contralateral side was generated during the acceleration phase, reaching a peak after BI at $25.4 \pm 9.2°$. The inclination remained between $-10°$ and $10°$ from the start of the serve to the end of the loading phase, then rapidly increased on the opposite side of the racket during the cocking and acceleration phases, with a peak value at BI ($29.0 \pm 9.3°$).

Figure 6 displays the intermediate REBA scores for both knees on a scale of 1 to 4. The values ranged from 1 to 4, with a mean value of 1.4 ± 0.6 for the front knee and 1.6 ± 0.8 for the back knee. A peak value was observed at TP (front knee: 3.0 ± 0.8; back knee: 2.9 ± 0.6). A second peak was observed at the end of the movement, with a higher mean value for the back knee (4.0 ± 0.8 vs. 3.0 ± 0.6). Increases in the scores were directly related to knee flexion. The peak value at the end of the serve for the back knee corresponds to significant flexion ($-146.1 \pm 32.7°$).

The REBA score for the intermediate shoulder (score between 1 and 6) is displayed in Figure 7. The values ranged from 1 to 4, with a mean value of 2.0 ± 0.6. The values were below 2 during the release backward phase and then increased to reach a maximum value of 3.8 ± 0.6 after BI. The values returned to 2 at the end of the follow-up phase. With regard to kinematics, a constant medial rotation of around $45°$ and a decrease ($40°$ to $10°$) in flexion were observed during the backward release phase. Abduction was zero during this phase. Axial rotation presented a wide angular variation. Lateral rotation increased sharply to reach a maximum lateral shoulder rotation of $-141.5 \pm 12.6°$ between RLP and

BI (acceleration phase) followed by significant medial rotation until the end of the serve (maximum shoulder medial rotation of 91.9 ± 20.6°).

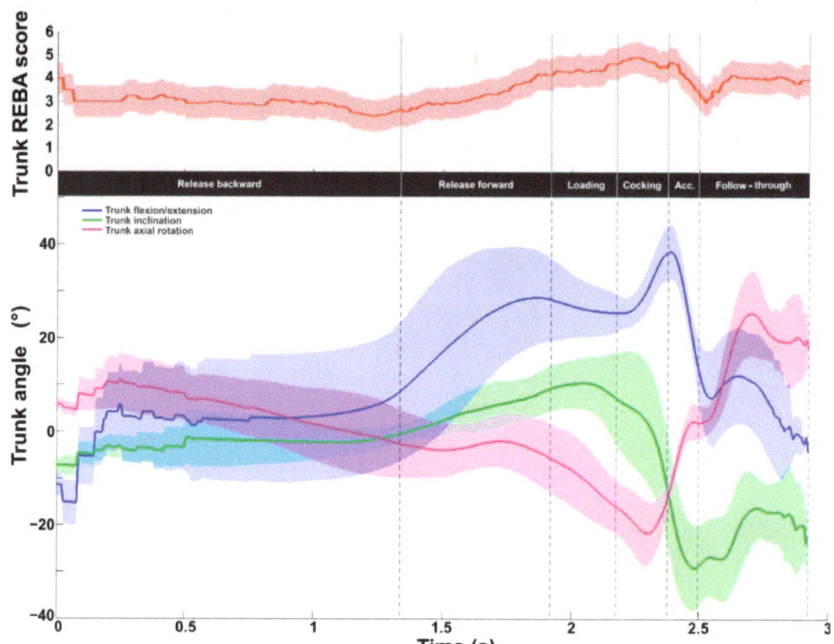

Figure 5. Trunk kinematic and ergonomic evaluations during the tennis serve. **Top panel**: Mean (±standard deviation) intermediate trunk REBA score. **Bottom panel**: Mean (±standard deviation) trunk flexion/extension, inclination, and axial rotation.

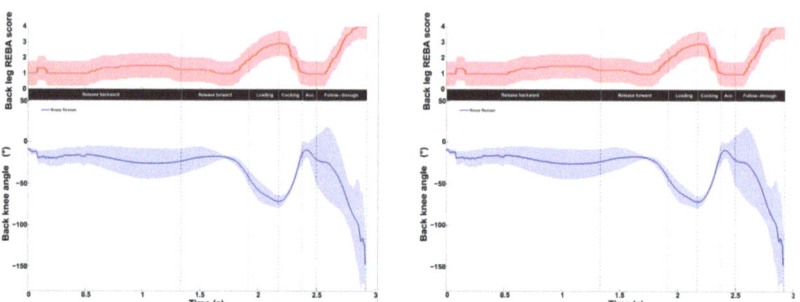

Figure 6. Knee kinematic and ergonomic evaluations during the tennis serve. **Top panels**: Mean (±standard deviation) intermediate leg REBA score. **Bottom panels**: Mean (±standard deviation) knee flexion.

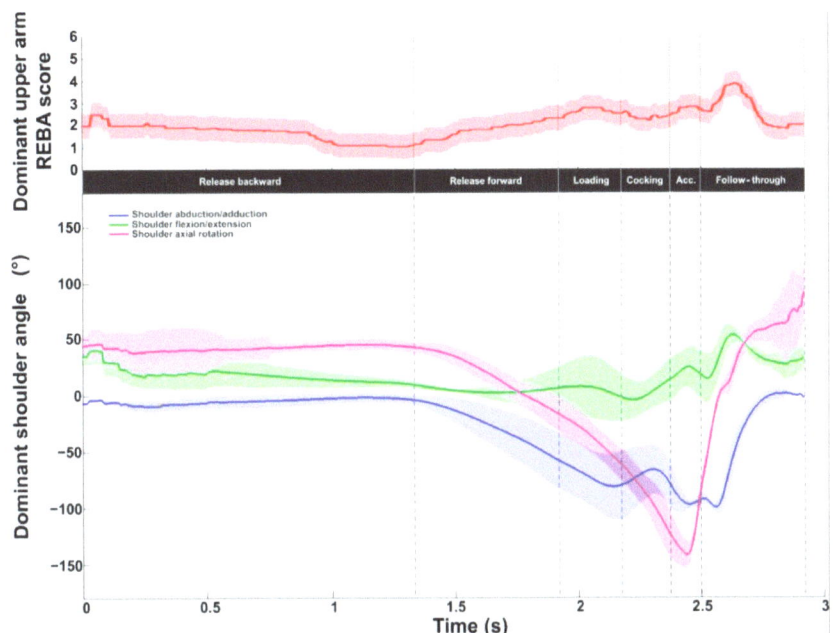

Figure 7. Shoulder kinematic and ergonomic evaluations during the tennis serve. **Top panel**: Mean (±standard deviation) intermediate shoulder REBA score. **Bottom panel**: Mean (±standard deviation) shoulder abduction/adduction, flexion/extension, and axial rotation.

Abduction increased smoothly during the release forward and loading phases and then slightly before BI (peak value: $-99.7 \pm 5.7°$). Abduction decreased during the follow-up phase, reaching values close to zero. As with flexion, values increased during the cocking and acceleration phases, with a peak during the follow-up phase ($53.3 \pm 9.0°$), then decreased slightly until the end of serve.

At the elbow, the average intermediate REBA score was 1.8 ± 0.3, with values ranging from 1 to 2 (on a scale of 1 to 3, Figure 8). A score of 2 was observed throughout the release and cocking phases. The lowest values (close to 1) were obtained during the loading and acceleration phases and at the end of the follow-through phase. Flexion values began at around 50°, decreasing during release forward. From halfway through release forward, the flexion values increased to reach a peak during the cocking phase (just before RLP). A sharp decrease was observed during the acceleration phase, with a minimum of $25.6 \pm 11.1°$ at BI, then flexion increased during the follow-through phase.

Figure 9 depicts the wrist intermediate REBA score. The values obtained during the serve averaged 2.0 ± 0.3 and covered the whole scale (between 1 and 3). The lowest values were found at the beginning and end. The maximum values were observed in the second half of the cocking phase and the acceleration phase, with a peak value of 2.9 ± 0.3 close to BI. In terms of kinematics, wrist flexion remained close to neutral until the end of the loading phase. Extension increased during the acceleration phase, with a peak value of $-12.0 \pm 6.9°$. After BI, a wrist flexion of around 5° was recorded. A radial deviation was observed in the first phase. From release forward, an ulnar deviation was present until the follow-through phase with a peak of $18.5 \pm 7.0°$ at BI. The RUD remained close to neutral during this last phase.

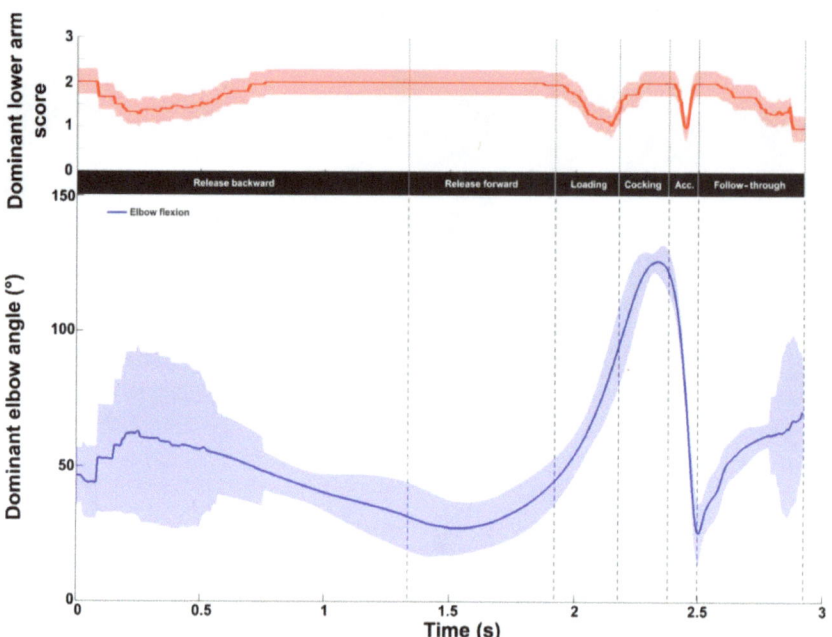

Figure 8. Elbow kinematic and ergonomic evaluations during the tennis serve. **Top panel**: Mean (±standard deviation) intermediate elbow REBA score. **Bottom panel**: Mean (±standard deviation) elbow flexion.

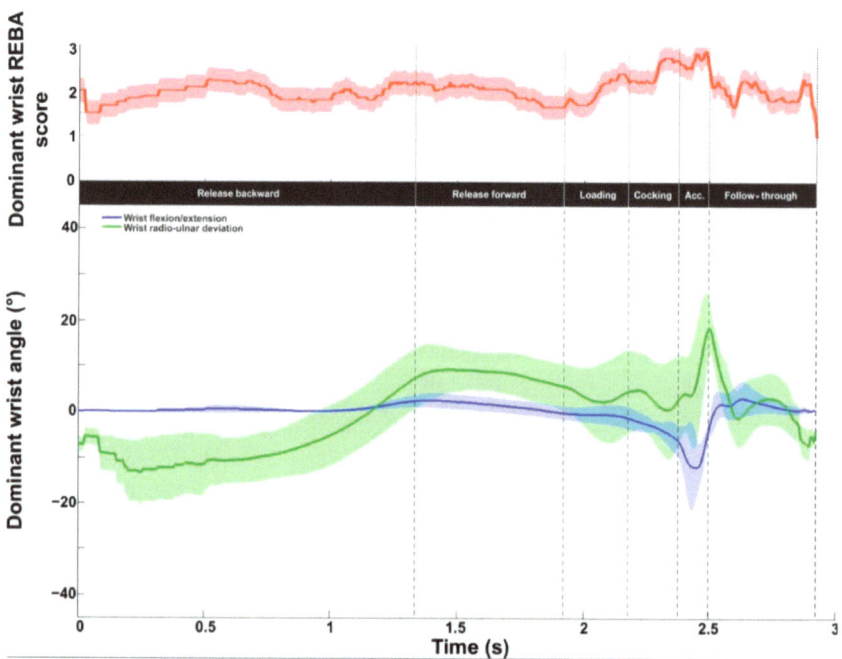

Figure 9. Wrist kinematic and ergonomic evaluations during the tennis serve. **Top panel**: Mean (±standard deviation) intermediate wrist REBA score. **Bottom panel**: Mean (±standard deviation) wrist flexion/extension and radioulnar deviation.

3.2. Performance and Prevention: Slow vs. Fast Serves

The REBA score profile was similar between the two serves, with some slight shifts in some stages (Figure 10). The respective REBA scores were 8.8 ± 3.7 and 8.4 ± 4.0 for slow and fast serves. It should be noted, however, that for the slow serve, the score fell sharply during release backward (REBA score of 5). In the acceleration stage, the fast serve showed higher values (peak value at 12), with a reduction in the value up to BI delayed compared with the slow serve. A difference also appeared in the middle of the follow-through stage, with a lower value for the fast serve (8 vs. 11).

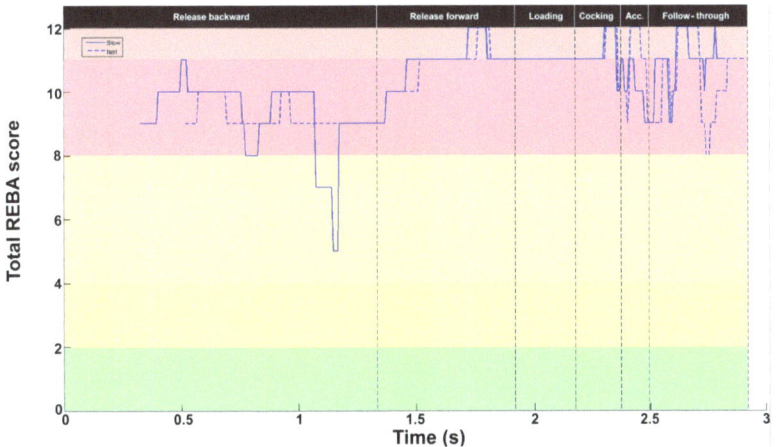

Figure 10. Evolution of the REBA score for slow (solid line) and fast (dotted line) serves. The background colors represent the REBA risk level (see last part of Figure 2).

Figures 11–16 show the intermediate ergonomic scores for each joint area in the REBA and the corresponding joint angles for the slow (solid line) and fast (dotted line) serves.

For the neck, the REBA profile presented two differences between the slow and fast serves. During the release backward stage, the score remained constant at 4 for the fast serve, while the slow serve dropped from 4 to 3 for a brief moment. During the following three stages, the profiles remained identical, with scores of 4. During the acceleration stage, the REBA score dropped to 2 at the start and then rose to 4 for the fast serve but only to 3 for the slow serve. Finally, in the follow-through stage, the profile was identical (the score oscillated between 3 and 4), but with a time lag. Regarding joint angles, the profiles were the same for flexion/extension, inclination, and axial rotation. It is interesting to note, however, that rotation was greater for the fast serve during the release and acceleration stages (slow: −2.7°; fast: −9.3°).

For the trunk, the REBA score showed an identical profile between the two serves (values oscillated between 1 and 5) with a time lag. With regard to angles, there were no major differences in the three trunk angles. The greatest difference was observed for inclination during loading (slow: 12.4°; fast: 8.3°) and during the follow-through, for flexion (slow: −11.4°; fast: −6.1°) and rotation (slow: 13°; fast: 20°), but with no impact on serve performance.

For the knees, the REBA scores were almost the same for both knees, with values varying between 1 and 4 for the back knee and 1 and 3 for the front knee. For flexion, no significant difference was observed in the front knee. On the other hand, for the back knee, flexion was slightly greater at TP and lower at BI.

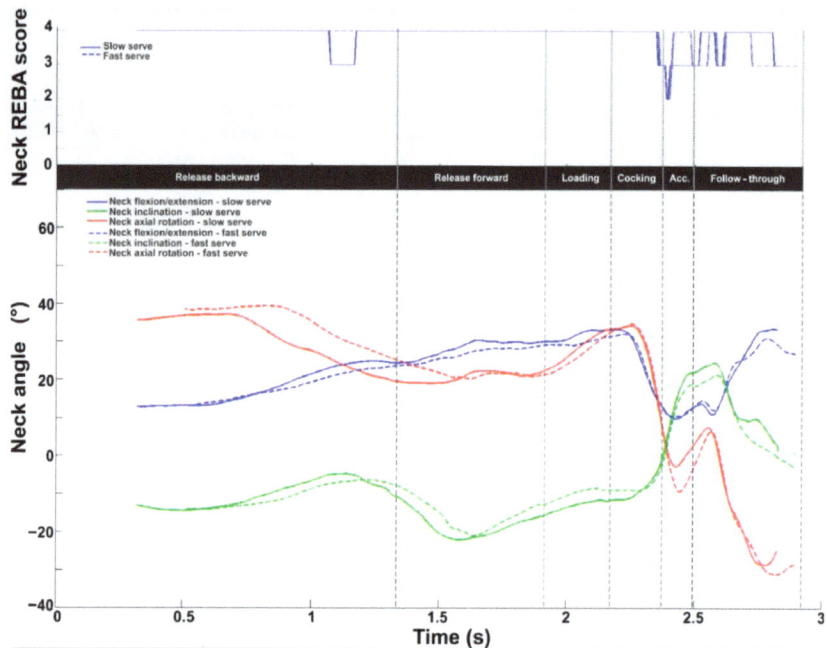

Figure 11. Neck kinematic and ergonomic evaluations for the slow (solid line) and fast (dotted line) serves. **Top panel**: Neck REBA score. **Bottom panel**: Neck flexion/extension (blue), inclination (green), and axial rotation (red).

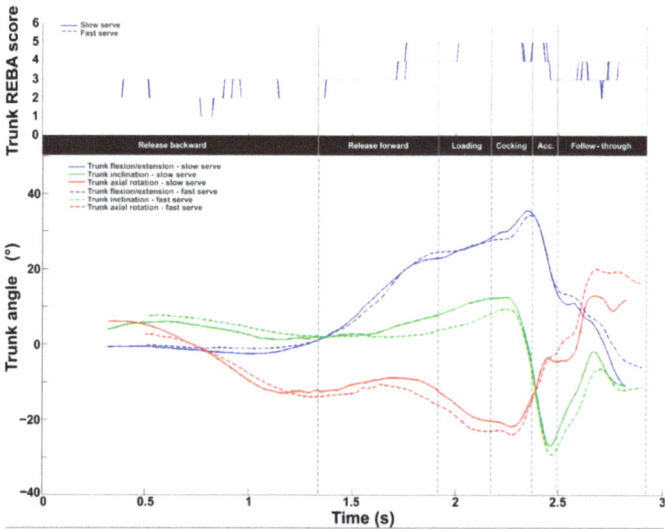

Figure 12. Trunk kinematic and ergonomic evaluations for the slow (solid line) and fast (dotted line) serves. **Top panel**: Trunk REBA score. **Bottom panel**: Trunk flexion/extension (blue), inclination (green), and axial rotation (red).

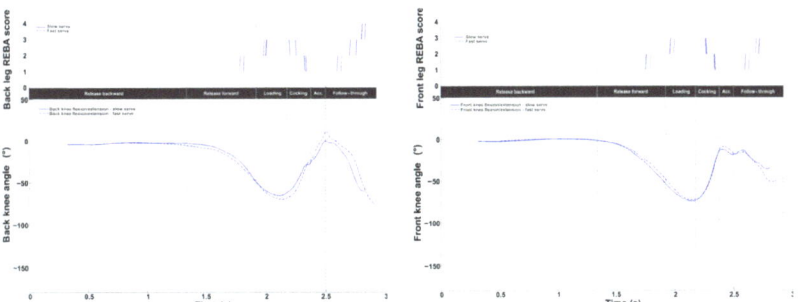

Figure 13. Back (left panels) and front (right panels) knee kinematic and ergonomic evaluations for the slow (solid line) and fast (dotted line) serves. **Top panels**: Knee REBA scores. **Bottom panels**: Knee flexion/extension (blue).

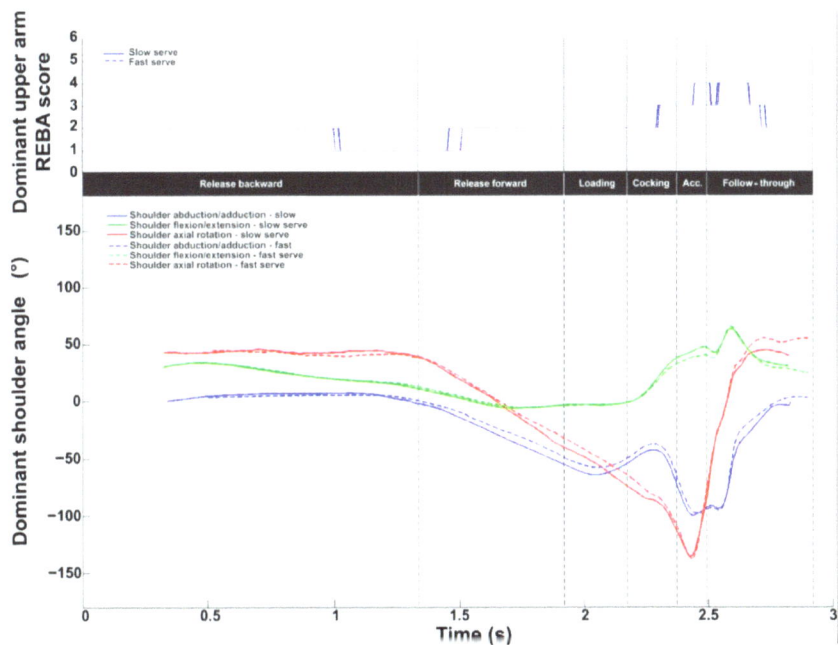

Figure 14. Dominant shoulder kinematic and ergonomic evaluations for the slow (solid line) and fast (dotted line) serves. **Top panel**: Dominant shoulder REBA score. **Bottom panel**: Dominant shoulder abduction/adduction (blue), flexion/extension (green), and axial rotation (red).

The REBA score profiles for the shoulder were very similar. The values ranged from 1 to 4. A difference was observed at BI. The score was lower (3 vs. 4) for the fast serve. The shoulder profiles in all three planes were very similar between the slow and fast serves.

For the elbow, no difference was observed in the REBA scores between the two serves. A difference of 12.6° was observed at BI. The elbow was less flexed for the fast serve (slow: 36.1°; fast: 23.7°).

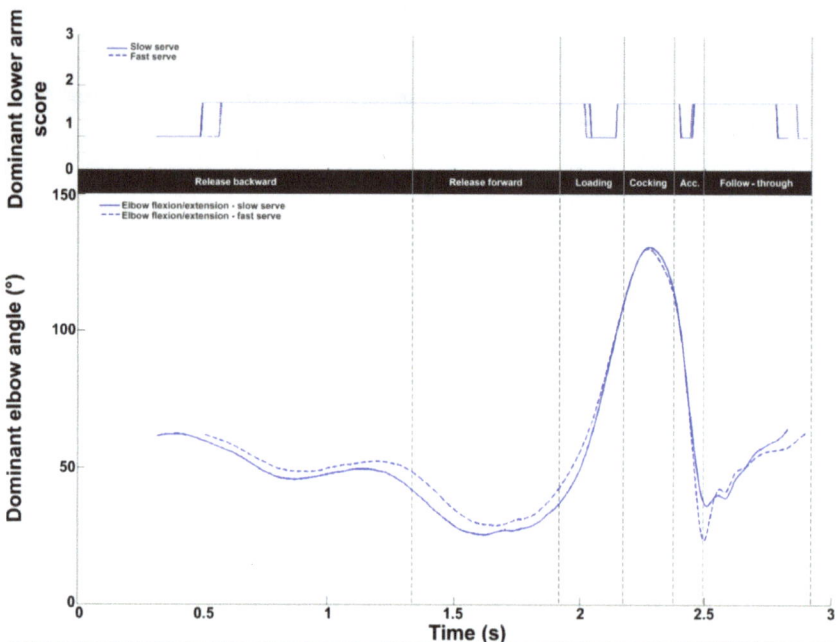

Figure 15. Dominant elbow kinematic and ergonomic evaluations for the slow (solid line) and fast (dotted line) serves. **Top panel**: Dominant elbow REBA score. **Bottom panel**: Dominant elbow flexion/extension (blue).

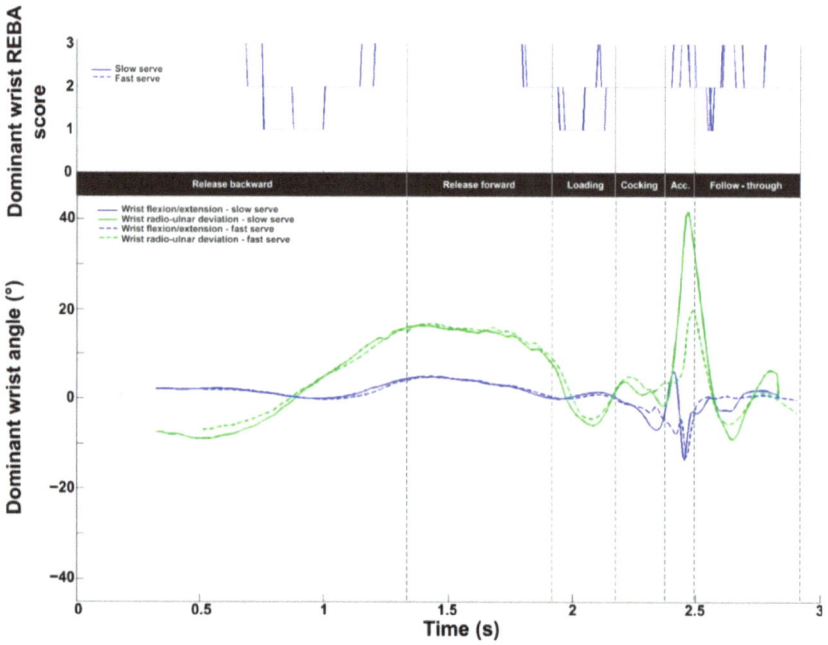

Figure 16. Dominant wrist kinematic and ergonomic evaluations for the slow (solid line) and fast (dotted line) serve. **Top panel**: Dominant wrist REBA score. **Bottom panel**: Dominant wrist flexion/extension (blue), and radioulnar deviation (green).

For the wrist, the REBA profiles remained close (the values oscillated between 1 and 3), with some shifts in the different phases. With regard to joint angles, significant differences were observed during acceleration. Wrist extension was lower and ulnar deviation was greater during the slow serve (slow: 41.7°; fast: 20.0°).

Table 3 summarizes the differences observed for one player in terms of kinematic variables and the associated risks of MSD occurrence. This information could subsequently be used by coaches or trainers to link MSD prevention and performance.

Table 3. Kinematic parameters that differ between the slow and fast serves and affect the MSD risk level.

Joint	Stage/Key Point		Comparison Slow vs. Fast
Neck	Acceleration	REBA	+1 for fast serve
		Axial rotation	+ 6.6°
Shoulder	Acceleration	REBA	−1 for fast serve
		Flexion	−7°
Elbow	BI	REBA	NS
		Flexion	−12.5° for fast serve
Wrist	BI	REBA	NS
		Ulnar deviation	−5.5° for fast serve

4. Discussion

The aim of this study was to evaluate tennis serve performance by considering the risk of MSD incurred by a player with regard to posture and the characteristics of the task, using the REBA tool. To address this original challenge, which has never been considered in the literature, a slow serve and a fast serve were compared. For this purpose, a 3D kinematic analysis of the serve was carried out. The body was modeled using 15 segments. Their displacements and relative joint angles were computed at each instant to obtain an evolution over time. The serves were divided into six stages using seven key points classically identified in the literature. Two force platforms were used to identify the flight phase and the number of feet on the ground during the support phase. All these data were used to quantify six intermediate REBA scores for six joint areas (neck, trunk, leg, shoulder, elbow, and wrist), as well as the total score reflecting the level of risk of MSD occurrence throughout the serve.

4.1. Tennis Serve and MSD Risk

Ergonomic analysis of the tennis serve revealed an average REBA score of 9.7 ± 1.1 across all stages, corresponding to "high-risk activity". Loading, cocking, and follow-through are the highest risk stages, with mean scores above 11, i.e., "very high-risk activity" [26]. This first result is in line with the literature and the number of injuries identified in tennis. The main injuries that affect the musculoskeletal system reported are as follows: shoulder (rotator cuff inflammation [38]), elbow (medial or lateral epicondylitis, i.e., tennis elbow [39]), wrist (tendonitis, e.g., De Quervain's tenosynovitis [40]), back (low back pain [41] due to lumbar disc degeneration and herniation [42]), knee (tendonitis, bursitis or meniscal lesion [43]), and ankle (sprain, plantar fasciitis or Achilles tendonitis [44]).

The temporal analysis proposed in this study highlighted the areas most exposed to MSD in relation to the six REBA joint areas, as well as the times when they were most exposed. For the neck, the REBA score was between 3 and 4 (out of 4), indicating a highly exposed area throughout the serve. The neck was continuously in rotation (+20° left or right) and in increasing extension throughout the six stages of the serve. These postures are the cause of a high intermediate ergonomic score throughout the serve. However, the risk level could be modulated. Indeed, during the release and cocking stages, movements are controlled and executed slowly, which would considerably reduce the risk of injury, according to Lee's study [45]. Conversely, fast neck rotation in extension during the second part of cocking and acceleration stages increases compressive and torsional stresses on spinal vertebrae and predisposes the neck to injury of an acute or chronic nature. In extension and rotation, the diameter of the intervertebra foramina through which nerve roots pass is decreased [46]. High ballistic, rotational forces passing through this area predispose the right zygapophysial joints and surrounding nerve and soft tissue to trauma [45]. The neck is therefore an area at risk of TMS because of its constant extension to maintain visual contact with the ball and the quick rotations caused by the high intermediate REBA score. Therefore, it is necessary to be aware of this joint, even if it has been considered not to be the most exposed area, especially considering the large number of serve repetitions in training and during matches in a year.

For the trunk, the intermediate score was between 2.5 and 5 (out of 6). The highest scores were observed for the loading and cocking stages (>4/6). With the exception of the follow-through stage, the trunk was in extension, with a value that increased from release to TP, where the peak value appeared. These values are in line with other studies on the trunk during the tennis serve [19,47]. This posture is already associated with the presence of an MSD risk in ergonomic tools [26–28]. On the other hand, during these two stages, the trunk was also rotated and inclined, which increased the risk of MSD with scores of 5/6. This usually translates into lower back pain associated with lumbar strain. The pain is partly muscular, involving the extensors, flexors, and rotators of the spine (multifidus).

The main cause would be alternating concentric/excentric contraction of these muscle groups to go from an extreme extension rotation to extreme flexion rotation during the serve [42]. These combined movements induce greater stress on the vertebrae than movements in a single plane, thus increasing the risk of pain and injury [48]. Moreover, as shown by Campbell et al. in elite adolescent tennis players, lumbar joint reaction moments during the acceleration phase (3 to 40 times greater than running) highlight the "high" loading conditions of the lumbar region, which could be at the origin of the development of low back pain during the repeated tennis serve [49].

For the shoulder, the intermediate REBA score was 2.0 ± 0.6 (on a scale of 1 to 6), reaching a peak of 3.8 ± 0.6 during the follow-through stage. This result does not directly indicate a significant risk of MSD during the serve. However, several studies have reported numerous shoulder injuries in tennis players. The main cause would be the large joint ranges in lateral rotation ($-141.5 \pm 12.6°$ in agreement with other studies [20,50]) and the high medial rotation velocities generated in the acceleration stage [19,21]. This overloading of the joints and muscles of the shoulder girdle would lead to inflammation of muscular tendons (biceps brachii and rotator cuff muscles) or joints (bursitis) or to deterioration of shoulder joint structures such as the ligament capsule or labrum [42,51,52]. This disparity between the low REBA intermediate score for the shoulder and the fact that the tennis serve is the cause of many injuries highlights the limitations of the REBA tool in sports. Indeed, the specificity and complexity of the serve impose shoulder motions that are not taken into account in the assessment of the intermediate score. The REBA assessment mainly dichotomizes the shoulder flexion–extension motion (five angular sectors), with a +1 increase in the case of rotation (with no precise value), whereas the tennis serve mainly involves rotational movement, which underestimates the REBA risk assessment.

For the elbow, the mean intermediate REBA score was 1.8 ± 0.3, with values ranging from 1 to 2 (on a scale of 1 to 3). This may translate into an intermediate risk of MSDs. However, as for the shoulder, the elbow is often affected by injuries. The origin can be found in the acceleration stage, where flexion decreases from $125.7 \pm 4.7°$ to $25.6 \pm 11.1°$ in 0.12 ± 0.01 s, which is in line with previous studies by Kibler et al. (extension from $116°$ to $20°$ of flexion within 0.21 s [53]) and Fett et al. (from $132.2 \pm 10.4°$ to $18.0 \pm 8.5°$ during acceleration stage [19]). Because of the combined rotation of the shoulder, this results in a double load on the elbow called "valgus extension overload", the cause of epicondylitis, in particular [54]. Lateral epicondylitis, or "tennis elbow" [55], is most common, affecting an average of one in two players [39,56]. The main causes are poor tennis technique [57], often observed in beginners, large racket size [58], and high repetition of the one-handed backhand [39]. Pain results from microtearing of the extensor carpi radialis brevis [39]. Nowadays, lateral epicondylitis prevalence has decreased because of improved technical outcomes and the two-handed backhand [55].

For the wrist, the intermediate REBA score was 2.0 ± 0.3 (maximum 3). The maximum score was reached during the second half of the cocking phase and the acceleration phase, with a peak value of 2.9 ± 0.3 close to BI. These values show that the maximum risk of MSD occurrence was reached for these stages. These high scores can be explained by a quick flexion movement from an extended position during the acceleration phase ($-12.0 \pm 6.9°$ to $4.2 \pm 2.5°$), coupled with a large ulnar deviation, particularly at BI ($18.5 \pm 6.9°$). Similar values have been reported in recent studies, notably for wrist flexion at BI by Wang et al. ($5.3 \pm 2.9°$ for expert players [9]) and Fleisig et al. ($15.0 \pm 8.0°$ for men and women [21]). These wrist joint angles are associated with injuries such as extensor carpi ulnaris tendinosis and instability, tenosynovitis, stress fractures, and injuries to the triangular fibrocartilage complex [59], which account for one-third of all upper limb injuries [60]. These harmful postures are exacerbated by internal forces (muscular forces and torques) and external forces (due to the interaction between the ball and the racket at BI) during the stroke [61]. Although torques are probably lower than the levels at which tissues sustain permanent structural damage, repetitive hitting with wrist angular configurations far from joint neutral would favor the development of wrist lesions in tennis players due to overuse [62]. In professional tennis players, over 1000 strokes can be recorded during a match lasting between 3 and 5 h, with several matches played with less than 48 rests during the Grand Slams [63].

Finally, for the knees, intermediate REBA scores were very similar between the front and back knees (front knee: 1.4 ± 0.6; back knee: 1.6 ± 0.8). The scores ranged from 1 to 3 for the front knee and from 1 to 4 (out of 4) for the back knee. The difference was observed during the follow-through stage and corresponded to greater knee flexion for the back knee. The angular variations observed between the moment of greatest knee flexion (TP back knee flexion: $-71.3 \pm 7.9°$; TP front knee flexion: $-66.6 \pm 4.7°$) and that of least flexion (during the acceleration phase, i.e., between RLP and BI, back knee flexion: $-9.5 \pm 9.3°$, front knee flexion: $-15.4 \pm 5.8°$) correspond to the values reported in the literature for these two moments. Several authors have found TP knee flexion values between 60 and 80° for different ages [12], serve types [13], and men and women [11]. Fleisig et al. reported a low front knee flexion of $13.0 \pm 8.0°$ at RLP [21]. Fett et al. [19] and Whiteside et al. [2] found similar values at BI between 5° and 20° for the back knee and between 15° and 30° for the front knee. These data are in line with the values measured in the present article. The knee is a highly solicited joint and ranks among the areas exposed to injury behind the shoulder and back, with a prevalence of around 20% [64]. The most commonly observed pathologies are patellofemoral dysfunction, jumper's knee, meniscal injuries, and bursitis [43]. These disorders affect the structural elements of the joint, i.e., alignment of the bony and muscular structures of the knee, in particular the extensor muscles, menisci, ligaments, and bursae, and are the result of overuse in flexion and torsion during stance [31,43].

In tennis, the risks are more related to angular variations during jump preparation (loading stage), fast extension during the cocking stage (extension velocities between 450 and $800°/s$ reported in the literature [19,21,65]), and high loading of the front lower limb joints during jump landing (follow-through stage). It was during these stages that the intermediate REBA scores were highest (>3 out of 4) and, therefore, the risk of MSD would be greatest (TP front knee: 3.0 ± 0.83; TP back knee: 2.9 ± 0.6; follow through front knee: 3.0 ± 0.6; follow through back knee: 4.0 ± 0.8).

The results presented were obtained for a group of young national-level players (17.8 ± 2.2 years). Wang et al. [9] showed that postures were affected by player level at different key points. The authors found differences in the trunk at trophy position and in the whole upper limb at ball impact. Whiteside et al. [2] found an effect of age on posture. A difference in peak trunk inclination was observed during trophy position between a group of children (10.6 ± 0.6 years) and a group of young people (14.8 ± 0.5 years). In a second study, Whiteside et al. [8] also showed an age effect on posture (trunk, pelvis, and upper limb) during trophy position and ball impact. These differences in joint angles as a function of age and level of expertise are important since they modify postures and consequently the results of the REBA ergonomic evaluation. It might therefore be appropriate to reproduce the ergonomic assessment at different ages and different levels to study the evolution of MSD risks during the tennis serve.

4.2. MSD Prevention and Performance

The comparison of a slow and fast serve for one player highlighted some differences between the performance achieved and the associated potential MSD risks. The overall assessment showed differences in MSD risk during the acceleration phase, with a total REBA score of at least one point for the fast serve. The following parameters were identified: neck axial rotation and shoulder flexion. For neck rotation, the intermediate REBA score was one point higher for the fast serve and could be linked to a more significant rotation than during the slow serve. On the other hand, for the shoulder, the risk of MSD was one point lower for the fast serve with less flexion than for the slow serve for the same stage.

On the other hand, joint angle differences were observed for elbow flexion and wrist ulnar deviation, but with no impact on the intermediate REBA score. This may be explained by the thresholds chosen at which the risks change. In the literature, it is known that level has an influence on MSD risk. Indeed, poor technique, often observed in beginners, has been associated with a higher risk of injury [31]. In training, this information could be used by coaches, trainers and players to improve performance while reducing MSD risks.

4.3. Application of Key Findings

The results presented in this work address our twofold objective to (1) carry out an ergonomic assessment of MSD risks and (2) associate this level of risk with the evaluation of performance during the tennis serve.

The first point proposed the temporal evolution of the kinematic variables of the following six joint areas included in the REBA tool: shoulder, elbow, wrist, neck, trunk, and legs (through the knee joint and the number of supports). Thanks to 3D analysis, all the joint angles of these joints were measured during the entire serve, divided into stages based on key points. This approach is totally original as, to our knowledge, no other study has proposed such a kinematic analysis of the serve. The majority of works proposed values at key instants without a temporal evaluation. The few works that proposed a temporal evaluation only considered a few body areas, such as the knee [3,5], or only the upper limb [66] or lower limb. A recent study investigated 28 joint angles of the upper and lower limbs and proposed a temporal evaluation of the 13 angles correlated with racket velocity, but only for the cocking and acceleration stages [34].

Kinematic evaluation was used to quantify postures in each step. These data were used as input to the REBA tool to qualify and quantify serve-related MSD risks based on posture and general task characteristics that had never been addressed before. Integrating this analysis into the performance analysis highlighted a number of differences that could lead to the medium-term consideration of player protection as part of performance optimization.

The results of our work enabled two ways to be identified. The first would be to modify the serve technique through the kinematic parameters involved in the high REBA score observed, in order to reduce the MSD risk while maintaining equivalent racket velocity. The second would be to propose muscle-strengthening or stretching exercises that would reduce the long-term occurrence of MSD throughout the player's career, despite the high REBA score (and, therefore, the risks). These two lines of action could be the subject of future research to protect athletes in the course of their sporting activities.

4.4. Limitations

Some limitations of this study could be addressed. This study was carried out on five serves per player and only for four players. In fact, this work is difficult to generalize to middle-aged and older tennis players. As the young players studied are not yet international players, the results are also difficult to transfer. Extending the analysis to a larger sample would enable generalizing the proposed results and studying the effect of different parameters (type of serve, stance style, age, expertise) on MSD risk.

The REBA tool is a generic ergonomic tool that was developed primarily for the assessment of work-related postures, with a predominantly analysis-based design. However, the tennis serve is a complex gesture involving numerous rotations in different planes. As a result, some risks are probably underestimated. At present, there are no ergonomic tools linked to the sport, and REBA is the one that takes into account the most elements of the activity in assessing risk. Future work on more suitable tools could be carried out in order to propose an MSD assessment more specific to sports.

5. Conclusions

The present study proposed a kinematic analysis of the six major joint areas of the body during the tennis serve. Joint angular evolutions were presented as a function of time for each stage of the serve in relation to the various key points of interest identified in the literature. These full-body kinematic data were used to perform an ergonomic assessment using the REBA tool at each point in time. The results showed that tennis serve is a high-risk activity that varies according to phase, with the greatest risk during the loading and cocking stages. The causes of these risks were expressed with reference to kinematic variations. An analysis of the slow and fast serves and associated performance values was proposed. The REBA profiles were similar, with an average score of 8.8 ± 3.7 and 8.4 ± 4.0, respectively, for the slow and fast serves. The maximum REBA score (12/12) was reached during the acceleration phase. The fast serve showed a one-point increase in the intermediate neck REBA score with an increase in axial rotation of $+6.6°$ and a one-point decrease in the intermediate shoulder REBA score with a reduction in flexion of $7°$ during the acceleration phase. The data can be used by coaches and athletes to improve performance while trying to prevent the occurrence of MSDs.

Author Contributions: Conceptualization, P.G. and J.J.-B.; methodology, P.G. and J.J.-B.; software, P.G. and J.J.-B.; validation, P.G. and J.J.-B.; formal analysis, P.G. and J.J.-B.; investigation, P.G. and J.J.-B.; resources, P.G. and J.J.-B.; data curation, P.G. and J.J.-B.; writing—original draft preparation, P.G. and J.J.-B.; writing—review and editing, P.G. and J.J.-B.; visualization, P.G. and J.J.-B.; supervision, P.G.; project administration, P.G.; funding acquisition, P.G. All authors have read and agreed to the published version of the manuscript.

Funding: This work was financially supported by the ErBio Association (grant agreement number 2023-054).

Institutional Review Board Statement: This study was conducted in accordance with the Declaration of Helsinki and approved by the International Institute of Biomechanics and Occupational Ergonomics (IIBOE23-E54) on 1 June 2023.

Informed Consent Statement: Informed consent was obtained from all subjects involved in this study.

Data Availability Statement: Data are available upon request.

Conflicts of Interest: The authors declare no conflicts of interest.

Appendix A

REBA grid adapted from Hignett et al. [26] for computing MSD risk associated with the tennis serve (extracted from Raman et al. [37]).

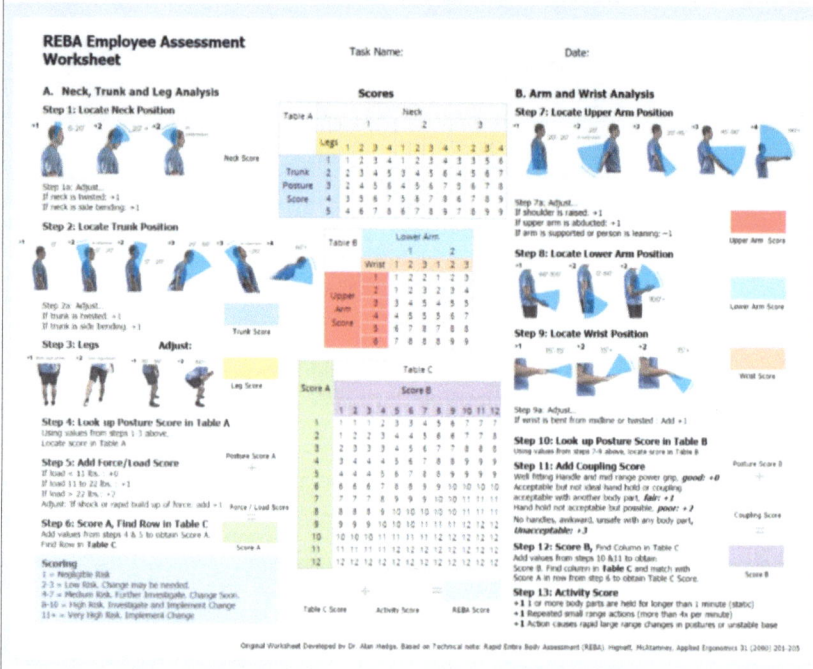

Figure A1. REBA method summary sheet. The left and right columns show the method for computing the intermediate scores, while the middle section contains the conversion charts for obtaining the final REBA score.

References

1. Kovacs, M.; Ellenbecker, T. An 8-Stage Model for Evaluating the Tennis Serve:Implications for Performance Enhancement and Injury Prevention. *Sports Health* **2011**, *3*, 504–513. [CrossRef] [PubMed]
2. Whiteside, D.; Elliott, B.; Lay, B.; Reid, M. A kinematic comparison of successful and unsuccessful tennis serves across the elite development pathway. *Hum. Mov. Sci.* **2013**, *32*, 822–835. [CrossRef]
3. Reid, M.; Elliott, B.; Alderson, J. Lower-limb coordination and shoulder joint mechanics in the tennis serve. *Med. Sci. Sports Exerc.* **2008**, *40*, 308–315. [CrossRef] [PubMed]
4. Elliott, B.; Wood, G. The biomechanics of the foot-up and foot-back tennis service techniques. *Aust. J. Sci. Med. Sport* **1983**, *3*, 3–6.
5. Hornestam, J.F.; Souza, T.R.; Magalhaes, F.A.; Begon, M.; Santos, T.R.T.; Fonseca, S.T. The Effects of Knee Flexion on Tennis Serve Performance of Intermediate Level Tennis Players. *Sensors* **2021**, *21*, 5254. [CrossRef]
6. Reid, M.; Elliott, B.; Alderson, J. Shoulder joint loading in the high performance flat and kick tennis serves. *Br. J. Sports Med.* **2007**, *41*, 884–889. [CrossRef] [PubMed]
7. Jacquier-Bret, J.; Gorce, P. Kinematics characteristics of key point of interest during tennis serve among tennis players: A systematic review and meta-analysis. *Front. Sports Act. Living* **2024**, *6*, 1432030. [CrossRef]
8. Whiteside, D.; Elliott, B.; Lay, B.; Reid, M. The effect of age on discrete kinematics of the elite female tennis serve. *J. Appl. Biomech.* **2013**, *29*, 573–582. [CrossRef]
9. Wang, L.H.; Lo, K.C.; Su, F.C. Skill level and forearm muscle fatigue effects on ball speed in tennis serve. *Sports Biomech.* **2021**, *20*, 419–430. [CrossRef]
10. Brocherie, F.; Dinu, D. Biomechanical estimation of tennis serve using inertial sensors: A case study. *Front. Sports Act. Living* **2022**, *4*, 962941. [CrossRef]
11. Elliott, B.; Marsh, T.; Blanksby, B. A Three-Dimensional Cinematographic Analysis of the Tennis Serve. *Int. J. Sport Biomech.* **1986**, *2*, 260–271. [CrossRef]
12. Tubez, F.; Schwartz, C.; Croisier, J.-L.; Brüls, O.; Denoël, V.; Paulus, J.; Forthomme, B. Evolution of the trophy position along the tennis serve player's development. *Sports Biomech.* **2021**, *20*, 431–443. [CrossRef] [PubMed]
13. Mourtzios, C.; Athanailidis, I.; Arvanitidou, V.; Kellis, E. Ankle and Knee Joint Kinematics Differ between Flat, Slice and Topspin Serves in Young Tennis Players. *Eur. J. Sport Sci.* **2022**, *1*, 16–22. [CrossRef]

14. Touzard, P.; Lecomte, C.; Bideau, B.; Kulpa, R.; Fourel, L.; Fadier, M.; Cantin, N.; Martin, C. There is no rush to upgrade the tennis racket in young intermediate competitive players: The effects of scaling racket on serve biomechanics and performance. *Front. Psychol.* **2023**, *14*, 1104146. [CrossRef] [PubMed]
15. Fadier, M.; Touzard, P.; Martin, C. Preliminary kinematic analysis of the serve in 10 and under players. *Coach. Sport Sci. Rev.* **2021**, *29*, 12–14. [CrossRef]
16. Gillet, B.; Rogowski, I.; Monga-Dubreuil, E.; Begon, M. Lower Trapezius Weakness and Shoulder Complex Biomechanics during the Tennis Serve. *Med. Sci. Sports Exerc.* **2019**, *51*, 2531–2539. [CrossRef]
17. Rogowski, I.; Creveaux, T.; Sevrez, V.; Cheze, L.; Dumas, R. How Does the Scapula Move during the Tennis Serve? *Med. Sci. Sports Exerc.* **2015**, *47*, 1444–1449. [CrossRef] [PubMed]
18. Abrams, G.D.; Harris, A.H.; Andriacchi, T.P.; Safran, M.R. Biomechanical analysis of three tennis serve types using a markerless system. *Br. J. Sports Med.* **2014**, *48*, 339–342. [CrossRef]
19. Fett, J.; Oberschelp, N.; Vuong, J.L.; Wiewelhove, T.; Ferrauti, A. Kinematic characteristics of the tennis serve from the ad and deuce court service positions in elite junior players. *PLoS ONE* **2021**, *16*, e0252650. [CrossRef]
20. Reid, M.; Giblin, G.; Whiteside, D. A kinematic comparison of the overhand throw and tennis serve in tennis players: How similar are they really? *J. Sports Sci.* **2014**, *33*, 713–723. [CrossRef]
21. Fleisig, G.; Nicholls, R.; Elliott, B.; Escamilla, R. Kinematics used by world class tennis players to produce high-velocity serves. *Sports Biomech.* **2003**, *2*, 51–64. [CrossRef]
22. Gomez-Galan, M.; Perez-Alonso, J.; Callejon-Ferre, A.J.; Lopez-Martinez, J. Musculoskeletal disorders: OWAS review. *Ind. Health* **2017**, *55*, 314–337. [CrossRef] [PubMed]
23. Rothrauff, B.B.; Pirosa, A.; Lin, H.; Sohn, J.; Langhans, M.T.; Tuan, R.S. Chapter 54—Stem Cell Therapy for Musculoskeletal Diseases. In *Principles of Regenerative Medicine*, 3rd ed.; Atala, A., Lanza, R., Mikos, A.G., Nerem, R., Eds.; Academic Press: Boston, MA, USA, 2019; pp. 953–970.
24. Martin, C.; Kulpa, R.; Ropars, M.; Delamarche, P.; Bideau, B. Identification of temporal pathomechanical factors during the tennis serve. *Med. Sci. Sports Exerc.* **2013**, *45*, 2113–2119. [CrossRef] [PubMed]
25. Gomez-Galan, M.; Callejon-Ferre, A.J.; Perez-Alonso, J.; Diaz-Perez, M.; Carrillo-Castrillo, J.A. Musculoskeletal Risks: RULA Bibliometric Review. *Int. J. Environ. Res. Public Health* **2020**, *17*, 4354. [CrossRef]
26. Hignett, S.; McAtamney, L. Rapid Entire Body Assessment (REBA). *Appl. Ergon.* **2000**, *31*, 201–205. [CrossRef]
27. McAtamney, L.; Corlett, N.E. RULA: A survey method for the investigation of work-related upper limb disorders. *Appl. Ergon.* **1993**, *24*, 91–99. [CrossRef]
28. Kee, D.; Karwowski, W. LUBA: An assessment technique for postural loading on the upper body based on joint motion discomfort and maximum holding time. *Appl. Ergon.* **2001**, *32*, 357–366. [CrossRef]
29. Karhu, O.; Kansi, P.; Kuorinka, I. Correcting working postures in industry: A practical method for analysis. *Appl. Ergon.* **1977**, *8*, 199–201. [CrossRef] [PubMed]
30. Rose, L.M.; Eklund, J.; Nord Nilsson, L.; Barman, L.; Lind, C.M. The RAMP package for MSD risk management in manual handling—A freely accessible tool, with website and training courses. *Appl. Ergon.* **2020**, *86*, 103101. [CrossRef]
31. Perkins, R.H.; Davis, D. Musculoskeletal injuries in tennis. *Phys. Med. Rehabil. Clin. N. Am.* **2006**, *17*, 609–631. [CrossRef]
32. Wu, G.; Siegler, S.; Allard, P.; Kirtley, C.; Leardini, A.; Rosenbaum, D.; Whittle, M.; D'Lima, D.D.; Cristofolini, L.; Witte, H.; et al. ISB recommendation on definitions of joint coordinate system of various joints for the reporting of human joint motion—Part I: Ankle, hip, and spine. *J. Biomech.* **2002**, *35*, 543–548. [CrossRef] [PubMed]
33. Wu, G.; van der Helm, F.C.T.; Veeger, H.E.J.; Makhsous, M.; Van Roy, P.; Anglin, C.; Nagels, J.; Karduna, A.R.; McQuade, K.; Wang, X.; et al. ISB recommendation on definitions of joint coordinate systems of various joints for the reporting of human joint motion—Part II: Shoulder, elbow, wrist and hand. *J. Biomech.* **2005**, *38*, 981–992. [CrossRef] [PubMed]
34. Jacquier-Bret, J.; Gorce, P. Kinematics of the Tennis Serve Using an Optoelectronic Motion Capture System: Are There Correlations between Joint Angles and Racket Velocity? *Sensors* **2024**, *24*, 3292. [CrossRef] [PubMed]
35. Lu, T.-W.; O'Connor, J.J. Bone position estimation from skin marker co-ordinates using global optimisation with joint constraints. *J. Biomech.* **1999**, *32*, 129–134. [CrossRef] [PubMed]
36. Bonnefoy-Mazure, A.; Slawinski, J.; Riquet, A.; Leveque, J.M.; Miller, C.; Cheze, L. Rotation sequence is an important factor in shoulder kinematics. Application to the elite players' flat serves. *J. Biomech.* **2010**, *43*, 2022–2025. [CrossRef]
37. Raman, V.; Ramlogan, S.; Sweet, J.; Sweet, D. Application of the Rapid Entire Body Assessment (REBA) in assessing chairside ergonomic risk of dental students. *Br. Dent. J.* **2020**; *online publication*. [CrossRef]
38. Bylak, J.; Hutchinson, M.R. Common sports injuries in young tennis players. *Sports Med.* **1998**, *26*, 119–132. [CrossRef]
39. Peters, T.; Baker, C.L., Jr. Lateral epicondylitis. *Clin. Sports Med.* **2001**, *20*, 549–563. [CrossRef] [PubMed]
40. Rettig, A.C. Wrist problems in the tennis player. *Med. Sci. Sports Exerc.* **1994**, *26*, 1207–1212. [CrossRef]
41. Marks, M.R.; Haas, S.S.; Wiesel, S.W. Low back pain in the competitive tennis player. *Clin. Sports Med.* **1988**, *7*, 277–287. [CrossRef]
42. Hainline, B. Low back injury. *Clin. Sports Med.* **1995**, *14*, 241–265. [CrossRef]
43. Gecha, S.R.; Torg, E. Knee injuries in tennis. *Clin. Sports Med.* **1988**, *7*, 435–452. [CrossRef] [PubMed]
44. Zecher, S.B.; Leach, R.E. Lower leg and foot injuries in tennis and other racquet sports. *Clin. Sports Med.* **1995**, *14*, 223–239. [CrossRef] [PubMed]

45. Lee, H.W. Mechanisms of neck and shoulder injuries in tennis players. *J. Orthop. Sports Phys. Ther.* **1995**, *21*, 28–37. [CrossRef] [PubMed]
46. Grieve, G.P. *Common Vertebral Joint Problems*; Churchill Livingstone: London, UK, 1988; p. 804.
47. Wagner, H.; Pfusterschmied, J.; Tilp, M.; Landlinger, J.; von Duvillard, S.P.; Muller, E. Upper-body kinematics in team-handball throw, tennis serve, and volleyball spike. *Scand. J. Med. Sci. Sports* **2014**, *24*, 345–354. [CrossRef] [PubMed]
48. Haberl, H.; Cripton, P.A.; Orr, T.E.; Beutler, T.; Frei, H.; Lanksch, W.R.; Nolte, L.P. Kinematic response of lumbar functional spinal units to axial torsion with and without superimposed compression and flexion/extension. *Eur. Spine J.* **2004**, *13*, 560–566. [CrossRef]
49. Campbell, A.; Straker, L.; O'Sullivan, P.; Elliott, B.; Reid, M. Lumbar loading in the elite adolescent tennis serve: Link to low back pain. *Med. Sci. Sports Exerc.* **2013**, *45*, 1562–1568. [CrossRef]
50. Konda, S.; Yanai, T.; Sakurai, S. Scapular rotation to attain the peak shoulder external rotation in tennis serve. *Med. Sci. Sports Exerc.* **2010**, *42*, 1745–1753. [CrossRef]
51. Jobe, F.W.; Bradley, J.P. The diagnosis and nonoperative treatment of shoulder injuries in athletes. *Clin. Sports Med.* **1989**, *8*, 419–438. [CrossRef]
52. van der Hoeven, H.; Kibler, W.B. Shoulder injuries in tennis players. *Br. J. Sports Med.* **2006**, *40*, 435–440; discussion 440. [CrossRef]
53. Kibler, W.B. Clinical biomechanics of the elbow in tennis: Implications for evaluation and diagnosis. *Med. Sci. Sports Exerc.* **1994**, *26*, 1203–1206. [CrossRef]
54. Eygendaal, D.; Rahussen, F.T.; Diercks, R.L. Biomechanics of the elbow joint in tennis players and relation to pathology. *Br. J. Sports Med.* **2007**, *41*, 820–823. [CrossRef] [PubMed]
55. De Smedt, T.; de Jong, A.; Van Leemput, W.; Lieven, D.; Van Glabbeek, F. Lateral epicondylitis in tennis: Update on aetiology, biomechanics and treatment. *Br. J. Sports Med.* **2007**, *41*, 816–819. [CrossRef] [PubMed]
56. Kekelekis, A.; Nikolaidis, P.T.; Moore, I.S.; Rosemann, T.; Knechtle, B. Risk Factors for Upper Limb Injury in Tennis Players: A Systematic Review. *Int. J. Environ. Res. Public Health* **2020**, *17*, 2744. [CrossRef] [PubMed]
57. Hennig, E.M.; Rosenbaum, D.; Milani, T.L. Transfer of tennis racket vibrations onto the human forearm. *Med. Sci. Sports Exerc.* **1992**, *24*, 1134–1140. [CrossRef] [PubMed]
58. Marx, R.G.; Sperling, J.W.; Cordasco, F.A. Overuse injuries of the upper extremity in tennis players. *Clin. Sports Med.* **2001**, *20*, 439–451. [CrossRef] [PubMed]
59. Patel, H.; Lala, S.; Helfner, B.; Wong, T.T. Tennis overuse injuries in the upper extremity. *Skelet. Radiol.* **2021**, *50*, 629–644. [CrossRef]
60. Kibler, W.B.; Safran, M. Tennis injuries. *Med. Sport Sci.* **2005**, *48*, 120–137. [CrossRef]
61. Bahamonde, R.E.; Knudson, D. Kinetics of the upper extremity in the open and square stance tennis forehand. *J. Sci. Med. Sport* **2003**, *6*, 88–101. [CrossRef]
62. Pluim, B.M.; Staal, J.B.; Windler, G.E.; Jayanthi, N. Tennis injuries: Occurrence, aetiology, and prevention. *Br. J. Sports Med.* **2006**, *40*, 415–423. [CrossRef]
63. Reid, M.; Duffield, R. The development of fatigue during match-play tennis. *Br. J. Sports Med.* **2014**, *48* (Suppl. 1), i7–i11. [CrossRef]
64. Renstrom, A.F. Knee pain in tennis players. *Clin. Sports Med.* **1995**, *14*, 163–175. [CrossRef] [PubMed]
65. Reid, M.; Giblin, G. Another day, another tennis coaching intervention, but does this one do what coaches purport? *Sports Biomech.* **2015**, *14*, 180–189. [CrossRef] [PubMed]
66. Shafizadeh, M.; Bonner, S.; Barnes, A.; Fraser, J. Effects of task and environmental constraints on axial kinematic synergies during the tennis service in expert players. *Eur. J. Sport. Sci.* **2019**, *20*, 1178–1186. [CrossRef] [PubMed]

Disclaimer/Publisher's Note: The statements, opinions and data contained in all publications are solely those of the individual author(s) and contributor(s) and not of MDPI and/or the editor(s). MDPI and/or the editor(s) disclaim responsibility for any injury to people or property resulting from any ideas, methods, instructions or products referred to in the content.

Article

Biomechanical Effects of the Badminton Split-Step on Forecourt Lunging Footwork

Yile Wang [1], Liu Xu [1], Hanhui Jiang [1], Lin Yu [1,*], Hanzhang Wu [1] and Qichang Mei [1,2,*]

[1] Faculty of Sports Science, Ningbo University, Ningbo 315211, China
[2] Auckland Bioengineering Institute, University of Auckland, Auckland 1010, New Zealand
* Correspondence: yulin@nbu.edu.cn (L.Y.); qmei907@aucklanduni.ac.nz (Q.M.)

Abstract: Background: This research investigates the biomechanical impact of the split-step technique on forehand and backhand lunges in badminton, aiming to enhance players' on-court movement efficiency. Despite the importance of agile positioning in badminton, the specific contributions of the split-step to the biomechanical impact of lunging footwork still need to be determined. Methods: This study examined the lower limb kinematics and ground reaction forces of 18 male badminton players performing forehand and backhand lunges. Data were collected using the VICON motion capture system and Kistler force platforms. Variability in biomechanical characteristics was assessed using paired-sample *t*-tests and Statistical Parametric Mapping 1D (SPM1D). Results: The study demonstrates that the split-step technique in badminton lunges significantly affects lower limb biomechanics. During forehand lunges, the split-step increases hip abduction and rotation while decreasing knee flexion at foot contact. In backhand lunges, it increases knee rotation and decreases ankle rotation. Additionally, the split-step enhances the loading rate of the initial ground reaction force peak and narrows the time gap between the first two peaks. Conclusions: These findings underscore the split-step's potential in optimizing lunging techniques, improving performance and reducing injury risks in badminton athletes.

Keywords: badminton; split-step; lunge; biomechanics; lower limb

1. Introduction

Badminton, as a widely popular sport globally, attracts numerous enthusiasts and professional athletes due to its fast-paced, agile, and highly skilled nature [1–3]. In badminton matches, athletes are required to swiftly react to the opponents' shots and quickly maneuver to appropriate positions for a counterattack. Efficient badminton footwork techniques, such as jump landing, split-step, forehand and backhand lunging steps, cross steps, lateral shuffles, rapid net shots, and turning, play a crucial role in athletes' movement efficiency and shot quality [1,4,5]. In this process, athletes must rapidly initiate and adeptly employ a series of complex footwork combinations, such as initiating with small steps followed by cross steps, adjustment steps, large strides, propulsion steps, jump steps, and take-off steps, to swiftly react to the incoming shuttlecock. This technique, known as the split-step, involves utilizing leg strength to pre-step in the initial phase of executing movement footwork to enhance the quality of movement footwork [6].

In badminton singles, players frequently lunge forward to hit the shuttlecock, accounting for approximately 37% of all movements [1,7–9], which require athletes to possess rapid mobility, as well as excellent coordination and strength control, to ensure stability upon reaching the striking position for accurate shot execution. Athletes typically employ the split-step during forecourt lunges to attain better initial velocity and advantageous positioning. The split-step is a crucial preparatory action, aiding athletes in swiftly transitioning from a stationary to a dynamic state, providing impetus and direction for subsequent lunging movements.

The biomechanical characteristics of lunging steps and their impact on athletes' performance have been widely discussed. Yu et al. (2021) further investigated the effects of different lunge step directions (such as left forward, right forward, left backward, and right backward) on patellofemoral joint load, revealing that left backward lunging exhibited higher contact pressure and von Mises stress, particularly on the patellar cartilage. These studies provide crucial insights into understanding the biomechanical properties of lunging steps [10]. Mei et al. (2017) explored the biomechanical characteristics of badminton players with different skill levels during right-forward lunging, finding significant differences in knee joint moments and ground reaction forces between professional and amateur players [11]. Additionally, Lam et al. (2017) indicated that heel design influences ground reaction forces and knee joint moments during maximum lunge steps for elite and intermediate badminton players, suggesting that athletes' skill levels and footwear design may affect the biomechanical characteristics of lunging steps [12]. Kuntze et al. (2010) examined the mechanical attributes of top male badminton players during specific movement techniques such as lunging, stepping, and shuffling through video analysis and biomechanical methods [13].

The split-step technique is common in racket sports such as tennis and badminton. Aviles et al. (2002) found in their study that high-level tennis players always execute a split-step (preparatory movement) before serving or receiving serves [6]. According to Phomsoupha et al. (2018), the split-step enables athletes to effectively utilize elastic energy in subsequent movements through the stretch-shortening cycle (SSC) mechanism of muscles [14]. Furthermore, Filipčič et al. (2017) conducted a comparative analysis of professional and junior badminton players and observed that professional players demonstrate more significant pre-activation of lower limb muscles during the execution of the split-step, facilitating faster initiation and higher acceleration in subsequent movements [15]. Uzu et al. (2009) analyzed the timing and frequency of split-steps in badminton matches and found that executing the split-step immediately after the opponent's shot is most effective, aiding athletes in adjusting to optimal positions in the shortest time possible [16]. Hsueh et al. (2016) pointed out that due to immature physical development and neuromuscular control, the efficiency of split-step execution in adolescent athletes is generally lower compared to adult professional athletes [17]. Regarding gender differences, Mecheri et al. (2019) discovered in their study that male athletes outperform females in generating power during the split-step, while females exhibit better flexibility in footwork [18].

Despite the valuable insights provided by previous research on badminton footwork techniques, the significance of the split-step as the initiating phase of footwork execution is undeniable. However, there remains limited research on the specific influence of the split-step on the biomechanical characteristics of lunging steps. This necessitates a deeper understanding of the mechanism behind the split-step technique. Therefore, this study aims to conduct detailed measurements and analysis of badminton players' kinematic parameters and ground reaction forces during lunging steps with and without the split-step technique through experimental methods. The objective is to elucidate the impact of the split-step technique on the lower limb biomechanical characteristics of athletes.

This study aims to investigate the biomechanical characteristics of the lower limbs of badminton players during forehand and backhand lunging steps with and without the split-step technique. By measuring and analyzing parameters such as kinematics and ground reaction forces during lunging steps in both scenarios, this research seeks to elucidate the mechanism of the split-step in badminton and how it affects athletes' movement efficiency and stability. Additionally, this study will explore the potential value of the split-step technique in preventing sports injuries, providing coaches and athletes with more scientific and rational training guidance.

2. Materials and Methods

2.1. Participants

The sample size was calculated using GPower v3.1 [19] with an ANOVA F test for repeated measures within factors of a lateral wedge with incremental hardness, with an effect size (f) of 0.5, a level of 0.05, and a power value of 0.996. This study recruited a total of 18 male participants who were university-level badminton players (age: 24.51 ± 1.30 years, mass: 66.47 ± 8.42 kg, height: 172.60 ± 7.65 cm, BMI: 22.31 ± 3.21 kg/m^2, years of playing: 7.07 ± 2.89 years). All participants were right-handed. They were required to meet the following criteria: (1) have a minimum of three years of experience in playing badminton, engaging in badminton training or competitive activities at least 2–3 times per week; (2) have no lower limb or whole-body deformities; and (3) have been free from injury or illness for the past six months prior to the start of the experiment, with no lower limb injuries. Participants provided informed consent before the experiment, demonstrating their understanding of the experimental procedures and objectives. Pre-experimental trials were conducted according to the experimental protocol.

Participants refrained from undertaking high-intensity training or competitive activities for two days preceding the experiment. To mitigate the potential confounding influence of footwear, each participant was provided with identical badminton shoes of the same brand and type [11,20].

The study was approved by the ethics committee of the research institute at the university, and all participants were informed of the test objectives, procedures, and requirements with written consent.

2.2. Experimental Protocol

Forward forehand (FH) and backhand lunges (BH) are two of the most critical forward lunge techniques [9,20,21]. Following previous research, the forehand lunge is characterized by moving in the direction of the racket hand, orienting the chest towards the net, executing a stroke with the racket, and promptly returning to the initial position [20]. Each lunge should ideally be accomplished within a 3 s timeframe, covering a distance approximately 1.5 times the length of the leg. On the other hand, the backhand lunge entails having the back oriented towards the net [11,12,20]. More specific details of the two footwork and lab setup are illustrated in Figure 1.

All participants were experienced players with right-sided dominance for racquet grasp and right leg performing lunges, as badminton footwork typically involves unilateral hand and foot [3,5,10]. Specifically, all badminton players initiated the FH and BH lunges with a split-step, stepping up the left foot, followed by the right leg and foot for lunges to the proper forecourt or the left forecourt. Then, all badminton players initiated an FH and BH lunge without making a split-step, followed by a right leg and foot lunge to either the right or left forecourt. Thus, the lower limb of interest for lunging footwork was the right side.

After determining the experimental test action, a lab-simulated badminton court facilitated with an 8-camera Vicon motion capture system and synchronously connected AMTI force plates was set up for the biomechanical experiment to record the markers' positions and ground reaction forces during badminton footwork [5,10,11]. The data collection frequencies were 200 Hz and 1000 Hz, respectively. The marker set model in this study included markers to both acromia of the torso, bilateral ASIS and PSIS of the pelvis, 3-marker cluster to the lateral aspect of both thighs, medial and lateral knee epicondyles, 3-marker cluster to the lateral aspect of both shank, medial, and lateral ankle malleoli, posterior calcaneus, anterior toe-tip, medial M1, and lateral M5 of the bilateral lower limb. The model was employed and validated in our previous study of badminton directional lunges [5,10].

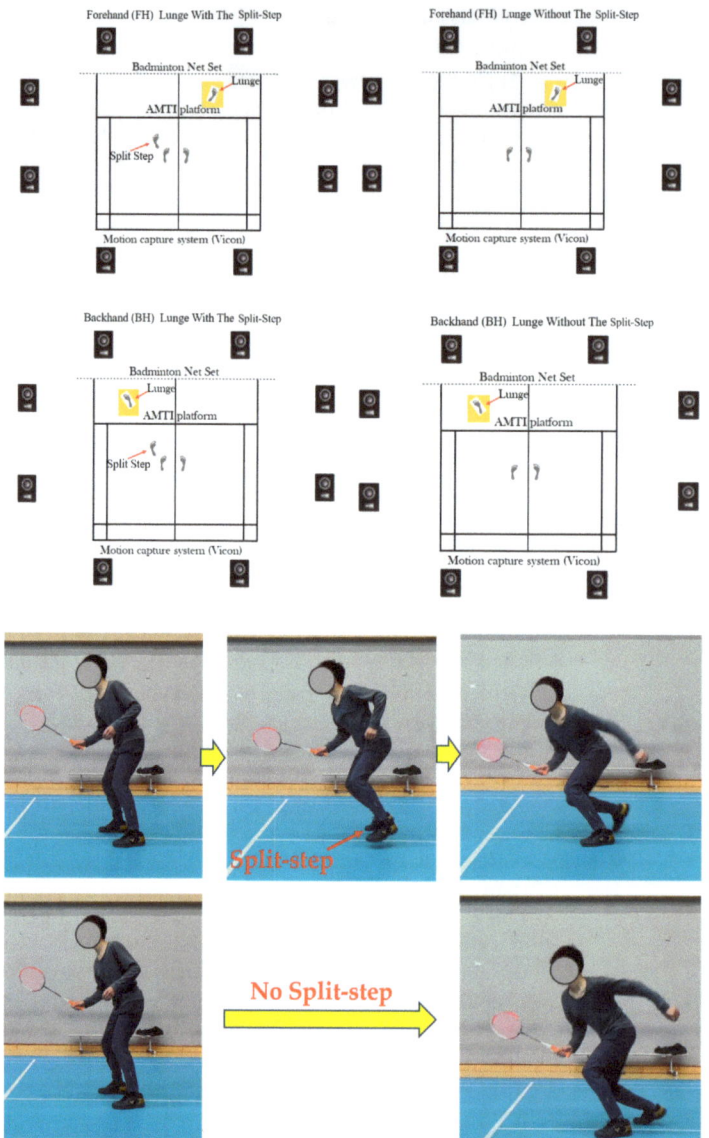

Figure 1. Illustration of experimental setup and the (non) split-step lunging footwork.

The lab setup included a badminton net and stick-hang shuttlecock in the target region for lunges to mimic real court situations. Before the data collection, badminton players were required to perform warm-up and lab court familiarization practice with randomly selected footwear for 10 min. Lunges were performed to standard and visually supervised by an experienced coach. Approach speed was defined as the speed from the initial position to force plate foot contact [22], which was manually controlled with a stopwatch by the coach.

2.3. Data Processing

The target limb for FH and BH footwork was the right limb. This study aimed to investigate the effect of the split-step on the performance of the badminton net lunge. Thus, as a close chain, the stance phase focused on analyzing the contact times, joint angles, and vertical ground reaction force (VGRF), defined from the threshold of 20 N in vertical ground reaction force [5,10]. Given their velocity sensitivity, the velocity was regulated utilizing a stopwatch to account for its impact on biomechanical parameters. Velocity was determined by computing the resultant speed derived from markers placed bilaterally on the anterior superior iliac spine (ASIS) and posterior superior iliac spine (PSIS) within the pelvis. More specific details of the marker's paste position are illustrated in Figure 2.

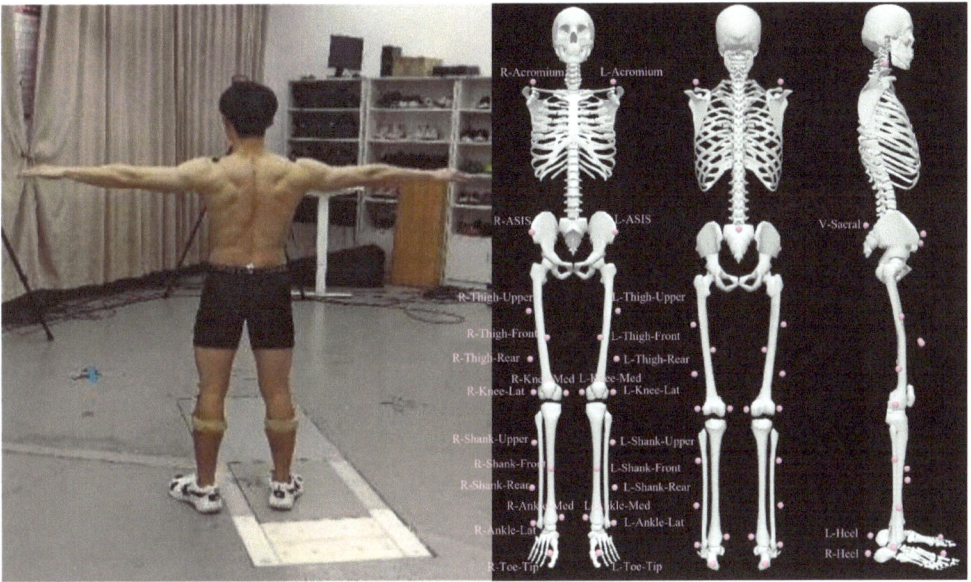

Figure 2. Diagram of marker set placement.

The marker trajectories and ground reaction force data were visually examined for quality, and any gaps in the data were filled using pattern fill functionality in an 8-camera Vicon motion capture system. Subsequently, the raw data were saved as C3D files for further processing utilizing a customized Matlab script. This processing involved generating "trc" and "mot" files, wherein the marker trajectories were filtered with a zero-phase fourth-order Butterworth low-pass filter set at a frequency of 6 Hz. The force data were filtered at 30 Hz [5,10,23]. Initially, the generic model underwent scaling procedures to align with the anthropometric dimensions of each participant, incorporating adjustments for anatomically relevant inertia and moment arms. Subsequently, inverse kinematics techniques were applied to compute the hip, knee, and ankle joint angles.

2.4. Statistical Analysis

This study aims to explore the biomechanical characteristics of badminton players during the propulsion step with and without a split-step, as well as the impact of these characteristics on performance efficiency and injury risk. It analyzes the lower limb kinematic characteristics and ground reaction force features during the landing cushioning phase and propulsion phase of the forehand and backhand propulsion steps with and without a split-step, based on the division of badminton textbook movement structures and the relevant literature in sports biomechanics. The landing cushioning and propulsion phases are delineated based on the ground reaction force data from a three-dimensional force plate, with the analysis focusing on the third trial out of five conducted.

Lower limb joint angle and range of motion, kinematic characteristics of the lower limbs at the moment of touchdown and during the contact phase, peak vertical GRF during the contact phase, first vertical peak loading rate, and difference in time to peak reaction force during support phase were chosen for statistical analyses based on the previous literature linked to impact injuries and quality in badminton lunges [12,13,22,24,25].

The foot contact time was defined as the duration from the initial contact to the final take-off of the lunging leg, as determined by the force plate [22,26]. The contact phase of the lunge step was delineated as the duration from the initial heel contact of the landing foot to toe-off, as ascertained through the force plate measurements. Specifically, heel contact and toe-off instances were identified as the moments when the vertical ground reaction force (VGRF) initially exceeded 10 N (heel contact) and subsequently reduced to 10 N (toe-off) [12].

The first vertical peak loading rate refers to the steepest slope observed on the vertical ground reaction force (VGRF) curve between consecutive data points from 20% to 80% before the initial peak impact [26–28]. The time difference in peak vertical reaction forces during the contact phase refers to the interval between observing three successive peaks in vertical reaction forces: from the first peak to the second peak and from the second peak to the third peak. These peaks correspond respectively to the instances of initial ground contact, support, and take-off phases in vertical reaction forces [22]. The definition of vertical ground reaction force is illustrated in Figure 3.

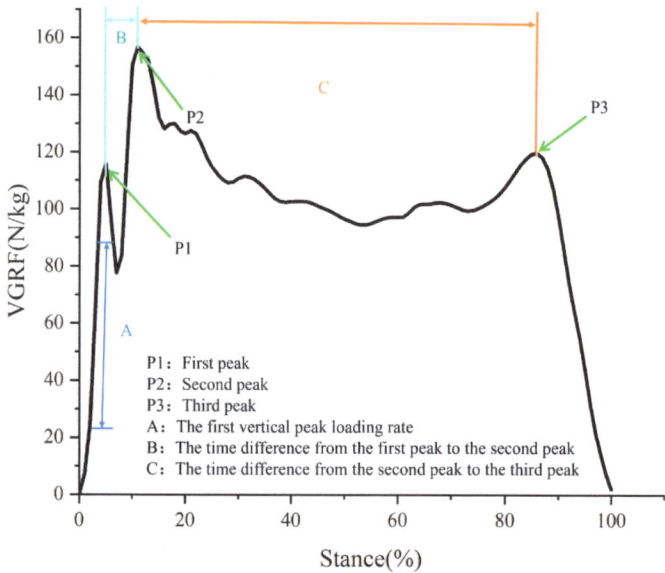

Figure 3. Illustrating the definition of vertical ground reaction force indicators.

Owing to their one-dimensional nature, the waveform data of joint angles and GRF were initially interpolated using a cubic spline, resulting in 101 data points representing the entirety of the stance phase (100%) [10]. Before statistical analysis, the normality of variables in this study was assessed using a Shapiro–Wilk test. Additionally, procedures were implemented to control the false discovery rate, particularly for the kinematic data of lower extremity joints. Due to the one-dimensional (1D) nature of joint kinematic trajectories [29,30], the Statistical Parametric Mapping 1D (SPM1D) was applied for the kinematics waveform data analysis of hip, knee, and ankle in three planes and vertical ground reaction force (VGRF) [11]. A paired-sample test was employed to compare the kinematic and ground reaction force data between the lunge steps with and without a split-step for both forehand and backhand movements in archery. All statistical analyses were performed with ORIGIN2022 (OriginLab Corporation, Northampton, MA, USA) and MATLAB R2016a with significance level settings at $p < 0.05$.

3. Results

3.1. Lower Limb Joint Angle and Range of Motion

Table 1 shows the angles of the hip, knee, and ankle at right foot contact during lunging with and without the split-step. In the FH lunge, the hip abduction and rotation angles in lunging with the split-step are significantly greater than in lunging without the split-step ($p < 0.05$). During the FH lunge, the knee flexion angle at foot contact in lunging with the split-step is significantly less than in lunging without the split-step ($p < 0.05$). In the BH lunge, the knee rotation angle at foot contact in lunging with the split-step is significantly greater than in lunging without the split-step ($p < 0.05$). In the BH lunge, the ankle rotation angle at foot contact in lunging with the split-step is significantly less than in lunging without the split-step ($p < 0.05$).

Table 1. The mean, standard deviation, and 95% confidence interval of the hip, knee, and ankle angles at the moment of right foot contact during FH and BH lunges with and without the split-step.

Joint	Variables	FH	FHS	95%CI	p	BH	BHS	95%CI	p
Hip	Flexion/Extension	25.85 ± 6.21	24.10 ± 6.48	[−0.21, 3.70]	0.08	23.68 ± 5.25	22.33 ± 5.28	[−1.31, 4.01]	0.30
	Abduction/Adduction	−31.34 ± 6.32	−33.40 ± 7.11	[0.73, 3.39]	0.004 *	−33.14 ± 4.54	−32.82 ± 4.98	[−2.27, 1.63]	0.74
	Internal/External rotation	−18.93 ± 13.64	−21.43 ± 14.50	[1.16, 3.84]	0.001 *	−14.32 ± 12.61	−20.80 ± 13.00	[−0.93, 13.89]	0.08
Knee	Flexion/Extension	−31.54 ± 9.11	−28.48 ± 6.16	[−5.39, −0.73]	0.01 *	−33.84 ± 8.44	−34.39 ± 8.09	[−2.07, 3.16]	0.06
	Abduction/Adduction	7.81 ± 4.73	7.82 ± 4.83	[−0.66, 0.65]	0.99	8.08 ± 5.55	6.15 ± 4.31	[−1.18, 5.04]	0.21
	Internal/External rotation	1.86 ± 7.67	1.68 ± 6.52	[−1.43, 1.80]	0.82	1.76 ± 1.79	1.20 ± 5.05	[−9.41, −1.47]	0.01 *
Ankle	Flexion/Extension	8.87 ± 8.05	8.09 ± 7.42	[−0.63, 2.20]	0.26	7.76 ± 10.68	7.19 ± 9.80	[−4.14, 5.29]	0.80
	Internal/External rotation	−1.74 ± 3.45	−1.36 ± 3.18	[−1.28, 0.51]	0.39	−2.25 ± 3.54	−0.52 ± 2.63	[−3.01, −0.43]	0.01 *

Note: * indicates significant difference ($p < 0.05$); FH represents forehand lunge without the split-step; FHS represents forehand lunge with the split-step; BH represents backhand lunge without the split-step; BHS represents backhand lunge with the split-step.

Figure 4 depicts the range of motion (ROM) of the hip, knee, and ankle angles during the right foot support phase of lunging with and without the split-step for badminton players. As shown, during the BH lunge, the ankle flexion–extension angle ROM in lunging with the split-step is significantly less than in lunging without the split-step ($p < 0.05$).

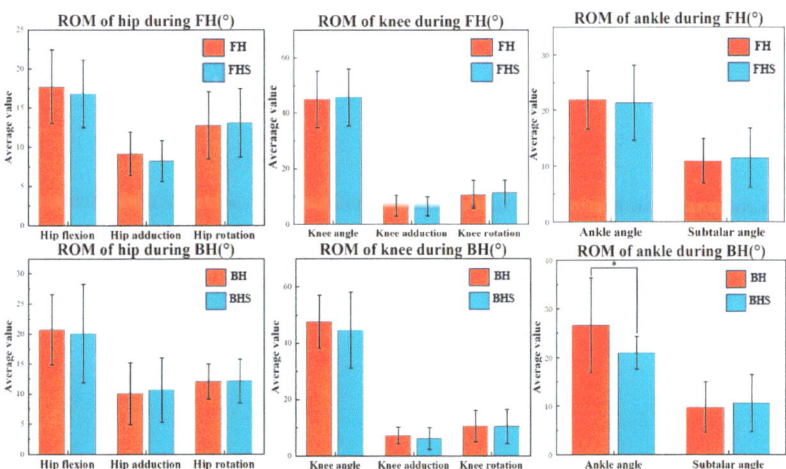

Figure 4. The mean and standard deviation of the range of motion (ROM) of the hip, knee, and ankle angles during the right foot support phase of the FH and BH lunges with and without the split-step. Notes: * indicates significant difference ($p < 0.05$); FH represents forehand lunge without the split-step; FHS represents forehand lunge with the split-step; BH represents backhand lunge without the split-step; BHS represents backhand lunge with the split-step.

Figure 5 illustrates the kinematic characteristics of the hip joint during the right foot support phase of the lunge for FH and BH strides. There were significant differences observed between the hip flexion angles of the FH lunges with and without the split-step at the 0–22% ($p = 0.015$) and 55–100% ($p < 0.001$) phases. Significant differences were found in the hip rotation angles between the FH lunges with and without the split-step at the 0–5% phase ($p = 0.044$).

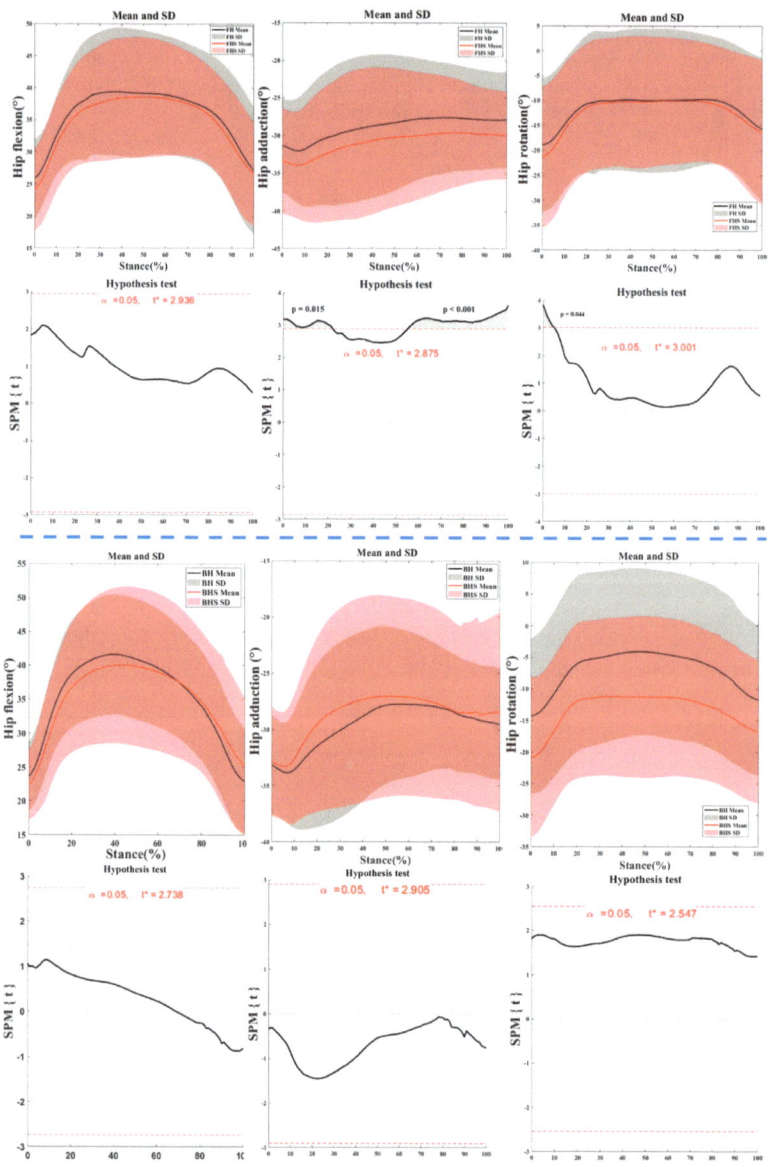

Figure 5. The kinematic characteristics of the hip joint during the right foot support phase of the lunge for FH and BH strides. Notes: FH represents forehand lunge without the split-step; FHS represents forehand lunge with the split-step; BH represents backhand lunge without the split-step; BHS represents backhand lunge with the split-step.

Figure 6 illustrates the kinematic characteristics of the knee joint during the right foot support phase of the lunge for FH and BH strides. The knee joint rotation angles for FH strides with and without the split-step show significant differences at the 2–23% ($p = 0.015$) and 84–95% ($p = 0.035$) phases. For BH strides, the knee joint flexion–extension angles during the right foot support phase of the lunge with and without the split-step exhibit significance at the 2–8% phase ($p = 0.040$).

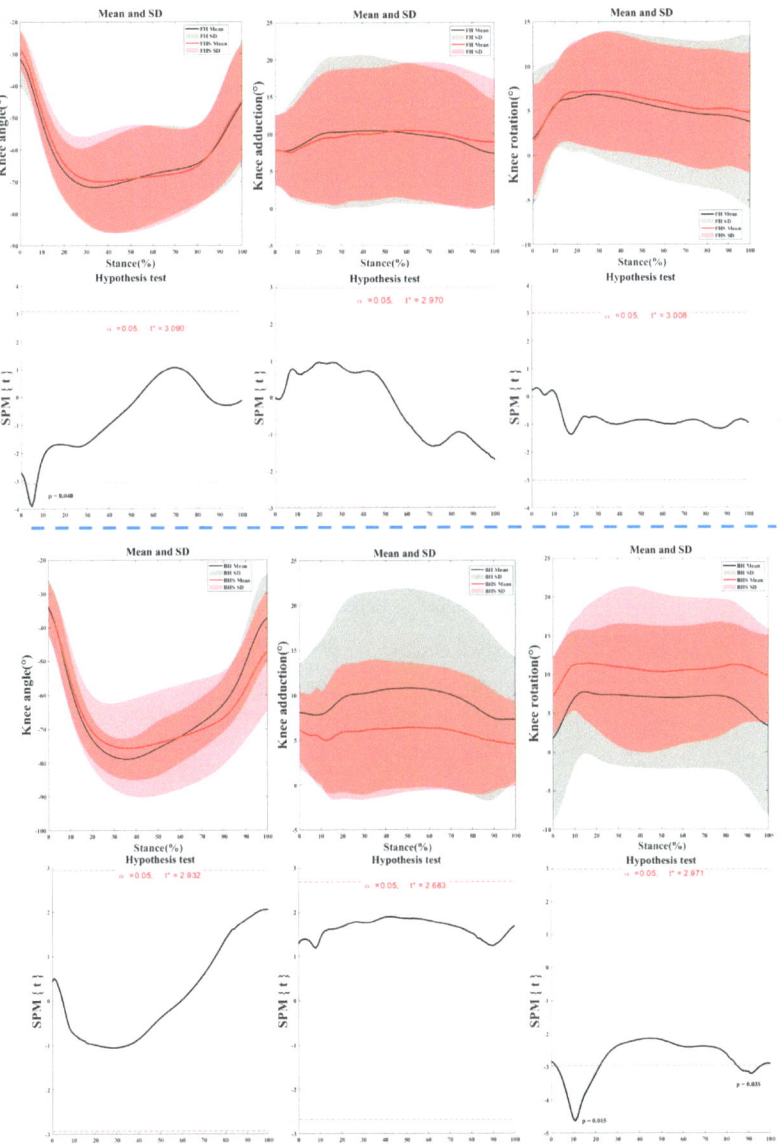

Figure 6. The kinematic characteristics of the knee joint during the right foot support phase of the lunge for FH and BH strides. Notes: FH represents forehand lunge without the split-step; FHS represents forehand lunge with the split-step; BH represents backhand lunge without the split-step; BHS represents backhand lunge with the split-step.

Figure 7 illustrates the kinematic characteristics of the ankle joint during the right foot support phase of the lunge for FH and BH strides.

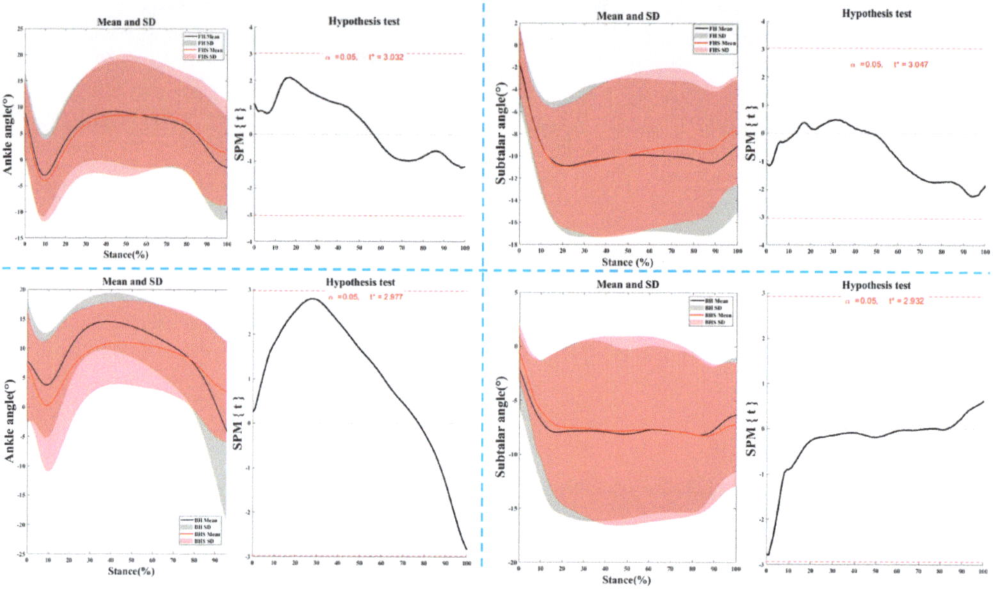

Figure 7. The kinematic characteristics of the ankle joint during the right foot support phase of the lunge for FH and BH strides. Notes: FH represents forehand lunge without the split-step; FHS represents forehand lunge with the split-step; BH represents backhand lunge without the split-step; BHS represents backhand lunge with the split-step.

3.2. Vertical Ground Reaction Force

Figure 8 illustrates the variations in vertical ground reaction force (VGRF) during the support phase of lunges for FH and BH strides. No statistically significant differences were observed.

Table 2 presents the characteristics of the first VGRF peak loading rate during the support phase of the lunge for FH and BH strides. There are differences in the first VGRF peak loading rate between strides with and without the split-step. During the forehand lunge, the first VGRF peak loading rate for strides with the split-step is significantly greater than for strides without the split-step ($p < 0.05$).

Table 2. The characteristics of the first VGRF peak loading rate during the support phase (unit: N/kg%).

Footwork	Mean ± SD	95%CI	p
FH	33.30 ± 13.40	[−13.67, 0.13]	0.04 *
FHS	40.06 ± 15.91		
BH	29.96 ± 15.23	[−5.37, 11.04]	0.48
BHS	29.24 ± 12.25		

Note: * indicates significant difference ($p < 0.05$); FH represents forehand lunge without the split-step; FHS represents forehand lunge with the split-step; BH represents backhand lunge without the split-step; BHS represents backhand lunge with the split-step.

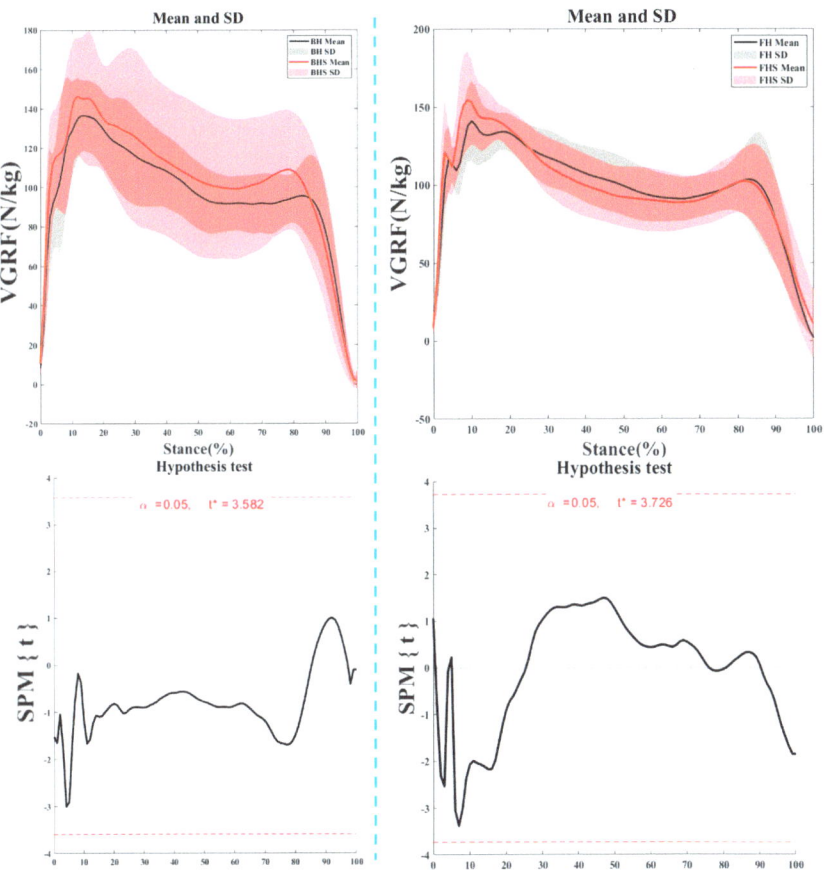

Figure 8. Vertical ground reaction force (VGRF) characteristics during the support phase. Notes: FH represents forehand lunge without the split-step; FHS represents forehand lunge with the split-step; BH represents backhand lunge without the split-step; BHS represents backhand lunge with the split-step.

Table 3 presents the characteristics of the time difference between the first and second peaks of the vertical ground reaction force (VGRF) during the support phase. For forehand lunges, the time difference between the first and second VGRF peaks was smaller in lunges with the split-step compared to lunges without the split-step, and this difference was statistically significant ($p < 0.05$).

Table 3. Time difference between the first and second VGRF peaks during the support phase (unit: %).

Footwork	Mean ± SD	95%CI	p
FH	9.9 ± 4.24	[0.21, 4.59]	0.03 *
FHS	7.5 ± 2.78		
BH	7.66 ± 2.38	[−2.29, 0.51]	0.12
BHS	8.55 ± 3.05		

Notes: * indicates significant difference ($p < 0.05$); FH represents forehand lunge without the split-step; FHS represents forehand lunge with the split-step; BH represents backhand lunge without the split-step; BHS represents backhand lunge with the split-step.

Table 4 presents the characteristics of the time difference between the second and third peaks of the vertical ground reaction force (VGRF) during the support phase. No statistically significant differences were observed.

Table 4. Time difference between the second and third GRF peaks during the support phase (unit: %).

Footwork	Mean ± SD	95%CI	p
FH	67.35 ± 10.79	[−9.95, 0.25]	0.06
FHS	72.2 ± 8.33		
BH	70.77 ± 7.97	[−2.66, 7.10]	0.35
BHS	68.56 ± 6.58		

Notes: FH represents forehand lunge without the split-step; FHS represents forehand lunge with the split-step; BH represents backhand lunge without the split-step; BHS represents backhand lunge with the split-step.

4. Discussion

This study aimed to investigate the biomechanical characteristics of the lower limbs of badminton players during forehand and backhand lunging steps with and without the split-step technique, as well as the impact of these characteristics on movement efficiency and sports injuries. Using a three-dimensional force plate and motion capture system, kinematic and ground reaction force parameters during lunging steps were measured and analyzed for 18 badminton players in both scenarios. The main findings of this study are as follows.

In this study, we observed a significant difference in the hip joint abduction/adduction angle and rotation angle between lunging steps with and without the split-step technique at the moment of right foot contact. This finding underscores the importance of the split-step in the footwork of badminton players [13,31], particularly in the kinematic characteristics of the hip joint. As a crucial pivot point for lower limb movement, variations in hip joint angles directly influence athletes' stride, speed, and stability. Introducing the split-step may provide athletes with greater stride length and faster movement speed by increasing the range of motion in the hip joint, thus offering an advantage in badminton matches [32]. The increase in hip joint abduction/adduction angle implies that athletes can utilize the hip muscles more effectively during lunging steps, which may be related to the pre-activation performed during the split-step [8]. Pre-activation enhances muscle readiness, allowing greater force production and faster speed during subsequent lunging steps. Additionally, the increase in the hip joint rotation angle may be associated with athletes adjusting their body orientation to adapt to the flight trajectory of the shuttlecock [33]. Rapid adjustments in body orientation are crucial for successful shuttlecock retrieval in badminton, and the flexible movement of the hip joint provides the necessary biomechanical foundation [34].

Regarding the ankle joint, we found that during the landing phase of the backhand lunges with the split-step, the rotation angle of the ankle joint was significantly smaller compared to backhand lunges without the split-step. Additionally, the ankle joint dorsiflexion angle's range of motion (ROM) was significantly smaller during backhand lunges with the split-step compared to those without the split-step. This suggests that during backhand lunges, the split-step may reduce the mobility of the ankle joint, thereby enhancing ankle joint stability and effectively preventing sports injuries [20,35]. Moreover, the stability and flexibility of the ankle joint are crucial for the coordinated movement of the entire lower limb chain [36,37]. Future research could further investigate the role of the ankle joint in different footwork patterns and explore methods to optimize ankle joint function through training.

Although significant differences were observed in the kinematic characteristics of the hip and ankle joint during the split-step, no significant changes were noted in the kinematic characteristics of the knee at the moment of ground contact. This may suggest that during the initial phase of lunging steps, the motion of the knee is primarily influenced by ground reaction forces and shifts in the body's center of mass rather than by the execution of the split-step. This finding is consistent with previous studies on the kinematics of lunging steps [10,31], indicating that the knee joints primarily serve a buffering and stabilizing role during stride transitions. In contrast, the hip joint plays a predominant role in dynamic stride adjustments [10].

In this study, we conducted a detailed analysis of badminton players' lower limb kinematic characteristics during forehand and backhand lunging steps, particularly during the right foot support phase, comparing the differences between lunging steps with and without the split-step technique. The results revealed significant effects of the split-step on athletes' lower limb kinematic characteristics, particularly at specific stages of hip and knee joint activity. Firstly, the hip joint abduction/adduction angle was significantly greater during forehand lunging steps with the split-step than without, especially during the movement's early (0–22%) and late (55–100%) phases. This suggests that the split-step may provide athletes with a greater range of motion in the hip joint, thereby aiding in increasing stride length and enhancing movement speed. Such kinematic characteristics of the hip joint are crucial for badminton players to adjust their body posture and prepare for hitting the shuttlecock during rapid movements. This advantage may directly impact their performance and match outcomes, particularly during critical game moments [13,38]. Secondly, the hip joint rotation angle was significantly smaller during forehand lunging steps with the split-step than without, especially during the movement's early (0–5%) phase. This may indicate that athletes are more inclined to adjust their body orientation through hip joint abduction/adduction movement rather than rotation during the split-step. This strategy may help athletes rapidly adapt to the optimal hitting position while maintaining stability [39].

Regarding the knee joint, the rotation angle during backhand lunging steps with the split-step was significantly greater than without at specific stages (2–23% and 84–95%). This suggests that the split-step may facilitate a larger range of rotation at the knee joint during the lunging step, which is crucial for athletes to maintain balance and adjust stride rhythm during movement [31,40]. The knee joint flexion/extension angle exhibited significant differences during forehand lunging steps, with the split-step at the 2–8% stage. This may reflect that the split-step provides additional propulsion for athletes during the initial push-off phase, resulting in greater torque during knee joint flexion [21,31].

In this study, we analyzed badminton players' ground reaction force (GRF) characteristics during forehand and backhand lunging steps with and without a split-step. The results revealed the impact of the preparatory step on the time difference between GRF peaks and loading rates, which holds significant implications for understanding the biomechanics of badminton footwork. Firstly, in forehand lunging steps, the time difference between the first and second GRF peaks was significantly shorter in steps with a split-step than those without. This suggests that the preparatory step facilitates a quicker transition from heel contact to full foot contact during the support phase, potentially enhancing the athlete's ability to efficiently absorb and transmit force, consequently generating greater propulsion during the push-off phase [10,11,41]. This ability to rapidly adjust footwork is crucial for swiftly reaching hitting positions and maintaining balance during badminton matches [5]. However, in forehand lunging steps, no significant difference was observed in the time difference between the second and third GRF peaks with and without a split-step. This suggests that the split-step may have a limited optimization effect on the time difference between GRF peaks during the push-off phase, potentially because the primary goal during this phase is to generate sufficient force to complete the step, and the time difference between GRF peaks may not be the primary determinant of performance during this phase.

Additionally, during forehand lunges, the first vertical GRF peak loading rate of lunges with the split-step was significantly greater than those without the split-step. This suggests that the split-step enhances the loading rate of vertical GRF upon foot contact, potentially aiding in shortening the duration of the lunge motion. This is consistent with findings from previous studies. Previous research has shown that the split-step can improve initial acceleration and stride efficiency in tennis players and reaction speed in soccer goalkeepers during penalty kicks [16,42].

When discussing the limitations of this study, it is essential to acknowledge that the sample size may affect the generalizability and reliability of the results. Due to the small sample size, our findings may only partially represent some biomechanical characteristics of lower limb movements during lunging steps in all badminton players. Additionally, individual differences among athletes, including skill level, training background, physical condition, and age, could significantly influence GRF characteristics, and these factors needed to be adequately considered in this study. Therefore, future research should aim to increase the sample size and account for individual differences among athletes to understand better the effects of preparatory steps on the biomechanical characteristics of lunging steps.

Furthermore, this study only focused on forehand and backhand lunging, while badminton players execute various steps during matches. To comprehensively understand the effects of split-steps, future research should include more types of steps, such as lateral steps and jumping steps, as well as different step executions in various match situations, such as fast counterattacks, defensive transitions, etc.

Moreover, this study primarily focused on the time difference between GRF peaks and loading rates without thoroughly analyzing the dynamic changes of GRF throughout the entire step cycle. Future research could investigate the effects of preparatory steps on the distribution and transmission of forces throughout the entire step cycle through finer temporal resolution and more comprehensive GRF analysis.

5. Conclusions

This study analyzed the biomechanical effects of incorporating the split-step in both forehand (FH) and backhand (BH) lunging steps in badminton. The results indicated that the split-step significantly improves the efficiency and velocity of the FH lunging step. This improvement is characterized by increased hip joint angles and decreased knee flexion angles at the moment of foot contact. Moreover, the study found an enhanced loading rate of the initial GRF peak and a reduced time interval between the first and second GRF peaks during the FH lunge with the split-step, further supporting the beneficial role of the split-step in enhancing stride efficiency. However, the impact of the split-step in the BH lunging step was not as pronounced, which may point to the influence of other factors on stride efficiency and stability. In summary, the split-step plays a vital role in optimizing performance for FH lunging actions. In contrast, the effectiveness of the split-step in BH actions warrants further exploration and refinement in training approaches. These insights offer a scientific foundation for athletes and coaches to improve technical training and movement efficiency in badminton.

Author Contributions: Conceptualization, Y.W. and L.Y.; methodology, Y.W. and L.X.; software, H.J. and L.Y.; validation, H.J., H.W. and L.Y.; formal analysis, Y.W. and L.Y.; investigation, Y.W., H.J. and H.W.; data curation, L.X. and L.Y.; writing original draft preparation, Y.W. and L.X.; writing review and editing, H.J., L.Y. and Q.M.; supervision, L.Y. and Q.M.; project administration, L.Y.; funding acquisition, L.Y. and Q.M. All authors have read and agreed to the published version of the manuscript.

Funding: This research was supported by the China National Higher Education Scientific Research and Planning project (23TY0209), the Scientific Research Fund of Zhejiang Provincial Education Department (Y202352339), the Badminton World Federation (BWF) sport science research project, the "Mechanics+" Interdisciplinary Top Innovative Youth Fund Project of Ningbo University (GC2024006), Ningbo University Teaching and Research project (JYXM2023051; JYXM2023123), and the K.C. Wong Magna Fund in Ningbo University.

Institutional Review Board Statement: The study was conducted in accordance with the Declaration of Helsinki, and approved by the Ethics Committee of Ningbo University (TY2024007).

Informed Consent Statement: Informed consent was obtained from all participants involved in the study.

Data Availability Statement: The data related to the results and findings of this study will be available upon reasonable request to the corresponding author.

Acknowledgments: The authors acknowledge the kind collaboration of all participants in this study.

Conflicts of Interest: The authors declare no conflicts of interest.

References

1. Phomsoupha, M.; Laffaye, G. The Science of Badminton: Game Characteristics, Anthropometry, Physiology, Visual Fitness and Biomechanics. *Sports Med.* **2015**, *45*, 473–495. [CrossRef]
2. Kwan, M.; Cheng, C.L.; Tang, W.T.; Rasmussen, J. Measurement of badminton racket deflection during a stroke. *Sports Eng.* **2010**, *12*, 143–153. [CrossRef]
3. Yu, L.; Mohamad, N.I. Development of Badminton-specific Footwork Training from Traditional Physical Exercise to Novel Intervention Approaches. *Phys. Act. Health* **2022**, *6*, 219–225. [CrossRef]
4. Valldecabres, R.; Casal, C.A.; Chiminazzo, J.G.C.; De Benito, A.M. Players' on-court movements and contextual variables in badminton world championship. *Front. Psychol.* **2020**, *11*, 508842. [CrossRef]
5. Yu, L.; Wang, Y.; Fernandez, J.; Mei, Q.; Zhao, J.; Yang, F.; Gu, Y. Dose–response effect of incremental lateral-wedge hardness on the lower limb Biomechanics during typical badminton footwork. *J. Sports Sci.* **2023**, *41*, 972–989. [CrossRef]
6. Aviles, C.; Benguigui, N.; Beaudoin, E.; Godart, F. Developing early perception and getting ready for action on the return of serve. *ITF Coach. Sport Sci. Rev.* **2002**, *28*, 8.
7. Park, S.-K.; Lam, W.-K.; Yoon, S.; Lee, K.-K.; Ryu, J. Effects of forefoot bending stiffness of badminton shoes on agility, comfort perception and lower leg kinematics during typical badminton movements. *Sports Biomech.* **2017**, *16*, 374–386. [CrossRef]
8. Cronin, J.; McNair, P.J.; Marshall, R.N. Lunge performance and its determinants. *J. Sports Sci.* **2003**, *21*, 49–57. [CrossRef]
9. Hu, X.; Li, J.X.; Hong, Y.; Wang, L. Characteristics of plantar loads in maximum forward lunge tasks in badminton. *PLoS ONE* **2015**, *10*, e0137558. [CrossRef]
10. Yu, L.; Mei, Q.; Mohamad, N.I.; Gu, Y.; Fernandez, J. An exploratory investigation of patellofemoral joint loadings during directional lunges in badminton. *Comput. Biol. Med.* **2021**, *132*, 104302. [CrossRef]
11. Mei, Q.; Gu, Y.; Fu, F.; Fernandez, J. A biomechanical investigation of right-forward lunging step among badminton players. *J. Sports Sci.* **2016**, *35*, 457–462. [CrossRef] [PubMed]
12. Lam, W.-K.; Lee, K.-K.; Park, S.-K.; Ryue, J.; Yoon, S.-H.; Ryu, J. Understanding the impact loading characteristics of a badminton lunge among badminton players. *PLoS ONE* **2018**, *13*, e0205800. [CrossRef] [PubMed]
13. Kuntze, G.; Mansfield, N.; Sellers, W. A biomechanical analysis of common lunge tasks in badminton. *J. Sports Sci.* **2010**, *28*, 183–191. [CrossRef]
14. Phomsoupha, M.; Berger, Q.; Laffaye, G. Multiple Repeated Sprint Ability Test for Badminton Players Involving Four Changes of Direction: Validity and Reliability (Part 1). *J. Strength Cond. Res.* **2018**, *32*, 423–431. [CrossRef] [PubMed]
15. Filipčič, A.; Leskošek, B.; Munivrana, G.; Ochiana, G.; Filipčič, T. Differences in Movement Speed Before and After a Split-Step Between Professional and Junior Tennis Players. *J. Hum. Kinet.* **2017**, *55*, 117–125. [CrossRef] [PubMed]
16. Uzu, R.; Shinya, M.; Oda, S. A split-step shortens the time to perform a choice reaction step-and-reach movement in a simulated tennis task. *J. Sports Sci.* **2009**, *27*, 1233–1240. [CrossRef] [PubMed]
17. Hsueh, Y.-C.; Pan, K.-M.; Tsai, C.-L. Hop Llmlng of Spllt Step and Kinetics Analysis of Lower Extremities in Badminton Start Footwork. In Proceedings of the 34th International Conference of Biomechanics in Sport, Tsukuba, Japan, 18–22 July 2016; pp. 640–643.
18. Mecheri, S.; Laffaye, G.; Triolet, C.; Leroy, D.; Dicks, M.; Choukou, M.A.; Benguigui, N. Relationship between split-step timing and leg stiffness in world-class tennis players when returning fast serves. *J. Sports Sci.* **2019**, *37*, 1962–1971. [CrossRef] [PubMed]
19. Faul, F.; Erdfelder, E.; Lang, A.-G.; Buchner, A. G* Power 3: A flexible statistical power analysis program for the social, behavioral, and biomedical sciences. *Behav. Res. Methods* **2007**, *39*, 175–191. [CrossRef] [PubMed]
20. Tong, J.; Lu, Z.; Cen, X.; Chen, C.; Ugbolue, U.C.; Gu, Y. The effects of ankle dorsiflexor fatigue on lower limb biomechanics during badminton forward forehand and backhand lunge. *Front. Bioeng. Biotechnol.* **2023**, *11*, 1013100. [CrossRef]
21. Hong, Y.; Wang, S.J.; Lam, W.K.; Cheung, J.T.-M. Kinetics of badminton lunges in four directions. *J. Appl. Biomech.* **2014**, *30*, 113–118. [CrossRef]
22. Lam, W.K.; Ding, R.; Qu, Y. Ground reaction forces and knee kinetics during single and repeated badminton lunges. *J. Sports Sci.* **2017**, *35*, 587–592. [CrossRef] [PubMed]
23. Mei, Q.; Gu, Y.; Xiang, L.; Yu, P.; Gao, Z.; Shim, V.; Fernandez, J. Foot shape and plantar pressure relationships in shod and barefoot populations. *Biomech. Model. Mechanobiol.* **2019**, *19*, 1211–1224. [CrossRef] [PubMed]
24. Cong, Y.; Lam, W.K.; Cheung, J.T.-M.; Zhang, M. In-shoe plantar tri-axial stress profiles during maximum-effort cutting maneuvers. *J. Biomech.* **2014**, *47*, 3799–3806. [CrossRef] [PubMed]
25. Fahlström, M.; Björnstig, U.; Lorentzon, R. Acute Achilles Tendon Rupture in Badminton Players. *Am. J. Sports Med.* **1998**, *26*, 467–470. [CrossRef]

26. Lam, G.W.K.; Ryue, J.; Lee, K.-K.; Park, S.K.; Cheung, J.; Ryu, J. Does shoe heel design influence ground reaction forces and knee moments during maximum lunges in elite and intermediate badminton players? *PLoS ONE* **2017**, *12*, e0174604. [CrossRef] [PubMed]
27. Nin, D.Z.; Lam, W.K.; Kong, P.W. Effect of body mass and midsole hardness on kinetic and perceptual variables during basketball landing manoeuvres. *J. Sports Sci.* **2016**, *34*, 756–765. [CrossRef]
28. Schmida, E.A.; Wille, C.M.; Stiffler-Joachim, M.R.; Kliethermes, S.A.; Heiderscheit, B.C. Vertical Loading Rate Is Not Associated with Running Injury, Regardless of Calculation Method. *Med. Sci. Sports Exerc.* **2022**, *54*, 1382. [CrossRef] [PubMed]
29. Pataky, T.C.; Vanrenterghem, J.; Robinson, M.A. Zero- vs. one-dimensional, parametric vs. non-parametric, and confidence interval vs. hypothesis testing procedures in one-dimensional biomechanical trajectory analysis. *J. Biomech.* **2015**, *48*, 1277–1285. [CrossRef]
30. Pataky, T.C. Generalized n-dimensional biomechanical field analysis using statistical parametric mapping. *J. Biomech.* **2010**, *43*, 1976–1982. [CrossRef]
31. Huang, M.-T.; Lee, H.-H.; Lin, C.-F.; Tsai, Y.-J.; Liao, J.-C. How does knee pain affect trunk and knee motion during badminton forehand lunges? *J. Sports Sci.* **2014**, *32*, 690–700. [CrossRef]
32. Huang, P.; Fu, L.; Zhang, Y.; Fekete, G.; Ren, F.; Gu, Y.D. Biomechanical Analysis Methods to Assess Professional Badminton Players' Lunge Performance. *J. Vis. Exp.* **2019**, *148*, e58842.
33. Nadzalan, A.M.; Mohamad, N.I.; Lee, J.L.F.; Tan, K.; Janep, M.; Hamzah, S.; Chinnasee, C. Muscle activation analysis of step and jump forward lunge among badminton players. *Age* **2017**, *22*, 1–39.
34. Lund, J.N.; Lam, W.-K.; Nielsen, M.H.; Qu, Y.; Kersting, U. The effect of insole hardness distribution on calf muscle loading and energy return during a forward badminton lunge. *Footwear Sci.* **2017**, *9*, S136–S137. [CrossRef]
35. Chen, T.L.-W.; Wang, Y.; Wong, D.W.-C.; Lam, W.-K.; Zhang, M. Joint contact force and movement deceleration among badminton forward lunges: A musculoskeletal modelling study. *Sports Biomech.* **2020**, *21*, 1249–1261. [CrossRef]
36. Donovan, L.; Miklovic, T.; Feger, M. Step-Down Task Identifies Differences in Ankle Biomechanics Across Functional Activities. *Int. J. Sports Med.* **2018**, *39*, 846–852. [CrossRef] [PubMed]
37. Crenna, P.; Frigo, C. Dynamics of the ankle joint analyzed through moment–angle loops during human walking: Gender and age effects. *Hum. Mov. Sci.* **2011**, *30*, 1185–1198. [CrossRef] [PubMed]
38. Lam, W.-K.; Wong, D.W.-C.; Lee, W.C.-C. Biomechanics of lower limb in badminton lunge: A systematic scoping review. *PeerJ* **2020**, *8*, e10300. [CrossRef] [PubMed]
39. Lee, J.J.J.; Loh, W.P. A state-of-the-art review on badminton lunge attributes. *Comput. Biol. Med.* **2019**, *108*, 213–222. [CrossRef] [PubMed]
40. Lin, C.-F.; Hua, S.-H.; Huang, M.-T.; Lee, H.-H.; Liao, J.-C. Biomechanical analysis of knee and trunk in badminton players with and without knee pain during backhand diagonal lunges. *J. Sports Sci.* **2015**, *33*, 1429–1439. [CrossRef]
41. Yu, L.; Jiang, H.; Mei, Q.; Mohamad, N.I.; Fernandez, J.; Gu, Y. Intelligent prediction of lower extremity loadings during badminton lunge footwork in a lab-simulated court. *Front. Bioeng. Biotechnol.* **2023**, *11*, 1229574. [CrossRef]
42. Dicks, M.; Davids, K.; Button, C. Individual differences in the visual control of intercepting a penalty kick in association football. *Hum. Mov. Sci.* **2010**, *29*, 401–411. [CrossRef] [PubMed]

Disclaimer/Publisher's Note: The statements, opinions and data contained in all publications are solely those of the individual author(s) and contributor(s) and not of MDPI and/or the editor(s). MDPI and/or the editor(s) disclaim responsibility for any injury to people or property resulting from any ideas, methods, instructions or products referred to in the content.

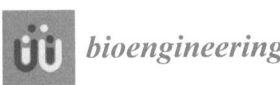

Article

The Influence of Dynamic Taping on Landing Biomechanics after Fatigue in Young Football Athletes: A Randomized, Sham-Controlled Crossover Trial

Chih-Kuan Wu [1,2,3], Yin-Chou Lin [1,2,4], Ya-Lin Chen [5], Yi-Ping Chao [6] and Tsung-Hsun Hsieh [3,7,8,*]

1. Department of Physical Medicine and Rehabilitation, Chang Gung Memorial Hospital, Linkou, Taoyuan 33305, Taiwan; a9227@adm.cgmh.org.tw (C.-K.W.); sirius@adm.cgmh.org.tw (Y.-C.L.)
2. Center of Comprehensive Sports Medicine, Chang Gung Memorial Hospital, Linkou, Taoyuan 33305, Taiwan
3. School of Physical Therapy and Graduate Institute of Rehabilitation Science, Chang Gung University, Taoyuan 33302, Taiwan
4. Department of Health Management and Enhancement, Open University of Kaohsiung, Kaohsiung 81249, Taiwan
5. Department of Athletic Training & Health, National Taiwan Sport University, Taoyuan 33301, Taiwan; eileen@ntsu.edu.tw
6. Department of Computer Science and Information Engineering, Chang Gung University, Taoyuan 33302, Taiwan; yiping@mail.cgu.edu.tw
7. Neuroscience Research Center, Chang Gung Memorial Hospital, Linkou, Taoyuan 33305, Taiwan
8. Healthy Aging Research Center, Chang Gung University, Taoyuan 33305, Taiwan
* Correspondence: hsiehth@mail.cgu.edu.tw

Abstract: Fatigue is believed to increase the risk of anterior cruciate ligament (ACL) injury by directly promoting high-risk biomechanics in the lower limbs. Studies have shown that dynamic taping can help normalize inadequate biomechanics during landings. This study aims to examine the effects of dynamic taping on landing biomechanics in fatigued football athletes. Twenty-seven high-school football athletes were recruited and randomly allocated to groups of either active taping or sham taping, with a crossover allocation two weeks later. In each group, the participants underwent a functional agility short-term fatigue protocol and were evaluated using the landing error scoring system before and after the fatigue protocol. The landing error scoring system (LESS) scores in the sham taping group increased from 4.24 ± 1.83 to 5.36 ± 2.00 ($t = -2.07$, $p = 0.04$, effect size = 0.61). In contrast, the pre–post difference did not reach statistical significance in the active taping group (from 4.24 ± 1.69 to 4.52 ± 1.69, $t = -1.50$, $p = 0.15$, effect size 0.46). Furthermore, the pre–post changes between the sham and active taping groups were statistically significant (sham taping: 1.12 ± 1.20; active taping: 0.28 ± 0.94, $p = 0.007$). Dynamic taping, particularly using the spiral technique, appeared to mitigate faulty landing biomechanics in the fatigued athletes by reducing hip and knee flexion and increasing hip internal rotation during landing. These results suggest that dynamic taping can potentially offer protective benefits in landing mechanics, which could further be applied to prevent ACL injuries in fatigued athletes.

Keywords: dynamic taping; landing biomechanics; fatigue; athletes

1. Introduction

An anterior cruciate ligament (ACL) injury presents a significant setback for competitive athletes. Studies indicate that even after surgery and extensive rehabilitation, only 55% of athletes return to competitive sports [1], with two-thirds playing at their pre-injury level post-ACL reconstruction surgery [2]. The ensuing functional limitations, financial burdens, and rehabilitation programs compound the stress for injured athletes. Non-contact ACL injuries often occur during movements involving cutting, deceleration, and landing, with the highest incidence rates seen in basketball, handball, and football [3–5]. Moreover, research has identified variations in ACL injuries across genders, ages, and ethnicities; for instance, a study in Asia found peak injury rates among high-school male and female athletes in the 11th grade [3].

ACL injuries are influenced by both extrinsic and intrinsic factors. Extrinsic factors, which are modifiable, encompass the type of sport, level of competition, playing environment, and equipment [6]. Intrinsic factors can be further categorized as non-modifiable (e.g., genetics, anatomical characteristics, female gender) or modifiable (e.g., biomechanical factors like muscle strengthening, jumping, and landing techniques) [7–13]. Various biomechanical risk factors have been identified, including increased knee and hip joint internal rotation, hip adduction, anterior tibial shear force, decreased knee flexion during landing, and increased knee valgus [14–19].

Fatigue has been found to alter lower-limb biomechanics, decreasing hip and knee flexion, increasing anterior tibial shear force, and altering the knee valgus and internal rotation angles, thereby increasing the load on the ACL [20–22]. To investigate fatigue's effect on lower-limb biomechanics, researchers have devised several protocols, such as the functional agility short-term fatigue protocol, which employs football-specific drills to induce fatigue. This protocol has shown alterations in landing biomechanics during stop jumping tests, including decreased hip and knee flexion, increased hip internal rotation at initial contact, and reduced knee flexion coupled with increased knee internal rotation at the peak of knee flexion [23–27].

Three-dimensional motion analysis is a comprehensive method for identifying landing risk factors; however, its extensive time requirements and higher costs limit its practicality. In contrast, the landing error scoring system (LESS) evaluates landing techniques using two-dimensional video images, making it clinically feasible and cost-effective. As a screening tool for ACL injury, the LESS demonstrates good sensitivity (86%) and specificity (64%) [18,28]. It identifies high-risk movement patterns and faulty landing biomechanics, such as increased hip internal rotation and adduction during initial contact, increased knee valgus, and reduced hip and knee flexion. An LESS score of 5 or more indicates a poor jump landing technique, correlating with a higher ACL injury risk ratio of 10.7 [28]. Previous studies have shown an increase in LESS scores for both sexes following functional exercise protocols, indicating a poorer landing technique [29]. Additionally, research by Van Melick et al. and Gokeler et al. revealed increased LESS scores after fatigue protocols, particularly in high-risk individuals such as those with an ACL reconstruction history [30,31].

Dynamic tape, developed by Ryan Kendrick, offers greater elasticity and resistance compared to rigid or Kinesio tape without restricting joint movement [32]. These characteristics allow for its use in daily activities or competitive games without restricting joint movement. Robinson et al.'s study shows its potential to reduce hip adduction moments and angles in patients with greater trochanteric pain syndrome [33]. However, clinical research on dynamic tape is extremely limited. Our previous research indicates that dynamic taping, especially with the spiral technique, reduces LESS scores in high-school volleyball athletes, particularly those at high risk [34]. Thus, dynamic taping holds promise for influencing lower-limb biomechanics. This study aims to investigate the effects of dynamic taping on landing biomechanics in fatigued athletes. We hypothesize that dynamic taping can mitigate adverse changes in lower-limb biomechanics following fatigue. Insights from this study may provide a novel approach to improving lower-limb biomechanics and reducing ACL injury rates.

2. Materials and Methods

2.1. Participants

Twenty-seven high-school football athletes were recruited for this study between January and November 2022. The sample size for this study was calculated using an a priori power analysis conducted with the G*Power software (Version 3.1.9.6; Heinrich-Heine-Universität Düsseldorf, Düsseldorf, Germany) based on our previous research that demonstrated an effect size of 0.75 with dynamic taping [34]. Given this effect size, an alpha level of 0.05, and a desired power of 0.8, we determined that a minimum of 16 participants were required. The inclusion criteria for this study were as follows: (1) high-school football athletes competing in Taiwan's Division One league; and (2) aged between 15 and 18 years. The exclusion criteria included the following: (1) participants who had received lower-limb surgery within the past year; (2) participants with acute medical conditions that would preclude participation in football training and competition; (3) participants who had sustained a traumatic brain injury within the past six months; (4) participants who had experienced vestibular impairments in the past six months; (5) participants with allergies to dynamic tape; and (6) pregnancy. The study's protocol was approved by the Chang Gung Memorial Hospital Institutional Review Board (approval no. 202002434B0) and registered with the Clinical Trial Registry (https://clinicaltrials.gov/—U.S. National Library of Medicine #NCT05288296). All participants and their legal guardians provided written informed assent and consent.

2.2. Dynamic Taping

The active and sham dynamic taping methods were used by the same experienced athletic trainer and applied directly to the skin (Figure 1). In the active taping method, a spiral double layer of 7.5 cm (Powerband) Dynamic tape® (Posture Pals Pty LTD, Hangzhou, China) was applied to the bilateral hips with the hips positioned in a 40° abduction, 20° extension, and full external rotation. This was aimed at resisting hip adduction, flexion, and internal rotation. Sham taping, on the other hand, was applied without inducing hip abduction and external rotation. The dynamic tape was applied bilaterally to evaluate LESS items such as stance width, lateral trunk flexion, and overall impression. The powerband was created by applying additional lengths of dynamic tape in parallel [32].

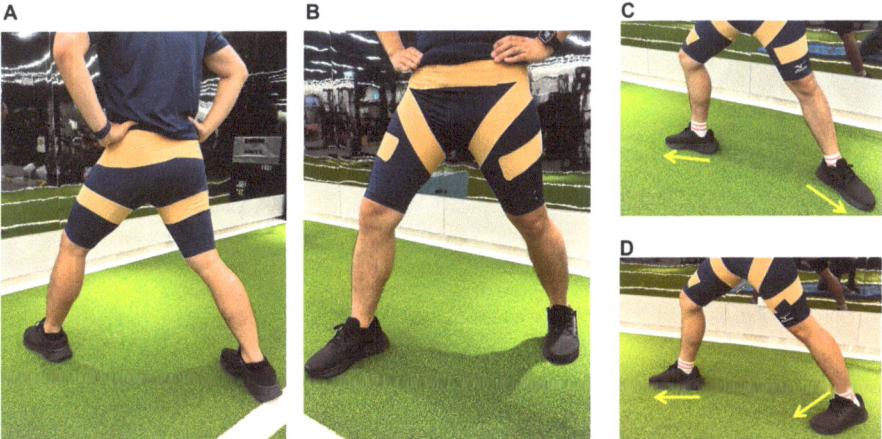

Figure 1. Demonstration of the dynamic tape applied to the bilateral hip. (**A**) Posterior view, (**B**) frontal view, (**C,D**) comparison of active and sham taping. The active and sham dynamic taping was applied directly to the skin over both hip joints. Starting from the anterior middle thigh, it wrapped around the thigh in an upper lateral direction to the posterior thigh, then continued to the proximal medial thigh, and subsequently wrapped below the anterior superior iliac crest in an upper lateral direction. After that, the tape crossed the lower back to the contralateral lower quarter of the abdomen. In active taping, the hip was positioned in 40° abduction, 20° extension, and full external rotation (**C**). In contrast, the hip was positioned without abduction and external rotation during sham taping (**D**).

2.3. Landing Error Scoring System

The LESS is a field screening field test designed to evaluate individual landing techniques through 17 items [28]. Before the task, all the participants were allowed as many practice trials as needed, but no feedback or coaching on their landing strategy was provided during the task. For the task, the participants jumped from a 30 cm high box to a designated landing area, a distance equivalent to 50% of their body height, and they immediately performed a vertical jump as high as possible. All the subjects completed three trials of the jump landing task before and after the fatigue protocol.

Two standard Handycams (DCR-CX900, Sony Group Corporation, Tokyo, Japan) captured the frontal and lateral views of the entire jump landing test. To rate the LESS scores, we reviewed the frontal and sagittal views frame by frame. These frames included the lower limb position, posture, and foot position at initial foot contact (Items 1–8), maximal knee flexion (Items 9 and 10), and the symmetry of landing (Item 11). Next, the trunk and lower-limb joint displacement from initial contact to maximal knee flexion were assessed (Items 12–15). Finally, the joint displacement and the overall impression of the entire landing task were evaluated (Items 16 and 17). Participants who scored an error in more than two of the three trials were marked with an error; otherwise, the individual item was coded as no error. The LESS scores were rated independently by an experienced rater, focusing primarily on the dominant leg. This rater, a physical medicine and rehabilitation physician, had over 10 years of experience in sports medicine and functional movement evaluation. The intra-rater reliability of this rater was high ($(ICC)_{2,1} = 0.916$). The rater was blinded to the randomized allocation of the active and sham taping.

2.4. Functional Agility Short-Term Fatigue Protocol

The functional agility short-term fatigue protocol (Figure 2) consists of the following series of agility drills selected for their relevance to common athletic skills in football [25]: (1) Step-ups: The participants performed step-ups on a 30 cm box for 20 s at a pace set by a metronome at 200 beats per minute. (2) L-drill: Three cones were arranged to form an 'L' shape with each cone 4.11 m apart. The participants sprinted to one cone, returned to the starting cone, and repeated the sprint before running around the second cone, cutting left to the third cone. They then circled the third cone, ran around the second cone, and sprinted back to the start. (3) Countermovement jump (CMJ): The participants performed five consecutive CMJs, aiming to reach 80% of their maximum jump height with each leap. (4) Agility ladder drill: Using a 6 m ladder, the participants performed the drill to the rhythm of a metronome set at 200 beats per minute. For the first and third run, they began at one end, facing the ladder, and quickly stepped into and out of the rungs with alternating feet, repeating this pattern until they reached the other end and then reversing direction. For the second and fourth run, the participants started perpendicular to the ladder and stepped laterally into and out of the rungs, again with alternating feet, until they reached the end and then returned. According to previous research, the participants had to complete all four sets of the protocol consecutively to reach fatigue status, with the entire sequence lasting approximately 6 min [25,27,35,36].

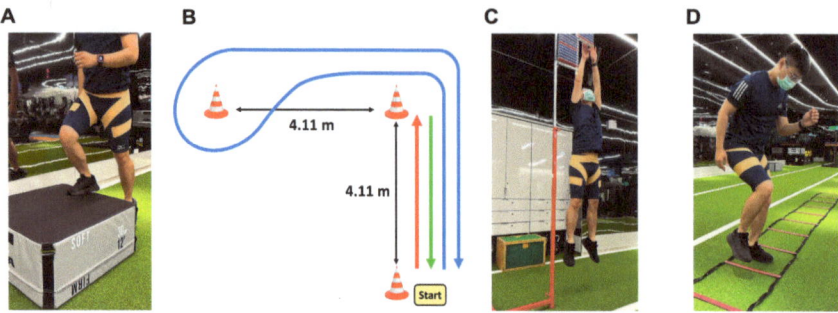

Figure 2. Functional agility short-term fatigue protocol. The participants performed four exercises consecutively without rest: (**A**) step-ups, (**B**) L-drill, (**C**) countermovement jump, and (**D**) agility ladder drill. They had to complete a total of four sets.

2.5. Research Design

This was a single-blind, randomized controlled crossover trial adhering to the CONSORT 2010 guidelines (Figure 3). After a comprehensive physical assessment, two participants were excluded due to ankle and knee injuries. Twenty-five participants were included in the study and randomly allocated via simple randomization by drawing lots to two sequences: (A) active taping followed by sham taping; and (B) sham taping followed by active taping. Opaque sealed envelopes were utilized to ensure allocation concealment. After taping, the participants underwent a fatigue protocol and were evaluated using the LESS before and after the protocol. Each taping session was separated by a two-week period to prevent interference from discomfort following the fatigue protocol and the effects of dynamic taping. Ultimately, all 25 participants completed the study without any loss to follow-up or discontinuation of the intervention (Table 1). The LESS scores were independently rated by an experienced rater. The sum and individual items of the LESS, along with subgroup analyses for high- and low-risk participants, were further analyzed.

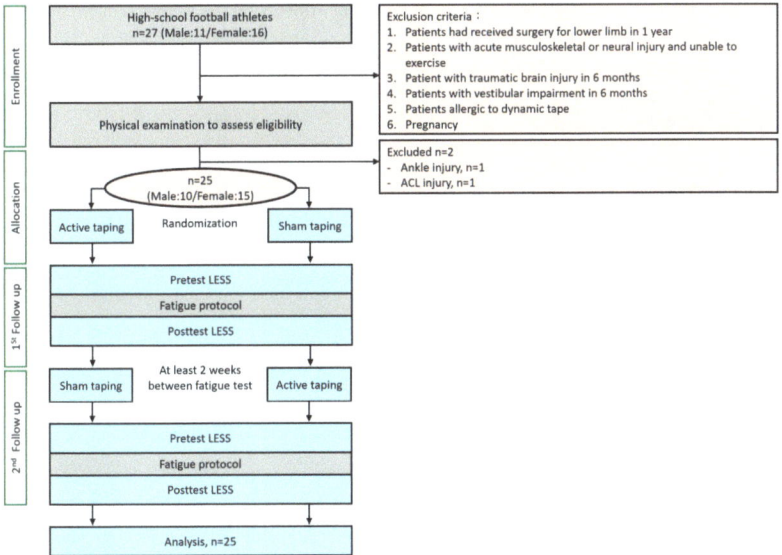

Figure 3. Experiment flowchart.

Table 1. Demographic data of participants.

	Male (n = 10)	Female (n = 15)	p-Value
Age (Year)	16.40 ± 0.51	16.40 ± 0.52	1
Body Height (cm)	173.70 ± 3.16	161.43 ± 4.40	<0.001 *
Body Weight (Kg)	59.30 ± 5.33	55.92 ± 4.66	0.11
BMI (Kg/cm^2)	19.67 ± 1.93	21.52 ± 2.30	0.048 *
Dominant Leg (Right/Left)	9/1	15/0	

BMI = body mass index. * Significant difference ($p < 0.05$) between male and female athletes. All data are reported as mean ± SD.

2.6. Statistical Analyses

A Shapiro–Wilk test was conducted to assess the normality of the measurements in the LESS. The results confirmed that the LESS scores for both the active and sham taping groups were normally distributed. We employed the paired *t*-test to compare the effects of the fatigue protocol on the LESS total score and each specific scoring item both before and after the sham and active dynamic taping. We also used independent *t*-tests to compare the pre–post difference between the sham and active groups. All statistical awere performed using IBM SPSS (Version 24.0; IBM Corporation, Armonk, NY, USA). Cohen's d effect sizes were calculated using G*Power to aid in interpreting the results. The magnitudes of the effect sizes were categorized using Cohen's thresholds: 0.0 to 0.19 as trivial; 0.20 to 0.49 as small; 0.50 to 0.79 as moderate; and above 0.80 as large [37]. The level of significance for all statistical tests was set at 0.05.

3. Results

After the fatigue protocol, the LESS scores of the athletes who received the sham taping increased from 4.24 ± 1.83 to 5.36 ± 2.00 (t = -2.07, $p = 0.04$, effect size = 0.61). In contrast, the active taping group did not show a significant statistical change following the fatigue protocol. Furthermore, the difference in the LESS scores between the sham and active taping groups following the fatigue protocol was statistically significant (sham taping: 1.12 ± 1.20; active taping: 0.28 ± 0.94, p = 0.007) (Table 2, Figure 4).

Table 2. The LESS scores of athletes between sham and active dynamic taping following a fatigue protocol.

LESS	Sham Taping (n = 25)	p-Value	t-Value	Effect Size	Active Taping (n = 25)	p-Value	t-Value	Effect Size	Δ (Post–Pre) between Groups p-Value
Pretest	4.24 ± 1.83	0.04 *	-2.07	0.61	4.24 ± 1.69	0.15	-1.50	0.46	
Posttest	5.36 ± 2.00				4.52 ± 1.69				
Δ (Post–pre)	1.12 ± 1.20				0.28 ± 0.94				0.007 †

Δ: Difference between pre and posttest. * Significant difference ($p < 0.05$) between pretest and posttest. † Significant difference ($p < 0.01$) of Δ between sham and active taping group. All data are reported as mean ± SD.

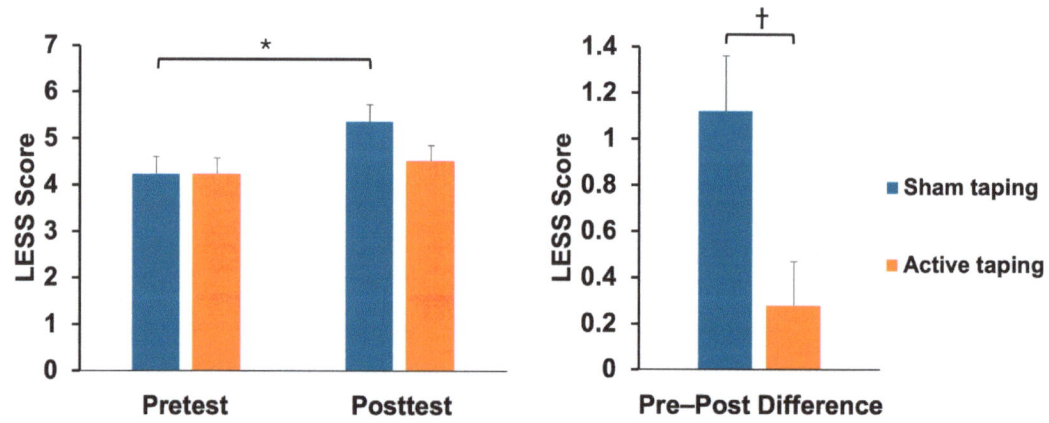

Figure 4. Comparison of LESS scores between sham and active dynamic taping following a fatigue protocol (mean ± SE). * = $p < 0.05$, † = $p < 0.01$.

For the specific LESS items, the frequency of a faulty landing strategy in the sham taping group increased for trunk flexion displacement and joint displacement (Items 14 and 16) after the fatigue protocol. In contrast, the active taping group did not exhibit any statistically significant changes (Table 3). Additionally, the difference in the medial knee position at initial contact (Item 5) between the sham and active taping groups following the fatigue protocol reached statistical significance (sham taping: $+0.16 \pm 0.47$; active taping: -0.12 ± 0.44, p = 0.04).

Table 3. The difference in individual items between sham and active dynamic taping following fatigue protocol.

LESS	Sham Taping				Active Taping				Δ (Post–Pre) between Groups p-Value
	Pretest (n = 25)	Posttest (n = 25)	Δ (Post–Pre)	p-Value	Pretest (n = 25)	Posttest (n = 25)	Δ (Post–Pre)	p-Value	
#1	0.64 ± 0.49	0.56 ± 0.51	−0.08 ± 0.49	0.43	0.40 ± 0.50	0.40 ± 0.50	0.00 ± 0.29	1.00	0.48
#2	0.00 ± 0.00	0.00 ± 0.00	0.00 ± 0.00	N/A	0.00 ± 0.00	0.00 ± 0.00	0.00 ± 0.00	N/A	N/A
#3	0.00 ± 0.00	0.04 ± 0.20	0.04 ± 0.20	0.33	0.00 ± 0.00	0.00 ± 0.00	0.00 ± 0.00	N/A	0.32
#4	0.64 ± 0.49	0.68 ± 0.48	0.04 ± 0.35	0.57	0.64 ± 0.49	0.52 ± 0.51	−0.12 ± 0.44	0.18	0.16
#5	0.24 ± 0.44	0.40 ± 0.50	0.16 ± 0.47	0.10	0.24 ± 0.44	0.12 ± 0.33	−0.12 ± 0.44	0.18	0.04 †
#6	0.04 ± 0.20	0.00 ± 0.00	−0.04 ± 0.20	0.33	0.00 ± 0.00	0.00 ± 0.00	0.00 ± 0.00	N/A	0.32
#7	0.00 ± 0.00	0.04 ± 0.20	0.04 ± 0.20	0.33	0.04 ± 0.20	0.04 ± 0.20	0.00 ± 0.00	1.00	0.32
#8	0.48 ± 0.51	0.52 ± 0.51	0.04 ± 0.45	0.66	0.60 ± 0.50	0.52 ± 0.51	−0.08 ± 0.49	0.42	0.38
#9	0.00 ± 0.00	0.00 ± 0.00	0.00 ± 0.00	N/A	0.00 ± 0.00	0.00 ± 0.00	0.00 ± 0.00	N/A	N/A
#10	0.08 ± 0.28	0.12 ± 0.33	0.04 ± 0.35	0.57	0.12 ± 0.33	0.08 ± 0.28	−0.04 ± 0.20	0.32	0.33
#11	0.16 ± 0.37	0.28 ± 0.46	0.12 ± 0.60	0.33	0.32 ± 0.48	0.40 ± 0.50	0.08 ± 0.57	0.49	0.81
#12	0.00 ± 0.00	0.00 ± 0.00	0.00 ± 0.00	N/A	0.00 ± 0.00	0.00 ± 0.00	0.00 ± 0.00	N/A	N/A
#13	0.00 ± 0.00	0.00 ± 0.00	0.00 ± 0.00	N/A	0.00 ± 0.00	0.00 ± 0.00	0.00 ± 0.00	N/A	N/A
#14	0.28 ± 0.46	0.52 ± 0.51	0.24 ± 0.44	0.01 *	0.28 ± 0.46	0.40 ± 0.50	0.12 ± 0.33	0.08	0.28
#15	0.64 ± 0.49	0.80 ± 0.41	0.16 ± 0.47	0.10	0.56 ± 0.51	0.68 ± 0.48	0.12 ± 0.33	0.08	0.73
#16	0.32 ± 0.48	0.60 ± 0.50	0.28 ± 0.54	0.02 *	0.32 ± 0.48	0.52 ± 0.51	0.20 ± 0.50	0.06	0.59
#17	0.72 ± 0.46	0.80 ± 0.41	0.08 ± 0.40	0.33	0.72 ± 0.46	0.84 ± 0.37	0.12 ± 0.53	0.27	0.76

N/A = not applicable. Δ: Difference between pretest and posttest. * Significant difference ($p < 0.05$) between pretest and posttest. † Significant difference ($p < 0.05$) between sham and active taping group. Item 1: knee flexion: initial contact, Item 2: hip flexion: initial contact, Item 3: trunk flexion: initial contact, Item 4: ankle plantar flexion: initial contact, Item 5: medial knee position: initial contact, Item 6: lateral trunk flexion: initial contact, Item 7: stance width: wide, Item 8: stance width: narrow, Item 9: foot position: external rotation, Item 10: foot position: internal rotation, Item 11: symmetric initial foot contact: initial contact, Item 12: knee flexion displacement, Item 13: hip flexion displacement, Item 14: trunk flexion displacement, Item 15: medial knee displacement, Item 16: joint displacement, Item 17: overall impression. All data are reported as mean ± SD.

In the high-risk group (LESS ≥ 6), the LESS scores for the athletes who received sham taping increased from 6.50 ± 0.84 to 7.67 ± 1.03 ($t = -2.91$, $p = 0.03$, effect size = 1.63). In the low-risk group (LESS ≤ 5), the LESS scores for the athletes who received sham taping also rose from 3.53 ± 1.43 to 4.63 ± 1.67 ($t = -4.59$, $p < 0.001$, effect size = 1.15). Conversely, the active taping group did not demonstrate a significant statistical change following the fatigue protocol. Furthermore, in the low-risk group, the pre–post difference between the sham and active taping groups following the fatigue protocol was statistically significant, with the sham taping group showing an increase of 1.11 ± 1.50 compared to 0.35 ± 1.27 in the active taping group ($p = 0.03$) (Table 4, Figure 5).

Table 4. Subgroup analysis of the high- and low-risk groups after sham and active taping.

LESS	Sham Taping (n = 25)	p-Value	t-Value	Effect Size	Active Taping (n = 25)	p-Value	t-Value	Effect Size	Δ (Post–Pre) between Groups p-Value
LESS ≥ 6									
Pretest	6.50 ± 0.84	0.03 *	−2.91	1.63	6.60 ± 0.86	1.00	0	N/A	
Posttest	7.67 ± 1.03				6.60 ± 1.14				
Δ (Post–pre)	1.17 ± 0.98				0.00 ± 1.00				0.08
LESS ≤ 5									
Pretest	3.53 ± 1.43	<0.001 ***	−4.59	1.15	3.65 ± 1.27	0.17	−1.73	0.51	
Posttest	4.63 ± 1.64				4.00 ± 1.38				
Δ (Post–pre)	1.11 ± 1.50				0.35 ± 1.27				0.03 †

Δ: Difference between pretest and posttest. * Significant difference (* = $p < 0.05$, *** = $p < 0.001$) between pretest and posttest. † Significant difference ($p < 0.05$) between pre–post difference of sham and active taping. All data are reported as mean ± SD.

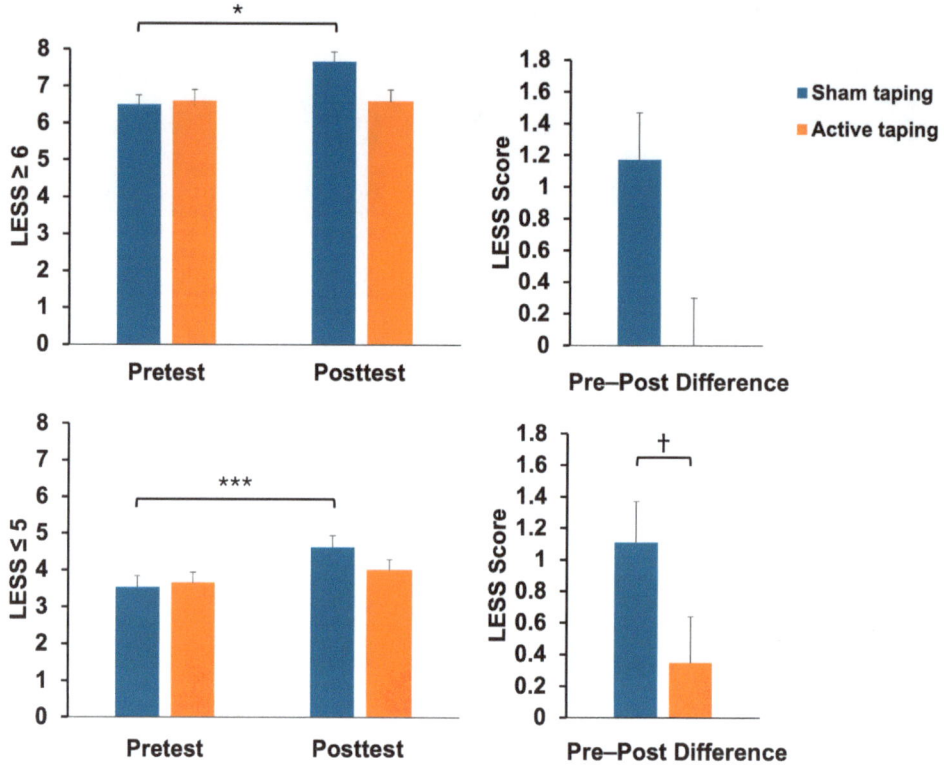

Figure 5. Comparison of LESS scores in high- and low-risk groups between sham and active dynamic taping following a fatigue protocol (mean ± SE). * = $p < 0.05$, *** = $p < 0.001$, † = $p < 0.05$.

4. Discussion

The results indicated a significant increase in the LESS score following the fatigue protocol. Additionally, dynamic taping using the spiral technique appeared to mitigate faulty landing biomechanics in the fatigued athletes, such as decreased hip and knee flexion and increased hip internal rotation during landing (Table 3). The impact of the dynamic taping was demonstrated across the high- and low-risk groups (Table 4). To our knowledge, this is the first study to explore the effects of dynamic taping on landing biomechanics before and after a fatigue protocol. Therefore, dynamic taping may potentially offer protective benefits in landing mechanics to prevent ACL injuries.

In a previous study [25], decreased hip and knee flexion were noted at initial contact during landing via motion analysis, resulting in a stiffer and more extended posture. This faulty posture is a risk factor for ACL injury due to increased anterior tibial translation and shear force, which strain the ACL [35]. In our study, the fatigued athletes who received sham taping also exhibited a stiffer posture upon landing, as evidenced by the increased trunk flexion displacement (Item 14) and joint displacement (Item 16). In contrast, these changes in landing biomechanics were not observed in the fatigued athletes who received active taping.

Fidai et al. demonstrated that the knee valgus increased during the drop jump test in youth athletes after a short-term fatigue protocol [38]. This increase in the knee valgus was noted at initial contact and at maximal knee flexion in the fatigued athletes [25,35]. In the current study, the difference in the medial knee position at initial contact (Item 5) between the active and sham taping groups reached statistical significance, but not in the medial knee displacement (Item 15), which shows the knee posture at maximal knee flexion. However, observational studies have shown that ACL injuries occur approximately 40 milliseconds after initial contact [39]. Therefore, dynamic taping could reduce the knee valgus at initial contact, potentially offering a protective effect.

Previous research has indicated that the minimal clinically important difference (MCID) for the LESS is approximately 1.16 [40]. In our study, the pre–post difference in the LESS scores in the sham taping group following the fatigue protocol was 1.12, which is very close to the MCID. In contrast, the difference in the LESS scores in the active taping group did not reach a significant change. Gokeler et al. reported that the LESS scores in both a healthy control group and high-risk patients, such as those who had undergone ACL reconstruction, increased after a fatigue protocol (from 2.5 to 6.0 in the control group; from 6.5 to 7.0 in the ACL reconstruction group) [30]. Our research presents similar results, with the LESS scores increasing significantly and closely approaching the MCID in both the high- and low-risk groups. However, compared to the low-risk group, the difference in LESS scores following the fatigue protocol in the high-risk group did not reach statistical significance. The possible explanations include the following: (1) a higher initial LESS score allows for less room for an increase, possibly creating a ceiling effect; (2) the small sample size in the high-risk group (only five participants) makes it difficult to achieve statistical significance.

A recent study showed that approximately two-thirds of ACL injuries occur in the first half of gameplay [41,42], suggesting that acute fatigue, typically resulting from high-intensity anaerobic exercise, may play a significant role [43]. In our current study, the functional agility short-term fatigue protocol, consisting of a series of agility drills in football, closely mimicked real game situations. Exercise training programs, such as the FIFA 11+ program for soccer athletes, have been proposed to prevent ACL injuries [44]. However, a meta-analysis revealed that while such programs decrease lower-limb injuries, they do not significantly reduce ACL injury rates. Additionally, compliance with ACL injury prevention programs among coaches and athletes has been found to be poor [45].

Biomechanical and neuromuscular factors are modifiable risk factors for ACL injuries and could be addressed through interventions such as Kinesio taping. However, studies have shown conflicting results. For instance, it was demonstrated that Kinesio taping did not reduce the knee valgus or lateral trunk lean during double-leg landings and jumps [46]. Conversely, another study found that Kinesio taping decreased the knee valgus at the initial contact of a double-leg landing in healthy male participants [47]. In our study, dynamic taping not only reduced the knee valgus at initial contact but also increased the trunk and joint displacement, particularly noted in Items 14 and 16 of our results, demonstrating its utility in correcting faulty landing biomechanics and potentially providing a supportive approach for athletes. Compared to Kinesio tape, dynamic taping is a relatively new technique with superior properties, including higher elasticity (dynamic tape: 200%; Kinesio tape: about 140%), multidirectional extensibility, absence of rigid endpoints, and stronger resistance and recoil [32]. Its application can produce a 'boomerang effect,' where potential elastic energy accumulated during concentric contraction is utilized as kinetic energy during the eccentric phase [48], making it a favorable option for correcting faulty landing biomechanics.

The strengths of this randomized controlled trial include the design, in which the participants served as their own controls. A sham group was established to minimize the placebo effect, and the rater was blinded to the allocation of the participants. However, this study has several limitations. First, although a sham group was incorporated, the absence of a non-taping group means that the study could not assess the impacts of psychological factors and proprioception separately. Second, the reliability and validity of the findings may be limited by the use of only one rater; involving multiple raters could have enhanced these aspects. Third, the small sample size may have hindered the achievement of statistical significance. Fourth, the duration of the effects of dynamic taping remains unknown. We only observed the immediate effects after the fatigue protocol without considering the duration of these effects and environmental factors.

5. Conclusions

The application of dynamic tape to the hip joint improves landing biomechanics by particularly reducing the knee valgus in initial contact and decreasing hip and knee extension during landing. This beneficial effect was observed in both the high- and low-risk athletes. Therefore, in clinical practice, dynamic tape could serve as a passive and supportive tool, providing protective benefits in landing mechanics to help prevent ACL injuries.

Author Contributions: Conceptualization, C.-K.W., Y.-L.C. and T.-H.H.; methodology, Y.-P.C. and T.-H.H.; validation, C.-K.W. and T.-H.H.; formal analysis, C.-K.W.; investigation, C.-K.W.; resources, Y.-L.C. and T.-H.H.; data curation, C.-K.W. and T.-H.H.; writing—original draft preparation, C.-K.W. and T.-H.H.; writing—review and editing, C.-K.W. and T.-H.H.; supervision, Y.-C.L. and Y.-L.C.; project administration, C.-K.W. and Y.-L.C.; funding acquisition, C.-K.W., Y.-C.L. and T.-H.H. All authors contributed to the article and approved the submitted version. All authors have read and agreed to the published version of the manuscript.

Funding: The authors also express their gratitude for being granted from the National Science and Technology Council, Taiwan (MOST110-2410-H182A-004, NSTC 112-2314-B-182-022), Chang Gung University (UMRPD1P0161).

Institutional Review Board Statement: This study was conducted in accordance with the Declaration of Helsinki and approved by the Institutional Review Board of Chang Gung Medical Foundation (No.: 202002434B0). The approved protocol period is valid from 1 August 2021 to 31 July 2024.

Informed Consent Statement: All participants and their legal guardians provided written informed assent and consent.

Data Availability Statement: The data supporting the conclusion of this study are available from the corresponding author on reasonable request.

Conflicts of Interest: The authors declare no conflicts of interest.

References

1. Ardern, C.L.; Taylor, N.F.; Feller, J.A.; Webster, K.E. Fifty-five per cent return to competitive sport following anterior cruciate ligament reconstruction surgery: An updated systematic review and meta-analysis including aspects of physical functioning and contextual factors. *Br. J. Sports Med.* **2014**, *48*, 1543–1552. [CrossRef] [PubMed]
2. Ardern, C.L.; Taylor, N.F.; Feller, J.A.; Webster, K.E. Return-to-sport outcomes at 2 to 7 years after anterior cruciate ligament reconstruction surgery. *Am. J. Sports Med.* **2012**, *40*, 41–48. [CrossRef] [PubMed]
3. Takahashi, S.; Okuwaki, T. Epidemiological survey of anterior cruciate ligament injury in Japanese junior high school and high school athletes: Cross-sectional study. *Res. Sports Med.* **2017**, *25*, 266–276. [CrossRef] [PubMed]
4. Barber Foss, K.D.; Myer, G.D.; Hewett, T.E. Epidemiology of basketball, soccer, and volleyball injuries in middle-school female athletes. *Phys. Sportsmed.* **2014**, *42*, 146–153. [CrossRef] [PubMed]
5. Swenson, D.M.; Collins, C.L.; Best, T.M.; Flanigan, D.C.; Fields, S.K.; Comstock, R.D. Epidemiology of knee injuries among U.S. high school athletes, 2005/2006–2010/2011. *Med. Sci. Sports Exerc.* **2013**, *45*, 462–469. [CrossRef]
6. Acevedo, R.J.; Rivera-Vega, A.; Miranda, G.; Micheo, W. Anterior Cruciate Ligament Injury: Identification of Risk Factors and Prevention Strategies. *Curr. Sports Med. Rep.* **2014**, *13*, 186–191. [CrossRef]
7. Bell, R.D.; Shultz, S.J.; Wideman, L.; Henrich, V.C. Collagen gene variants previously associated with anterior cruciate ligament injury risk are also associated with joint laxity. *Sports Health* **2012**, *4*, 312–318. [CrossRef]
8. Magnusson, K.; Turkiewicz, A.; Hughes, V.; Frobell, R.; Englund, M. High genetic contribution to anterior cruciate ligament rupture: Heritability ~69. *Br. J. Sports Med.* **2020**, *55*, 385–389. [CrossRef] [PubMed]
9. Posthumus, M.; Collins, M.; van der Merwe, L.; O'Cuinneagain, D.; van der Merwe, W.; Ribbans, W.J.; Schwellnus, M.P.; Raleigh, S.M. Matrix metalloproteinase genes on chromosome 11q22 and the risk of anterior cruciate ligament (ACL) rupture. *Scand. J. Med. Sci. Sports* **2012**, *22*, 523–533. [CrossRef]
10. Shen, L.; Jin, Z.G.; Dong, Q.R.; Li, L.B. Anatomical Risk Factors of Anterior Cruciate Ligament Injury. *Chin. Med. J.* **2018**, *131*, 2960–2967. [CrossRef]
11. Li, F.; Qin, L.; Gong, X.; Huang, Z.; Wang, T.; Liu, Z.; Sandiford, S.; Yang, J.; Zhu, S.; Liang, X.; et al. The Chinese ACL injury population has a higher proportion of small ACL tibial insertion sizes than Western patients. *Knee Surg. Sports Traumatol. Arthrosc.* **2020**, *28*, 888–896. [CrossRef] [PubMed]
12. Kızılgöz, V.; Sivrioğlu, A.K.; Aydın, H.; Ulusoy, G.R.; Çetin, T.; Tuncer, K. The Combined Effect of Body Mass Index and Tibial Slope Angles on Anterior Cruciate Ligament Injury Risk in Male Knees: A Case-Control Study. *Clin. Med. Insights Arthritis Musculoskelet. Disord.* **2019**, *12*, 1–8. [CrossRef] [PubMed]

13. Konopka, J.A.; Hsue, L.; Chang, W.; Thio, T.; Dragoo, J.L. The Effect of Oral Contraceptive Hormones on Anterior Cruciate Ligament Strength. *Am. J. Sports Med.* **2020**, *48*, 85–92. [CrossRef] [PubMed]
14. Hewett, T.E.; Myer, G.D.; Ford, K.R.; Heidt, R.S., Jr.; Colosimo, A.J.; McLean, S.G.; van den Bogert, A.J.; Paterno, M.V.; Succop, P. Biomechanical measures of neuromuscular control and valgus loading of the knee predict anterior cruciate ligament injury risk in female athletes: A prospective study. *Am. J. Sports Med.* **2005**, *33*, 492–501. [CrossRef] [PubMed]
15. Malloy, P.J.; Morgan, A.M.; Meinerz, C.M.; Geiser, C.F.; Kipp, K. Hip External Rotator Strength Is Associated With Better Dynamic Control of the Lower Extremity During Landing Tasks. *J. Strength. Cond. Res.* **2016**, *30*, 282–291. [CrossRef] [PubMed]
16. Earl, J.E.; Monteiro, S.K.; Snyder, K.R. Differences in lower extremity kinematics between a bilateral drop-vertical jump and a single-leg step-down. *J. Orthop. Sports Phys. Ther.* **2007**, *37*, 245–252. [CrossRef] [PubMed]
17. Lawrence, R.K., 3rd; Kernozek, T.W.; Miller, E.J.; Torry, M.R.; Reuteman, P. Influences of hip external rotation strength on knee mechanics during single-leg drop landings in females. *Clin. Biomech.* **2008**, *23*, 806–813. [CrossRef] [PubMed]
18. Padua, D.A.; Marshall, S.W.; Boling, M.C.; Thigpen, C.A.; Garrett, W.E., Jr.; Beutler, A.I. The Landing Error Scoring System (LESS) Is a valid and reliable clinical assessment tool of jump-landing biomechanics: The JUMP-ACL study. *Am. J. Sports Med.* **2009**, *37*, 1996–2002. [CrossRef]
19. Shultz, S.J.; Beynnon, B.D.; Schmitz, R.J. Sex differences in coupled knee motions during the transition from non-weight bearing to weight bearing. *J. Orthop. Res.* **2009**, *27*, 717–723. [CrossRef]
20. Chappell, J.D.; Herman, D.C.; Knight, B.S.; Kirkendall, D.T.; Garrett, W.E.; Yu, B. Effect of fatigue on knee kinetics and kinematics in stop-jump tasks. *Am. J. Sports Med.* **2005**, *33*, 1022–1029. [CrossRef]
21. Hughes, G.; Watkins, J. A risk-factor model for anterior cruciate ligament injury. *Sports Med.* **2006**, *36*, 411–428. [CrossRef] [PubMed]
22. Sanna, G.; O'Connor, K.M. Fatigue-related changes in stance leg mechanics during sidestep cutting maneuvers. *Clin. Biomech.* **2008**, *23*, 946–954. [CrossRef] [PubMed]
23. McLean, S.G.; Samorezov, J.E. Fatigue-induced ACL injury risk stems from a degradation in central control. *Med. Sci. Sports Exerc.* **2009**, *41*, 1661–1672. [CrossRef]
24. McLean, S.G.; Fellin, R.E.; Suedekum, N.; Calabrese, G.; Passerallo, A.; Joy, S. Impact of fatigue on gender-based high-risk landing strategies. *Med. Sci. Sports Exerc.* **2007**, *39*, 502–514. [CrossRef] [PubMed]
25. Cortes, N.; Quammen, D.; Lucci, S.; Greska, E.; Onate, J. A functional agility short-term fatigue protocol changes lower extremity mechanics. *J. Sports Sci.* **2012**, *30*, 797–805. [CrossRef] [PubMed]
26. Lucci, S.; Cortes, N.; Van Lunen, B.; Ringleb, S.; Onate, J. Knee and hip sagittal and transverse plane changes after two fatigue protocols. *J. Sci. Med. Sport.* **2011**, *14*, 453–459. [CrossRef] [PubMed]
27. Quammen, D.; Cortes, N.; Van Lunen, B.L.; Lucci, S.; Ringleb, S.I.; Onate, J. Two different fatigue protocols and lower extremity motion patterns during a stop-jump task. *J. Athl. Train.* **2012**, *47*, 32–41. [CrossRef] [PubMed]
28. Padua, D.A.; DiStefano, L.J.; Beutler, A.I.; de la Motte, S.J.; DiStefano, M.J.; Marshall, S.W. The Landing Error Scoring System as a Screening Tool for an Anterior Cruciate Ligament Injury-Prevention Program in Elite-Youth Soccer Athletes. *J. Athl. Train.* **2015**, *50*, 589–595. [CrossRef]
29. Wesley, C.A.; Aronson, P.A.; Docherty, C.L. Lower Extremity Landing Biomechanics in Both Sexes After a Functional Exercise Protocol. *J. Athl. Train.* **2015**, *50*, 914–920. [CrossRef]
30. Gokeler, A.; Eppinga, P.; Dijkstra, P.U.; Welling, W.; Padua, D.A.; Otten, E.; Benjaminse, A. Effect of fatigue on landing performance assessed with the landing error scoring system (less) in patients after ACL reconstruction. A pilot study. *Int. J. Sports Phys. Ther.* **2014**, *9*, 302–311.
31. Van Melick, N.; van Rijn, L.; Nijhuis-van der Sanden, M.W.G.; Hoogeboom, T.J.; van Cingel, R.E.H. Fatigue affects quality of movement more in ACL-reconstructed soccer players than in healthy soccer players. *Knee Surg. Sports Traumatol. Arthrosc.* **2019**, *27*, 549–555. [CrossRef] [PubMed]
32. McNeill, W.; Pedersen, C. Dynamic tape. Is it all about controlling load? *J. Bodyw. Mov. Ther.* **2016**, *20*, 179–188. [CrossRef] [PubMed]
33. Robinson, N.A.; Spratford, W.; Welvaert, M.; Gaida, J.; Fearon, A.M. Does Dynamic Tape change the walking biomechanics of women with greater trochanteric pain syndrome? A blinded randomised controlled crossover trial. *Gait Posture* **2019**, *70*, 275–283. [CrossRef] [PubMed]
34. Wu, C.K.; Lin, Y.C.; Lai, C.P.; Wang, H.P.; Hsieh, T.H. Dynamic Taping Improves Landing Biomechanics in Young Volleyball Athletes. *Int. J. Environ. Res. Public Health* **2022**, *19*, 13716. [CrossRef] [PubMed]
35. Cortes, N.; Greska, E.; Kollock, R.; Ambegaonkar, J.; Onate, J.A. Changes in lower extremity biomechanics due to a short-term fatigue protocol. *J. Athl. Train.* **2013**, *48*, 306–313. [CrossRef]
36. Wilke, J.; Fleckenstein, J.; Krause, F.; Vogt, L.; Banzer, W. Sport-specific functional movement can simulate aspects of neuromuscular fatigue occurring in team sports. *Sports Biomech.* **2016**, *15*, 151–161. [CrossRef] [PubMed]
37. Cohen, J. *Statistical Power Analysis for the Behavioral Sciences*; Routledge: New York, NY, USA, 2013.
38. Fidai, M.S.; Okoroha, K.R.; Meldau, J.; Meta, F.; Lizzio, V.A.; Borowsky, P.; Redler, L.H.; Moutzouros, V.; Makhni, E.C. Fatigue Increases Dynamic Knee Valgus in Youth Athletes: Results From a Field-Based Drop-Jump Test. *Arthroscopy* **2020**, *36*, 214–222. [CrossRef] [PubMed]

39. Koga, H.; Nakamae, A.; Shima, Y.; Bahr, R.; Krosshaug, T. Hip and Ankle Kinematics in Noncontact Anterior Cruciate Ligament Injury Situations: Video Analysis Using Model-Based Image Matching. *Am. J. Sports Med.* **2018**, *46*, 333–340. [CrossRef] [PubMed]
40. Pointer, C.E.; Reems, T.D.; Hartley, E.M.; Hoch, J.M. The Ability of the Landing Error Scoring System to Detect Changes in Landing Mechanics: A Critically Appraised Topic. *Int. J. Athl. Ther. Train.* **2017**, *22*, 12–20. [CrossRef]
41. Della Villa, F.; Buckthorpe, M.; Grassi, A.; Nabiuzzi, A.; Tosarelli, F.; Zaffagnini, S.; Della Villa, S. Systematic video analysis of ACL injuries in professional male football (soccer): Injury mechanisms, situational patterns and biomechanics study on 134 consecutive cases. *Br. J. Sports Med.* **2020**, *54*, 1423–1432. [CrossRef]
42. Lucarno, S.; Zago, M.; Buckthorpe, M.; Grassi, A.; Tosarelli, F.; Smith, R.; Della Villa, F. Systematic Video Analysis of Anterior Cruciate Ligament Injuries in Professional Female Soccer Players. *Am. J. Sports Med.* **2021**, *49*, 1794–1802. [CrossRef] [PubMed]
43. Mohr, M.; Krustrup, P.; Bangsbo, J. Match performance of high-standard soccer players with special reference to development of fatigue. *J. Sports Sci.* **2003**, *21*, 519–528. [CrossRef] [PubMed]
44. Daneshjoo, A.; Mokhtar, A.H.; Rahnama, N.; Yusof, A. The effects of comprehensive warm-up programs on proprioception, static and dynamic balance on male soccer players. *PLoS ONE* **2012**, *7*, e51568. [CrossRef]
45. Joy, E.A.; Taylor, J.R.; Novak, M.A.; Chen, M.; Fink, B.P.; Porucznik, C.A. Factors influencing the implementation of anterior cruciate ligament injury prevention strategies by girls soccer coaches. *J. Strength. Cond. Res.* **2013**, *27*, 2263–2269. [CrossRef] [PubMed]
46. Sheikhi, B.; Letafatkar, A.; Hogg, J.; Naseri-Mobaraki, E. The influence of kinesio taping on trunk and lower extremity motions during different landing tasks: Implications for anterior cruciate ligament injury. *J. Exp. Orthop.* **2021**, *8*, 25. [CrossRef] [PubMed]
47. Limroongreungrat, W.; Boonkerd, C. Immediate effect of ACL kinesio taping technique on knee joint biomechanics during a drop vertical jump: A randomized crossover controlled trial. *BMC Sports Sci. Med. Rehabil.* **2019**, *11*, 32. [CrossRef]
48. Castro-Méndez, A.; Palomo-Toucedo, I.C.; Pabón-Carrasco, M.; Ortiz-Romero, M.; Fernández-Seguín, L.M. The Short-Term Effect of Dynamic Tape versus the Low-Dye Taping Technique in Plantar Fasciitis: A Randomized Clinical Trial. *Int. J. Environ. Res. Public Health* **2022**, *19*, 16536. [CrossRef]

Disclaimer/Publisher's Note: The statements, opinions and data contained in all publications are solely those of the individual author(s) and contributor(s) and not of MDPI and/or the editor(s). MDPI and/or the editor(s) disclaim responsibility for any injury to people or property resulting from any ideas, methods, instructions or products referred to in the content.

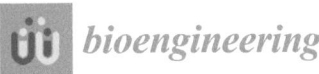

Article

Bilateral Asymmetries of Plantar Pressure and Foot Balance During Walking, Running, and Turning Gait in Typically Developing Children

Wei Liu [1,2], Liu Xu [1], Haidan Wu [1], Yile Wang [1], Hanhui Jiang [1], Zixiang Gao [1], Endre Jánosi [3], Gusztav Fekete [4,*], Qichang Mei [1,5] and Yaodong Gu [1,*]

1. Faculty of Sports Science, Ningbo University, Ningbo 315211, China; gaozixiang0111@outlook.com (Z.G.)
2. Faculty of Engineering, University of Pannonia, 8201 Veszprem, Hungary
3. Savaria Institute of Technology, Faculty of Informatics, Eötvös Loránd University, 9700 Szombathely, Hungary; je@inf.elte.hu
4. Department of Material Science and Technology, AUDI Hungária Faculty of Vehicle Engineering, Széchenyi István University, 9026 Győr, Hungary
5. Auckland Bioengineering Institute, The University of Auckland, Auckland 1010, New Zealand
* Correspondence: fekete.gusztav@sze.hu (G.F.); guyaodong@nbu.edu.cn (Y.G.); Tel.: +86-574-87600208 (Y.G.)

Abstract: Biomechanical asymmetries between children's left and right feet can affect stability and coordination, especially during dynamic movements. This study aimed to examine plantar pressure distribution, foot balance, and center of pressure (COP) trajectories in children during walking, running, and turning activities to understand how different movements influence these asymmetries. Fifteen children participated in the study, using a FootScan plantar pressure plate to capture detailed pressure and balance data. The parameters, including time-varying forces, COP, and Foot Balance Index (FBI), were analyzed through a one-dimensional Statistical Parametric Mapping (SPM1d) package. Results showed that asymmetries in COP and FBI became more pronounced, particularly during the tasks of running and directional turns. Regional plantar pressure analysis also revealed a more significant load on specific foot areas during these dynamic movements, indicating an increased reliance on one foot for stability and control. These findings suggest that early identification of asymmetrical loading patterns may be vital in promoting a balanced gait and preventing potential foot health issues in children. This study contributes to understanding pediatric foot biomechanics and provides insights for developing targeted interventions to support healthy physical development in children.

Keywords: children gait; plantar pressure distribution; foot balance; center of pressure; movement asymmetry; SPM1D

1. Introduction

The human foot has 28 bones, 33 joints, 112 ligaments, 13 extrinsic muscles, and 21 intrinsic muscles [1]. The foot is one of the most significant bodily elements and an essential component of locomotion [2]. The muscles, ligaments, and tendons associated with the foot bones are essential in maintaining overall form and ensuring function under static or dynamic conditions [3]. Differences in foot structure are associated with differences in foot function during static postures or dynamic movements. Many pathologies of the foot have a biomechanical origin and are usually related to foot type [4–6].

Intrinsic and extrinsic foot muscles control the arch [7] to respond to the increased load transport and running demands [8], suggesting that the arch is the "core" of the foot and is essential to normal foot function [9]. The foot of children develops quickly between the ages of 7 and 12 [9], and it has been reported that male arch height increases between ages 6 and 13 and female arch increases between ages 8 and 13 [10]. Previous findings demonstrated that child foot size and bone structure throughout average childhood growth are impacted by variations in gender and age. According to this biological nature, it has been shown that children's feet usually have a neutral and internally rotated foot posture, which frequently leads to aberrant foot morphology [11], thus affecting the daily location.

During walking and running, the arches of different morphologies and structures also cause changes in plantar pressure and load [12–15]. A study on preschool children found that the mean forces and pressures beneath the first and second metatarsals and the midfoot during the stance phase of walking were associated with the navicular heights and foot arch volumes [12]. Children's shoes with arch support are a non-surgical corrective method to affect the changes in plantar pressure caused by foot shape differences [11,13]. With the arch support structure, the average plantar contact area of the midfoot increased during running [13]. A recent study investigating gait turning with different angles [16], reporting that plantar pressure patterns shifted during the beginning of the approaching step. However, there are only a few studies focusing on biomechanics and plantar loadings while executing the walking, running, and turning tasks.

Although there has been much research on foot shape changes and growth patterns in children, there has yet to be research on the symmetry/asymmetry in plantar loading profiles between the right and left foot in children. Therefore, the purpose of this study was to explore the loading and COP differences between the left and right feet of children in completing four maneuvers: walking, walking turn, running, and running turn.

2. Materials and Methods

2.1. Participants

Fifteen healthy female children (average age: 7.0 ± 1.3 years; height: 128.4 ± 6.9 cm; weight: 23.2 ± 3.8 kg) participated in this study. All participants were free of lower-limb injuries or surgeries within the past six months. Each participant's dominant leg was identified based on their preferred kicking foot [17], with all participants being right-leg dominant. Before the study, both participants and their guardians received a thorough explanation of the procedures and provided informed consent. Ethical approval was obtained from the university's research ethics committee.

2.2. Test Protocol

Data were collected on a FootScan plantar pressure plate (RsScan International, Olen, Belgium) embedded in a 20-m walkway. The plate, measuring 2 m $\times$ 0.4 m $\times$ 0.02 m with a default sampling frequency of 480 Hz, was calibrated for each participant's weight before testing [18]. Each participant performed four tasks in a barefoot condition: straight walking, straight running, turning during walking (left and right), and turning during running (left and right). For turning tasks, the stance leg was analyzed (e.g., right foot for left turns, left foot for right turns) (Figure 1A,B). Participants performed a minimum of three successful trials per task, and any trials with incomplete steps on the pressure plate were excluded. Foot pressure data were collected from ten anatomical regions (Figure 1C), including the big toe (Toe 1), other toes (T2–5), metatarsals I–V (M1–M5), midfoot (MF), medial heel (MH), and lateral heel (LH).

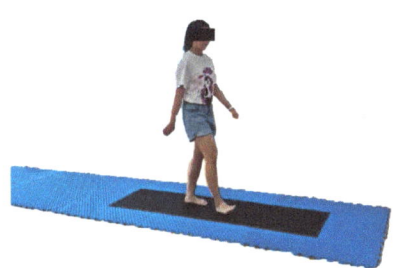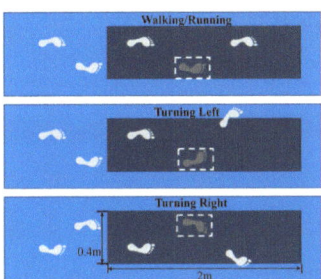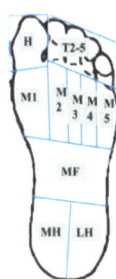

A. Experimental protocol   B. Acquisition of the plantar pressure C. Ten anatomic regions

Figure 1. Illustration of the test protocol of straight running (**A**), left and right turning (**B**), and division of anatomic regions (**C**).

2.3. Data Processing

Time series parameters for each stance phase were interpolated to 101 points using a cubic spline to ensure uniformity and represent 100% of the stance [19]. The Foot Balance Index (FBI), calculated from the average peak pressures of metatarsal and heel regions, indicated foot stability, with positive values denoting pronation and negative values denoting supination. The trajectory of the Center of Pressure (COP) during each stance phase was also interpolated to 101 data points for statistical comparison.

The Foot Balance Index (FBI) was calculated using the mean peak pressure values from the metatarsal and heel regions, as shown in Equation (1). M1, M2, M3, M4, and M5 represent the five metatarsal regions, and MH and LH represent the Medial Heel (MH) and Lateral Heel (LH) regions. F_{avg} means average force over the stance. The FBI provides a measure of overall foot stability:, where a positive value indicates pronation and a negative value indicates supination [18,20]:

$$\text{FBI} = \frac{(M1 + M2 + MH) - (M3 + M4 + M5 + LH)}{F_{avg}} \times 100\% \quad (1)$$

The Center of Pressure (COP) trajectory, a key indicator of gait characteristics, was analyzed for each stance phase across walking, running, and turning tasks [21–23]. Both the COP and FBI trajectories were interpolated to a standard length of 101 data points using a cubic spline method, ensuring consistency for statistical analysis.

2.4. Statistical Analysis

To capture consistent performance, three trials for each movement task—walking, running, turning while walking, and turning while running—were averaged per participant to reduce trial variability. Force data were then normalized by Z_{avg}, derived by dividing the total force by the sum of the original data frames [24–26]. Time-series data, including force, Center of Pressure (COP), and Foot Balance Index (FBI), were checked for normality before analysis. Statistical comparisons were conducted using the Statistical Parametric Mapping (SPM1d) method with independent sample t-tests based on random field theory [27,28]. All analyses were performed in MATLAB R2018a (The MathWorks, Natick, MA, USA), with results presented as mean values and standard deviations (SD). A two-tailed *p*-value of less than 0.05 was set as the threshold for statistical significance.

3. Results

3.1. Center of Pressure Trajectory

Figure 2 illustrates the differences in the center of pressure (COP) trajectory in the left foot and right foot during both walking and running. During the stance phase, the left foot's COP shifts toward pronation, while the right foot's COP shifts toward supination. Hypothesis testing reveals significant differences in COP distribution throughout the stance phase for walking and running ($p < 0.001$).

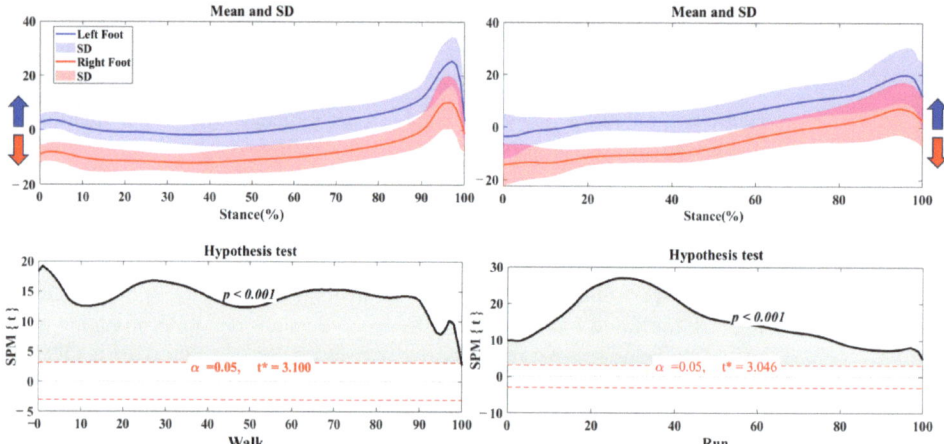

Figure 2. The COP of trajectory in the left and right foot during walking and running with the highlighted direction of pronation (Blue arrow) and supination (Red arrow). Note: Y-axis (%foot width).

Figure 3 illustrates the differences in the center of pressure (COP) trajectory when turning left versus right during walking and running. During the stance phase of children's gait, the COP shifts pronation when turning left and toward supination when turning right. The standard deviation highlights that this trend is especially noticeable in running conditions. The hypothesis test results confirm significant differences in COP distribution throughout the stance phase of children's gait for both walking and running ($p < 0.001$).

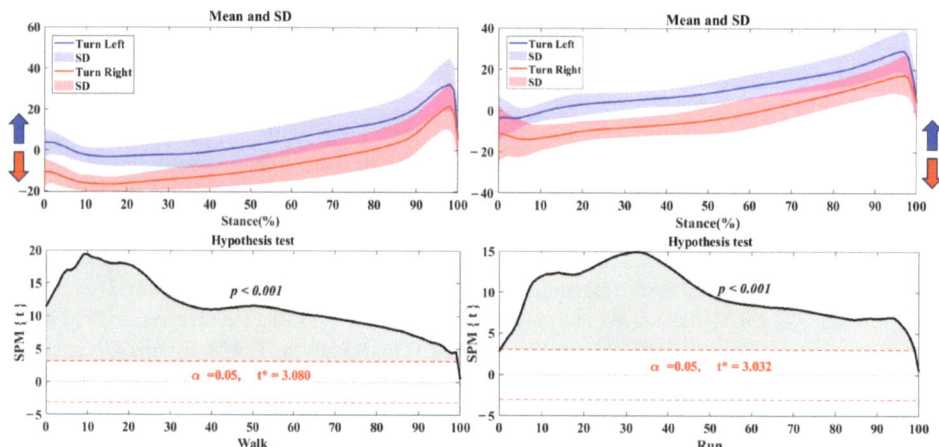

Figure 3. The COP of trajectory in the turning right/left during walking and running with the highlighted direction of pronation (Blue arrow) and supination (Red arrow). Note: Y-axis (%foot width).

3.2. Foot Balance Index

Figure 4 shows that there are distinct differences in the Foot Balance Index (FBI) between the left and right feet during both walking and running. The left foot tends toward pronation (negative FBI values), while the right foot shows a tendency for supination (positive FBI values). This imbalance is more pronounced during running, with wider variations in the FBI, particularly for the right foot. Statistical tests confirm these differences, showing a highly significant result ($p < 0.001$) during the 18%–53% phase of running, indicating an increased asymmetry in foot balance in this condition.

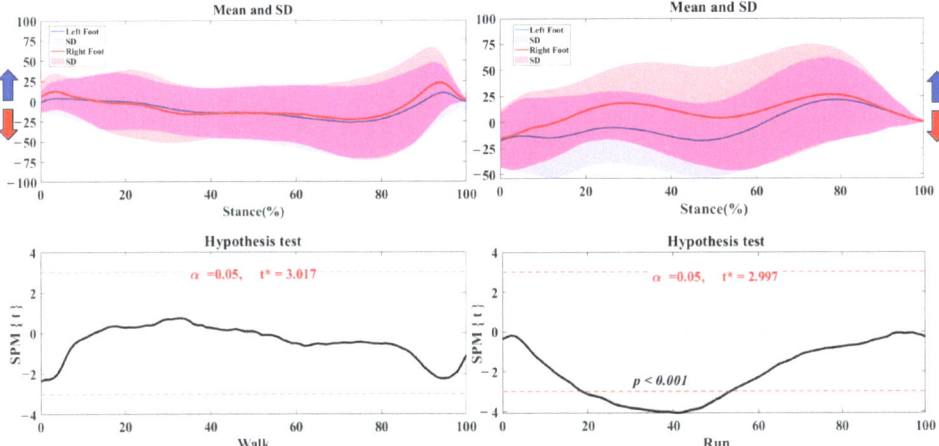

Figure 4. The FBI of trajectory in the left and right foot during walking and running with the highlighted direction of pronation (Blue arrow) and supination (Red arrow). Note: Y-axis (%).

Figure 5 shows the Foot Balance Index (FBI) results for left and right turns during walking and running. During left turns, the foot shifts towards pronation, while right turns shift towards supination. This pattern is more pronounced during running, particularly in the mid-stance phase, where deviations and variability are greater. However, no statistically significant differences between left and right turns in walking or running were found.

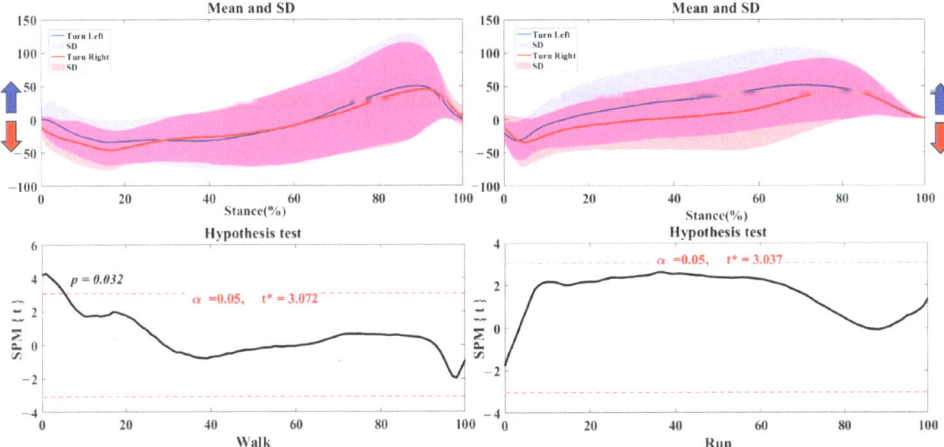

Figure 5. The FBI of trajectory in the turning right/left during walking and running with the highlighted direction of pronation (Blue arrow) and supination (Red arrow). Note: Y-axis (%).

3.3. Regional Plantar Forces

As shown in Figure 6, plantar pressure distribution testing revealed significant differences between the left and right sides during walking. The M2 region on the left side had notably lower pressure than the right side during 76%–95% of the contact phase ($p < 0.01$). No significant pressure differences were observed in other plantar regions.

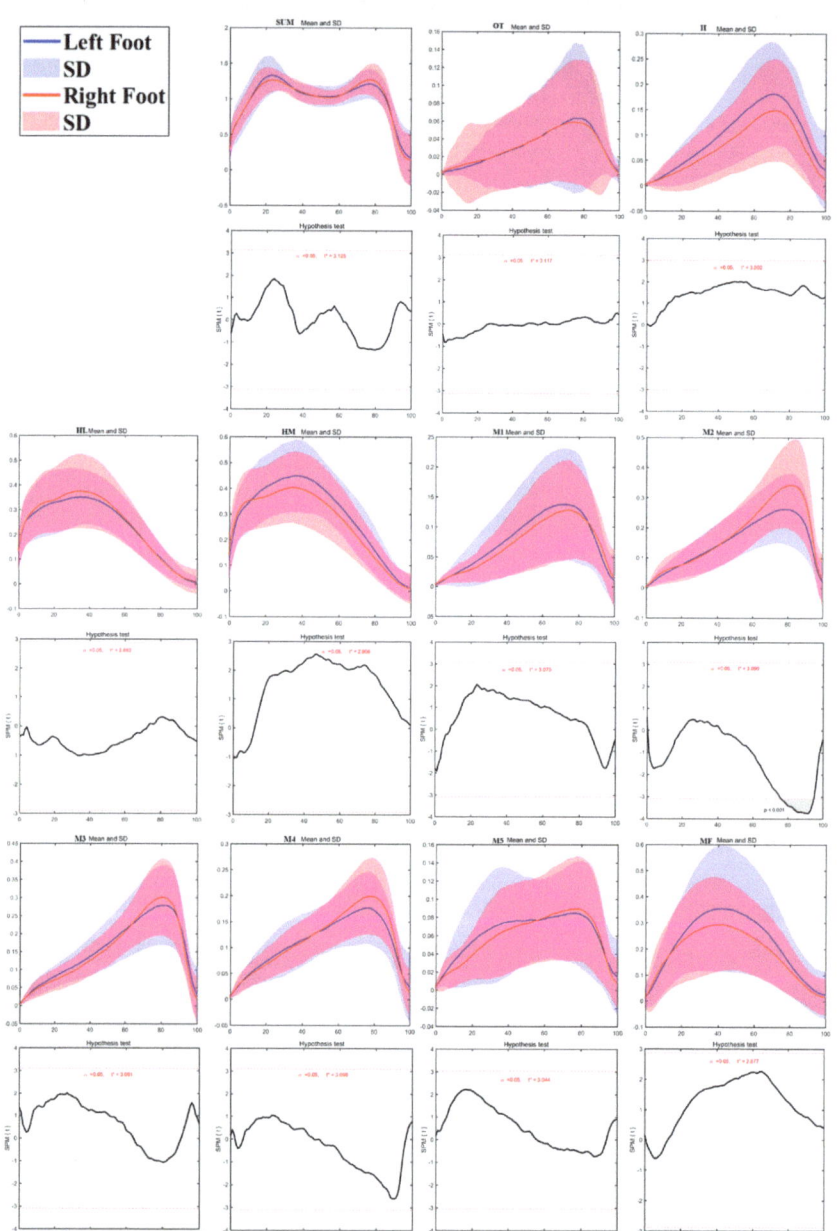

Figure 6. The sum of plantar pressure (SUM) and regional plantar forces during walking on the left foot and right foot with highlighted statistics. Note: Y-axis (normalized using Zavg).

As shown in Figure 7, plantar pressure distribution testing revealed significant differences between the left and right sides during running. The M1 region on the left side showed significantly lower pressure than the right side during 10%–54% of the contact phase ($p < 0.01$). In contrast, the M4 region on the left side exhibited significantly higher pressure than the right side from 16%–35% ($p < 0.01$), and the M5 region showed significantly higher pressure from 5%–78% of the contact phase ($p < 0.01$). No significant differences were found in the other plantar regions.

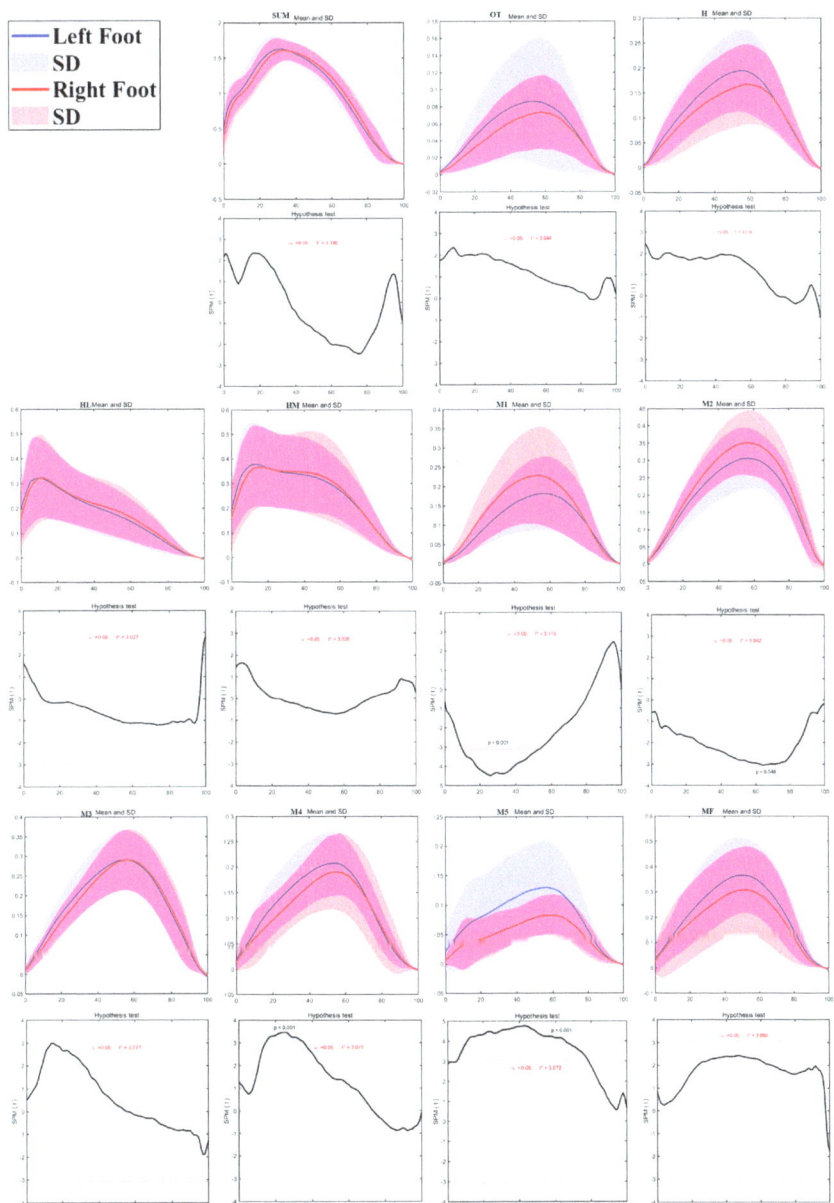

Figure 7. The sum of plantar pressure (SUM) and regional plantar forces during running in the left foot and right foot with highlighted statistics. Note: Y-axis (normalized using Zavg).

As shown in Figure 8, plantar pressure distribution testing revealed significant differences between the left and right sides during walking turns. The H region during the Turn Left task showed significantly lower pressure compared to the Turn Right task at 3%–4%

(p = 0.05), 8%–9% (p = 0.49), and 25%–38% of the contact phase (p < 0.01). In contrast, the M2 region during the Turn Left task exhibited significantly higher pressure than the Turn Right task from 76%–92% of the contact phase (p < 0.01). No significant differences were found in the other plantar regions.

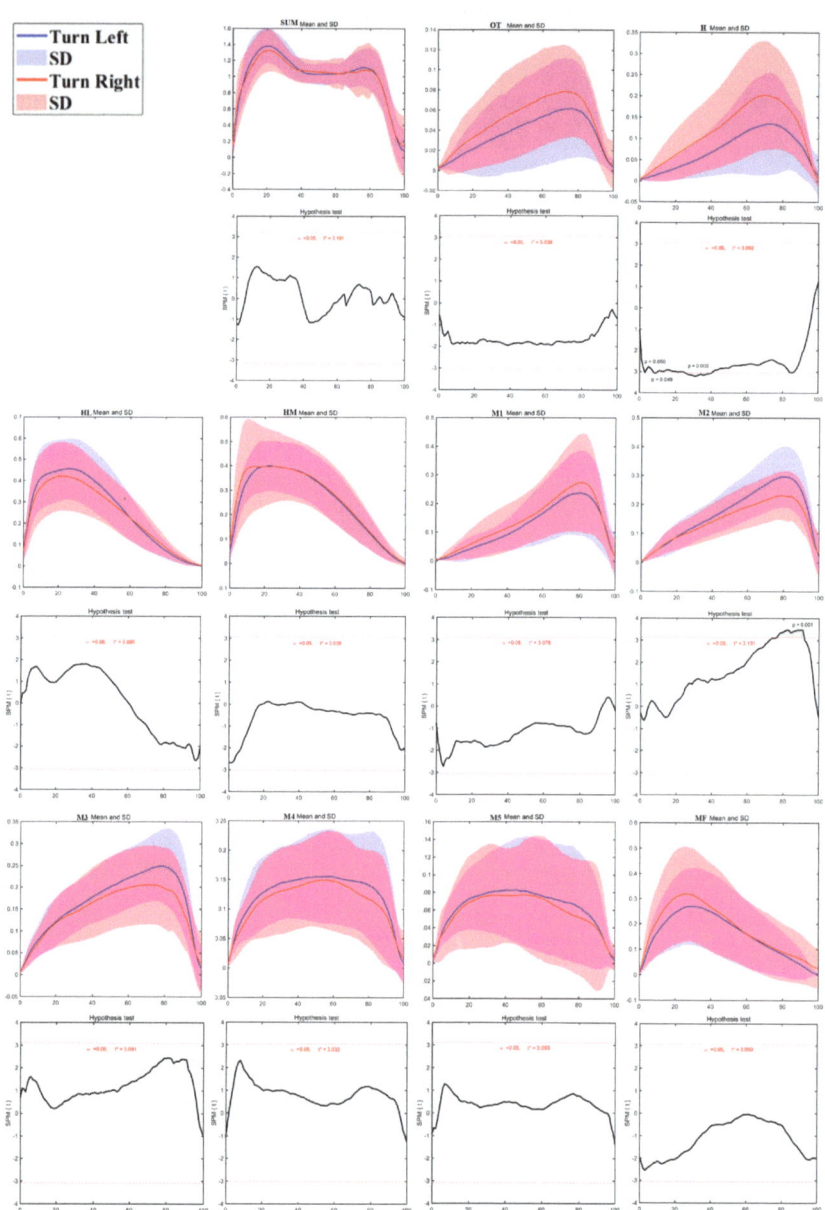

Figure 8. The sum of plantar pressure (SUM) and regional plantar forces during Turning Walking Tasks in the left turn and right turn with highlighted statistics. Note: Y-axis (normalized using Zavg).

As shown in Figure 9, plantar pressure distribution testing revealed significant differences between the left and right sides during the running turn. The M1 region during the True Left task showed significantly higher pressure than the True Right task from 9%–16% of the contact phase (p = 0.032). The M4 region exhibited significantly higher pressure from 46%–76% ($p < 0.01$), and the M5 region showed significantly higher pressure from 39%–88% of the contact phase ($p < 0.01$). Conversely, the M3 region during the True Left task demonstrated significantly lower pressure than the True Right task from 0%–9% ($p = 0.025$), and the M4 region showed lower pressure from 1%–5% of the stance phase ($p = 0.043$). No significant differences were found in the other plantar areas.

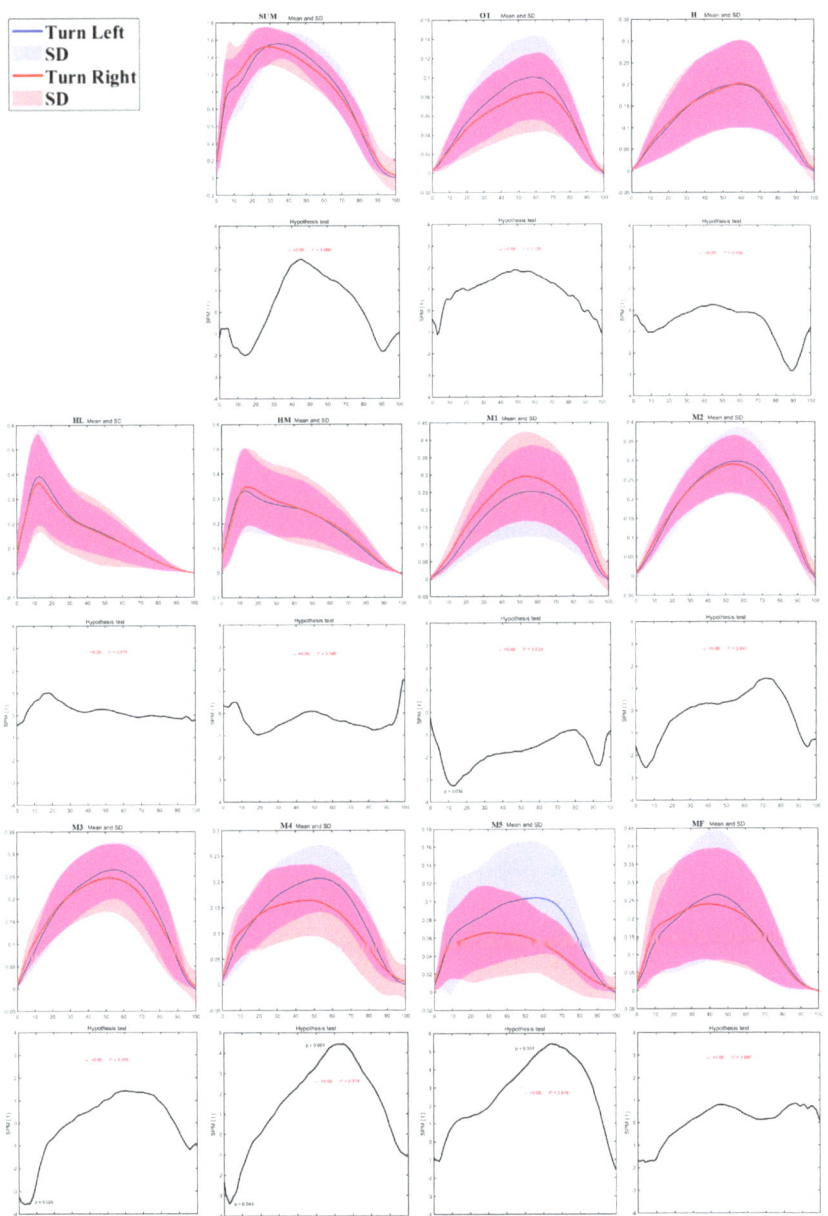

Figure 9. The sum of plantar pressure (SUM) and regional plantar forces during Turning running Tasks in the left turn and right turn with highlighted statistics. Note: Y-axis (normalized using Zavg).

4. Discussion

This study provides an in-depth examination of biomechanical differences between children's left and right feet across multiple movement tasks, specifically walking, running, walking turns, and running turns. Using metrics such as the center of pressure (COP) trajectory, Foot Balance Index (FBI), and regional plantar pressure, we identified that biomechanical asymmetries became prominent from walking and running to turning activities. These findings underscore the different demands placed on children's feet under varied movement conditions, highlighting how movement patterns shape foot biomechanics in dynamic activities. This has implications for understanding children's adaptation to loads and the potential risks of asymmetric load distribution.

The analysis of COP trajectories revealed substantial left-right differences in stability strategies, particularly noticeable during stance phases across different activities. For walking, COP showed a tendency for pronation in the left foot and supination in the right, reflecting a relatively balanced load distribution during this low-impact activity. This alignment suggests that, in a steady gait, children's feet exhibit minor asymmetries that still allow for balanced movement, likely due to the low speed and force requirements [29,30]. However, during running, COP trajectories diverged significantly between the left and right feet. The pronounced reliance on one foot to achieve stability at higher speeds reflects children's adaptation to the demands of rapid adjustments during high-impact activities [31]. This finding aligns with prior studies indicating that increased speed and load in movement often heighten asymmetries, as children may unconsciously favor their dominant foot for stabilization and control [32–34].

In directional turning tasks, COP trajectory analysis revealed distinct directional shifts, with COP in the left foot leaning toward pronation for left turns and COP in the right foot moving toward supination for right turns. This trend was particularly pronounced in running turns, likely due to the complex balancing requirements and redirecting momentum at high speeds. Turning demands rapid adjustments of the center of mass and increased stability from the support foot [35,36], and the observed COP shifts reflect children's adaptation to these demands. These findings indicate that children rely on specific foot regions to achieve stability during turns, especially during running. This reliance may reflect a developmental trend in which children's neuromuscular systems still adapt to managing balance during quick, dynamic shifts [26,37,38]. Notably, this also raises considerations for injury prevention, as the increased load on the support foot during turns could lead to overuse or strain if the foot consistently bears these loads asymmetrically.

FBI findings further substantiated the observed COP asymmetries, demonstrating that balance control differs substantially between the left and right feet in straight and turning movements. In walking, the left foot tended slightly toward pronation and the right toward supination, suggesting balanced but minor asymmetry. However, the FBI asymmetry became more significant during running, especially in the mid-stance phase, indicating that the feet adopt distinct balance strategies to manage the increased demands of running. This more significant divergence in FBI suggests that running requires elevated foot stability and control, which may lead to an overreliance on one foot to maintain balance [39,40]. Previous studies similarly report that running placed significant stress on stability and control, which could amplify existing foot asymmetries as load increases [24,41]. This finding implies that high-demand movements may increase the risk of imbalance-related foot health issues, underscoring the need for targeted interventions to enhance bilateral stability during running.

The regional plantar pressure analysis highlighted areas where pressure distribution differed markedly between the left and right feet, with these differences intensifying with activity demands. For instance, pressure in the left second metatarsal region (M2) was lower during walking than in the right, suggesting relatively balanced load distribution in low-impact movement. However, during running, the first metatarsal (M1) on the left side showed significantly lower pressure than the right, while pressure was notably higher in the fourth (M4) and fifth metatarsal (M5) regions of the left foot. In turning tasks, particularly running turns, the support foot bore more significant localized pressures, with higher loads concentrated in the first and fifth metatarsal regions. This uneven pressure distribution suggests that children may rely more on specific areas of the support foot to stabilize during high-speed directional changes [26,40,42]. Such a pattern indicates that, as movement demands increase, certain foot regions experience heightened pressure, likely to compensate for rapid shifts in momentum and direction. This has critical implications for children's foot health, as persistent asymmetric pressure distribution may predispose them to localized strain and injury [43,44].

These findings offer practical insights for supporting children's foot health. Identifying asymmetries in foot biomechanics across varied activities can guide targeted interventions to promote more balanced gait patterns. For instance, balance training exercises could focus on reducing reliance on one foot, potentially mitigating injury risks linked to prolonged asymmetric load distribution. Additionally, the observed COP and FBI asymmetries may serve as early indicators of developing gait imbalances, which could aid in detecting potential issues in children's foot development. Incorporating assessments of load distribution patterns into routine pediatric evaluations could allow for proactive management of foot health, particularly in children engaging in sports or other physically demanding activities.

This study has certain limitations. The relatively small sample size and focus on a specific age group may limit the generalizability of the findings. Further studies with more diverse samples, including gender, different age groups, and physical activity levels, would provide a more comprehensive understanding of these biomechanical patterns. Additionally, as the study was conducted in a controlled laboratory setting, future research could investigate these dynamics in real-world environments to improve the ecological validity of the results. Expanding research to consider footwear types and ground surfaces would offer deeper insights into how different conditions influence children's foot biomechanics.

5. Conclusions

This study identified biomechanical differences between children's left and right feet during walking, running, and turning tasks, showing that pressure is redistributed. Children may rely more heavily on either foot for stability and control, which became the dominant limb, as reflected in the center of pressure (COP), Foot Balance Index (FBI), and regional plantar pressure distributions. These findings highlight the importance of early identification and intervention for asymmetrical loading patterns to promote balance and reduce injury risk, providing valuable insights for future assessments and interventions in children's gait and foot health.

Author Contributions: Conceptualization, W.L., Q.M. and Y.G.; methodology, Y.W., L.X., H.W. and Q.M.; software, W.L., H.W. and Z.G.; validation, L.X., H.J., G.F. and Y.G.; formal analysis, W.L. and Y.W.; investigation, H.W., H.J. and Z.G.; data curation, L.X., H.W. and Z.G.; writing—original draft preparation, W.L., Y.W. and H.J.; writing—review and editing, G.F. and Q.M.; visualization, E.J.; supervision, G.F. and Y.G.; project administration, Y.G.; funding acquisition, Y.G. All authors have read and agreed to the published version of the manuscript.

Funding: This research received no external funding.

Institutional Review Board Statement: The study was conducted according to the guidelines of the Declaration of Helsinki and approved by the Ethics Committee in the Research Institute of Ningbo University (RAGH20201216).

Informed Consent Statement: Informed consent was obtained from all participants involved in the study.

Data Availability Statement: The data may be available upon reasonable request from the corresponding authors.

Acknowledgments: The authors would like to acknowledge all children and their parents for the participation and collaboration during this project.

Conflicts of Interest: The authors declare no conflicts of interest.

References

1. Levy, J.C.; Mizel, M.S.; Wilson, L.S.; Fox, W.; McHale, K.; Taylor, D.C.; Temple, T. Incidence of foot and ankle injuries in west point cadets with pes planus compared to the general cadet population. *Foot Ankle Int.* **2006**, *27*, 1060–1064. [CrossRef] [PubMed]
2. Mauch, M.; Grau, S.; Krauss, I.; Maiwald, C.; Horstmann, T. A new approach to children's footwear based on foot type classification. *Ergonomics* **2009**, *52*, 999–1008. [CrossRef] [PubMed]
3. Mauch, M.; Grau, S.; Krauss, I.; Maiwald, C.; Horstmann, T. Foot morphology of normal, underweight and overweight children. *Int. J. Obes.* **2008**, *32*, 1068–1075. [CrossRef] [PubMed]
4. Ledoux, W.R.; Shofer, J.B.; Ahroni, J.H.; Smith, D.G.; Sangeorzan, B.J.; Boyko, E.J. Biomechanical differences among pes cavus, neutrally aligned, and pes planus feet in subjects with diabetes. *Foot Ankle Int.* **2003**, *24*, 845–850. [CrossRef]
5. Naudi, S.; Dauplat, G.; Staquet, V.; Parent, S.; Mehdi, N.; Maynou, C. Anterior tarsectomy long-term results in adult pes cavus. *Orthop. Traumatol.-Surg. Res.* **2009**, *95*, 293–300. [CrossRef]
6. Sugathan, H.K.; Sherlock, D.A. A Modified Jones Procedure for Managing Clawing of Lesser Toes in Pes Cavus: Long-term Follow-up in 8 Patients. *J. Foot Ankle Surg.* **2009**, *48*, 637–641. [CrossRef]
7. Carvalho, B.K.G.d.; Penha, P.J.; Penha, N.L.J.; Andrade, R.M.; Ribeiro, A.P.; Joao, S.M.A. The influence of gender and body mass index on the FPI-6 evaluated foot posture of 10- to 14-year-old school children in Sao Paulo, Brazil: A cross-sectional study. *J. Foot Ankle Res.* **2017**, *10*, 1. [CrossRef]
8. Ferber, R.; Noehren, B.; Hamill, J.; Davis, I. Competitive Female Runners With a History of Iliotibial Band Syndrome Demonstrate Atypical Hip and Knee Kinematics. *J. Orthop. Sports Phys. Ther.* **2010**, *40*, 52–58. [CrossRef]
9. Bosch, K.; Nagel, A.; Weigend, L.; Rosenbaum, D. From "first" to "last" steps in life-Pressure patterns of three generations. *Clin. Biomech.* **2009**, *24*, 676–681. [CrossRef]
10. Szczepanowska-Wolowiec, B.; Sztandera, P.; Kotela, I.; Zak, M. Vulnerability of the foot's morphological structure to deformities caused by foot loading paradigm in school-aged children: A cross-sectional study. *Sci. Rep.* **2021**, *11*, 2749. [CrossRef]
11. Wang, Y.; Jiang, H.; Yu, L.; Gao, Z.; Liu, W.; Mei, Q.; Gu, Y. Understanding the Role of Children's Footwear on Children's Feet and Gait Development: A Systematic Scoping Review. *Healthcare* **2023**, *11*, 1418. [CrossRef] [PubMed]
12. Chow, J.Y.; Seifert, L.; Hérault, R.; Chia, S.J.Y.; Lee, M.C.Y. A dynamical system perspective to understanding badminton singles game play. *Hum. Mov. Sci.* **2014**, *33*, 70–84. [CrossRef] [PubMed]
13. Molloy, J.M.; Christie, D.S.; Teyhen, D.S.; Yeykal, N.S.; Tragord, B.S.; Neal, M.S.; Nelson, E.S.; McPoil, T. Effect of Running Shoe Type on the Distribution and Magnitude of Plantar Pressures in Individuals with Low- or High-Arched Feet. *J. Am. Podiatr. Med. Assoc.* **2009**, *99*, 330–338. [CrossRef] [PubMed]
14. Cen, X.Z.; Xu, D.T.; Baker, J.S.; Gu, Y.D. Association of Arch Stiffness with Plantar Impulse Distribution during Walking, Running, and Gait Termination. *Int. J. Environ. Res. Public Health* **2020**, *17*, 2090. [CrossRef] [PubMed]
15. Yu, P.M.; Cen, X.Z.; Xiang, L.L.; Mei, Q.C.; Wang, A.L.; Gu, Y.D.; Fernandez, J. Regional plantar forces and surface geometry variations of a chronic ankle instability population described by statistical shape modelling. *Gait Posture* **2023**, *106*, 11–17. [CrossRef]
16. Hu, X.Y.; Tang, J.P.; Cai, W.F.; Sun, Z.L.; Zhao, Z.; Qu, X.D. Characteristics of foot plantar pressure during turning in young male adults. *Gait Posture* **2023**, *101*, 1–7. [CrossRef]
17. Chapman, J.P.; Chapman, L.J.; Allen, J.J. The measurement of foot preference. *Neuropsychologia* **1987**, *25*, 579–584. [CrossRef]
18. Gao, Z.; Mei, Q.; Xiang, L.; Baker, J.S.; Fernandez, J.; Gu, Y. Effects of limb dominance on the symmetrical distribution of plantar loading during walking and running. *Proc. Inst. Mech. Eng. Part P J. Sports Eng. Technol.* **2022**, *236*, 17–23. [CrossRef]
19. Yu, L.; Yu, P.; Liu, W.; Gao, Z.; Sun, D.; Mei, Q.; Fernandez, J.; Gu, Y. Understanding foot loading and balance behavior of children with motor sensory processing disorder. *Children* **2022**, *9*, 379. [CrossRef]
20. Chang, W.-D.; Chang, N.-J.; Lin, H.-Y.; Lai, P.-T. Changes of plantar pressure and gait parameters in children with mild cerebral palsy who used a customized external strap orthosis: A crossover study. *BioMed Res. Int.* **2015**, *2015*, 813942. [CrossRef]
21. Mei, Q.; Gu, Y.; Fernandez, J. Alterations of pregnant gait during pregnancy and post-partum. *Sci. Rep.* **2018**, *8*, 2217. [CrossRef] [PubMed]

22. Carpinella, I.; Crenna, P.; Calabrese, E.; Rabuffetti, M.; Mazzoleni, P.; Nemni, R.; Ferrarin, M. Locomotor function in the early stage of Parkinson's disease. *IEEE Trans. Neural Syst. Rehabil. Eng.* **2007**, *15*, 543–551. [CrossRef] [PubMed]
23. Mei, Q.; Feng, N.; Ren, X.; Lake, M.; Gu, Y. Foot Loading patterns with different unstable soles structure. *J. Mech. Med. Biol.* **2015**, *15*, 1550014. [CrossRef]
24. Gao, Z.; Mei, Q.; Fekete, G.; Baker, J.S.; Gu, Y. The effect of prolonged running on the symmetry of biomechanical variables of the lower limb joints. *Symmetry* **2020**, *12*, 720. [CrossRef]
25. Wen, J.; Ding, Q.; Yu, Z.; Sun, W.; Wang, Q.; Wei, K. Adaptive changes of foot pressure in hallux valgus patients. *Gait Posture* **2012**, *36*, 344–349. [CrossRef]
26. Yu, L.; Mohamad, N.I. Development of badminton-specific footwork training from traditional physical exercise to novel intervention approaches. *Phys. Act. Health* **2022**, *6*, 219–225. [CrossRef]
27. Mei, Q.; Xiang, L.; Li, J.; Fernandez, J.; Gu, Y. Analysis of Running Ground Reaction Forces Using the One-Dimensional Statistical Parametric Mapping (SPM1d). *Yiyong Shengwu Lixue/J. Med. Biomech.* **2021**, *36*, 684–691. [CrossRef]
28. Pataky, T.C. One-dimensional statistical parametric mapping in Python. *Comput. Methods Biomech. Biomed. Eng.* **2012**, *15*, 295–301. [CrossRef]
29. Sadeghi, H.; Allard, P.; Prince, F.; Labelle, H. Symmetry and limb dominance in able-bodied gait: A review. *Gait Posture* **2000**, *12*, 34–45. [CrossRef]
30. Bosch, K.; Rosenbaum, D. Gait symmetry improves in childhood—A 4-year follow-up of foot loading data. *Gait Posture* **2010**, *32*, 464–468. [CrossRef]
31. Eshraghi, A.; Safaeepour, Z.; Geil, M.D.; Andrysek, J. Walking and balance in children and adolescents with lower-limb amputation: A review of literature. *Clin. Biomech.* **2018**, *59*, 181–198. [CrossRef] [PubMed]
32. Hsiang, S.M.; Chang, C. The effect of gait speed and load carrying on the reliability of ground reaction forces. *Saf. Sci.* **2002**, *40*, 639–657. [CrossRef]
33. Schaefer, S.; Jagenow, D.; Verrel, J.; Lindenberger, U. The influence of cognitive load and walking speed on gait regularity in children and young adults. *Gait Posture* **2015**, *41*, 258–262. [CrossRef] [PubMed]
34. Tajima, T.; Tateuchi, H.; Koyama, Y.; Ikezoe, T.; Ichihashi, N. Gait strategies to reduce the dynamic joint load in the lower limbs during a loading response in young healthy adults. *Hum. Mov. Sci.* **2018**, *58*, 260–267. [CrossRef]
35. Hase, K.; Stein, R.B. Turning strategies during human walking. *J. Neurophysiol.* **1999**, *81*, 2914–2922. [CrossRef]
36. Dixon, P.C.; Stebbins, J.; Theologis, T.; Zavatsky, A.B. Spatio-temporal parameters and lower-limb kinematics of turning gait in typically developing children. *Gait Posture* **2013**, *38*, 870–875. [CrossRef]
37. Ludwig, O.; Kelm, J.; Hammes, A.; Schmitt, E.; Fröhlich, M. Neuromuscular performance of balance and posture control in childhood and adolescence. *Heliyon* **2020**, *6*, e04541. [CrossRef]
38. Fong, S.S.M.; Chung, L.M.Y.; Bae, Y.-H.; Vackova, D.; Ma, A.W.W.; Liu, K.P.Y. Neuromuscular processes in the control of posture in children with developmental coordination disorder: Current evidence and future research directions. *Curr. Dev. Disord. Rep.* **2018**, *5*, 43–48. [CrossRef]
39. Daley, M.A.; Felix, G.; Biewener, A.A. Running stability is enhanced by a proximo-distal gradient in joint neuromechanical control. *J. Exp. Biol.* **2007**, *210*, 383–394. [CrossRef]
40. Spech, C.; Paponetti, M.; Mansfield, C.; Schmitt, L.; Briggs, M. Biomechanical variations in children who are overweight and obese during high-impact activities: A systematic review and meta-analysis. *Obes. Rev.* **2022**, *23*, e13431. [CrossRef]
41. Carpes, F.P.; Mota, C.B.; Faria, I.E. On the bilateral asymmetry during running and cycling—A review considering leg preference. *Phys. Ther. Sport* **2010**, *11*, 136–142. [CrossRef] [PubMed]
42. Yiou, E.; Caderby, T.; Delafontaine, A.; Fourcade, P.; Honeine, J.L. Balance control during gait initiation: State of the art and research perspectives. *World J. Orthop.* **2017**, *8*, 815. [CrossRef] [PubMed]
43. Keenan, B.E.; Evans, S.L.; Oomens, C.W.J. A review of foot finite element modelling for pressure ulcer prevention in bedrest: Current perspectives and future recommendations. *J. Tissue Viability* **2022**, *31*, 73–83. [CrossRef] [PubMed]
44. Ménard, A.L.; Begon, M.; Barrette, J.; Green, B.; Ballaz, L.; Nault, M.L. Plantar pressure analysis: Identifying risk of foot and ankle injury in soccer players. *Transl. Sports Med.* **2021**, *4*, 684–690. [CrossRef]

Disclaimer/Publisher's Note: The statements, opinions and data contained in all publications are solely those of the individual author(s) and contributor(s) and not of MDPI and/or the editor(s). MDPI and/or the editor(s) disclaim responsibility for any injury to people or property resulting from any ideas, methods, instructions or products referred to in the content.

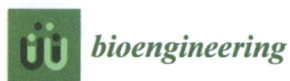

Article

Optimizing Fall Risk Diagnosis in Older Adults Using a Bayesian Classifier and Simulated Annealing

Enrique Hernandez-Laredo [1], Ángel Gabriel Estévez-Pedraza [1,*], Laura Mercedes Santiago-Fuentes [2] and Lorena Parra-Rodríguez [3]

[1] Tianguistenco Professional Academic Unit, Autonomous University of the State of Mexico, Tianguistenco 52640, Mexico; ehernandezl@uaemex.mx
[2] Health Science Department, Metropolitan Autonomous University, Mexico City 09310, Mexico; lmsf@xanum.uam.mx
[3] Research Department, National Institute of Geriatrics, Mexico City 10200, Mexico; lparra@inger.gob.mx
* Correspondence: aestevezp@uaemex.mx

Abstract: The aim of this study was to improve the diagnostic ability of fall risk classifiers using a Bayesian approach and the Simulated Annealing (SA) algorithm. A total of 47 features from 181 records (40 Center of Pressure (CoP) indices and 7 patient descriptive variables) were analyzed. The wrapper method of feature selection using the SA algorithm was applied to optimize the cost function based on the difference of the mean minus the standard deviation of the Area Under the Curve (AUC) of the fall risk classifiers across multiple dimensions. A stratified 60–20–20% hold-out method was used for train, test, and validation sets, respectively. The results showed that although the highest performance was observed with 31 features (0.815 ± 0.110), lower variability and higher explainability were achieved with only 15 features (0.780 ± 0.055). These findings suggest that the SA algorithm is a valuable tool for feature selection for acceptable fall risk diagnosis. This method offers an alternative or complementary resource in situations where clinical tools are difficult to apply.

Keywords: fall risk classification; simulated annealing algorithm; features selection; older adults; Center of Pressure (CoP) indices

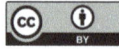

Citation: Hernandez-Laredo, E.; Estévez-Pedraza, Á.G.; Santiago-Fuentes, L.M.; Parra-Rodríguez, L. Optimizing Fall Risk Diagnosis in Older Adults Using a Bayesian Classifier and Simulated Annealing. *Bioengineering* **2024**, *11*, 908. https://doi.org/10.3390/bioengineering11090908

Academic Editor: Philippe Gorce

Received: 7 August 2024
Revised: 6 September 2024
Accepted: 6 September 2024
Published: 11 September 2024

Copyright: © 2024 by the authors. Licensee MDPI, Basel, Switzerland. This article is an open access article distributed under the terms and conditions of the Creative Commons Attribution (CC BY) license (https://creativecommons.org/licenses/by/4.0/).

1. Introduction

Globally, the World Health Organization (WHO) estimates that 684,000 fatal falls and 37.7 million falls serious enough to require medical attention occur annually, which involves various health problems and considerable economic costs at the public health, family, and personal levels [1]. About 35% of older adults have at least one fall per year [2,3], and this percentage increases to 32–42% for those over 70 years, making this population group one of the most vulnerable to injury or even death from a fall [1,3].

Given the relevance and implications of this public health problem in the adult population, it is important to make a correct and timely diagnosis. Balance assessment has been used to identify a possible fall risk, either through the use of technological systems [4] or by applying clinical tools based on questionnaires and standardized physical tests, such as Short Physical Performance Battery (SPPB), Timed Up and Go (TUG), Berg Balance Scale (BBS), Short Falls Efficacy Scale-International, Mini-Balance Evaluation Systems Test (Mini-BESTest), etc. [5]. However, the questionnaires have questionable accuracy and are not generalizable since they are susceptible to bias, as the evaluations are partially subjective and depend on the experience and ability of the evaluator [6]. Likewise, asking the fallers questions about the accidents they have had causes anxiety and stress due to the negative memories that are triggered, and at other times, they do not remember the fall or the number of falls [7,8]. These limitations can be reduced by using affordable technologies such as force platforms [9] and its low-cost alternatives [10,11]. These platforms allow for a quantitative study called stabilometry [12], from which Center of Pressure (CoP) indices can be obtained that allow for the characterization of the body sway by metrics and graphs [13,14].

The use of artificial intelligence techniques has made it possible to generate predictive or diagnostic models for balance alterations and/or fall risk based on sociodemographic, anthropometric, and CoP indices [15–22]. Specifically, it has been observed that Machine Learning algorithms based on Bayesian [22] and Decision Tree [15,23,24] classifiers, and Multi-Layer Perceptron [20] perform better in assessing fall risk compared with other techniques. On the other hand, Deep Learning techniques, particularly Neural Networks, are innovative methods that offer superior accuracy compared to traditional approaches [25]. However, these techniques often present challenges in interpretability, making it difficult to explain the studied phenomenon based on the input features. Furthermore, their performance may be compromised when trained on limited datasets [26,27]. This limitation is particularly relevant in the field of static stabilometry, where available data sources are often scarce [28].

Predicting an infrequent future event like falls is inherently challenging [28], so it is necessary to optimize feature selection to improve the performance of Machine Learning models [20] and provide a better explanation of which CoP indices best describe fall risk, as even with numerous research, it has been impossible to reach a consensus [29,30]. As such, this paper presents the Bayesian classification technique in combination with the heuristic approach of Simulated Annealing (SA) for feature selection to increase the diagnostic prediction of fall risk classifiers using human balance data from a sample of older adults. The current work could contribute to the production of an optimal computational model capable of predicting fall risk from quick stabilometric assessment.

2. Materials and Methods

2.1. Subjects and Preprocessing

For this study, a "public data set of human balance evaluations" database was used [31]. This includes information on 116 females and 47 males, aged 18 to 85 years. The participants were assessed repeatedly three times to obtain their stabilometric data using a force platform (OPT400600-1000; AMTI, Watertown, MA, USA), and their Short Falls Efficacy Scale-International (Short FES-I) scores were registered. Additionally, the dataset includes details such as sex, age, height, weight, body mass index (BMI), fall history, foot length, and polypharmacy.

Only information from older adults aged 60 years or older were used, who were labeled as Fall Risk if they recorded ≥ 1 fall in the previous 12 months and/or were rated as being of high concern in the Short FES-I. From each subject, 40 CoP indices were calculated according to Prieto [14]. To balance the dataset concerning the number of records per class, only the first set of repeated tests was selected for the Non-Fall Risk class, while for the Fall Risk class, 3 repeated tests were selected.

The CoP indices, age (years), weight (kilograms), height (centimeters), BMI (kilograms/meters^2), and foot length (centimeters) were also used as continuous variables, polypharmacy as a discrete variable, while sex was used as a dichotomic variable (man or woman).

2.2. Bayesian Classifier

2.2.1. Statistical Analysis

A descriptive analysis was performed. Continuous and discrete variables are presented as means and standard deviations, and sex as a number and percentage. The normality of the continuous variables was assessed using Kolmogorov–Smirnov test. Comparisons of Fall Risk versus Non-Fall Risk individuals were estimated through a T-test for parametric variables, a Mann–Whitney test for non-parametric variables, and a χ^2 test for categorical variables. The predictive validity of a Fall Risk for all continuous and discrete variables was assessed using the Hosmer–Lemeshow Goodness of Fit test and the Area Under the Curve (AUC).

2.2.2. Model Architecture

A Bayesian classifier was used to generate a fall risk model. According to Bayes' theorem, the probability of belonging to the Fall Risk class (P_{FR}) is given by Equation (1):

$$P_{FR} = P \times \left(\frac{1}{(2\pi)^{\frac{k}{2}} \times |S|^{\frac{1}{2}}} \right) \times e^{-\frac{1}{2}(\overline{X}-\mu)' \times \frac{(\overline{X}-\mu)}{S}} \quad (1)$$

where P denotes the a priori probability of the classes (equiprobability between classes), μ is the mean value of the class in the feature space, S is the covariance matrix of the features, $\overline{X}$ is the feature vector, and k is the number of features. On the other hand, the probability of the class Non-Fall Risk (P_{NFR}) is given by the complementary probability of P_{FR}, which is $P_{NFR} = 1 - P_{FR}$. Therefore, the classifier prediction rule is given by Equation (2):

$$\begin{cases} if\ P_{FR} > P_{NFR} & Fall\ Risk \\ else & Non\text{-}Fall\ Risk \end{cases} \quad (2)$$

All features' values were standardized to a zero mean and unit variance so that they are dimensionless and have the same scale. The Bayesian classifier was coded and executed in a script of MATLAB® version 2024A. For more details about the scripts, please refer to the link for the public repository on GitHub.

2.3. Feature Selection by the Simulated Annealing Algorithm

For the feature selection task, the SA algorithm was used to optimize the performance of the Bayesian classifier. In that sense, the problem was represented through an array with n available elements (n = Bayesian classifier number dimensions); to assign n, random indices of m features are available (m = total numbers of features). The initial solution was composed by 4 patient descriptive variables (sex, BMI, age, polypharmacy) [3,16] and 7 CoP indices (total length ML, total length AP, 95% conf. ellipse area, mean velocity, mean velocity-AP, mean frequency, and RMS distance), which have been shown to be associated with the fall risk in older adults [16,32–35]. For dimensions greater than 11 features, the initial solution was represented by the optimal feature combination from the SA optimization of the previous dimension and the addition of a random feature.

The cost function was integrated as the difference of the mean and standard deviation of the AUC of the train, test, and validation sets. On the other hand, for initial parameters, an initial temperature (T) of 0.5979 was calculated using an initial acceptance probability of 0.9 according to [36]. A stop temperature (Tmin) of 0.0232 [37], geometric cooling with an additive constant of 0.82 [36,38], and an adaptive steady state (Lk) with 30 iterations were used.

The original SA algorithm [39] was modified by adding two improvements. First, the cost function was penalized with a value equal to 0 when the sensitivity or specificity of the train, test, or validation set was less than 0.6. Second, the result of the cost function of each SA iteration was stored in a vector, with the purpose of finding the maximum value of the cost function at the end of all SA iterations. Algorithm 1 shows the pseudocode used.

Algorithm 1: Feature selection algorithm based on simulated annealing

Input: Training dataset
Output: Optimal Feature Combination = best_features
1. T = 0.5979
2. Tmin = 0.0232
3. Lk = 30
4. Initial solution is declared
5. C0 = the function cost value of initial solution
6. i = 1   %% number of iterations
7. n = 11   %% n = dimensions
8. Cp = 0   %% function cost value of current solution
9. do while (T > Tmin):
10.   Generate a n-dimension random solution array
11.   Training Bayesian classifier
12.   Calculate the Bayesian classifier's AUC for the train, test and validation sets.
13.   if ((sensibility or specificity) < 0.6):
14.   Cost_function [i] = 0
15.   else:
16.   Cost_function [i] = mean (AUC_train, AUC_test, AUC_validation) − std (AUC_train, AUC_test, AUC_validation)
17.   Cp = max (Cost_function)
18.   DeltaE = Cp − C0
19.   if (DeltaE >= 0):
20.   C0 = Cp
21.   features [i] = last n-dimension random solution array
22.   elseif exp(DeltaE/(T)) > rand(1,1):
23.   C0 = Cp
24.   features [i] = last n-dimension random solution array
25.   k = k + 1
26.   T = T * × 0.82
27.   Lk = Lk + Lk × (1 − exp(−1))
28. best_features [n] = features (find (max (Cost_function))
29. n = n + 1
30. Restart pseudocode

2.4. Validation Strategies and Evaluation Metrics

The most used validation method with stabilometric datasets has been the 80–20% hold-out method [15,20,23], and to ensure a better comparison, this method was selected. However, to decrease the probability of bias, the data were divided into the train, test, and validation sets, corresponding to 60%, 20%, and 20%, respectively [40], using the stratified hold-out method based on the fall risk label. The sensitivity, specificity, and AUC metrics were used to evaluate the performance of the Bayesian classifier's optimal feature combination.

To assess the robustness of the top five feature combinations with the highest AUC, 150 new training sets were generated using the bootstrap aggregation technique from the original set. This approach enabled the construction of an ensemble learning model composed of 150 Bayesian classifiers, with the objective of analyzing in detail the impact of the optimal features through the performance of the mean AUC for fall risk diagnosis.

In addition, a univariate logistic regression model was generated for each CoP index, and its AUC was compared with the performance of the Bayesian classifier. These models were also made in MATLAB® version 2024A.

3. Results

Information from 76 individuals was included in the study. The mean age of these participants was 71.31 ± 6.47 years, 78.94% of the sample was women, and 38.15% presented fall risk conditions. Due to the balance of the data described in Section 2.1, a total of

181 stabilometric assessments were included, of which 94 records corresponded to the Non-Fall Risk class and 87 to the Fall Risk class. Features such as sex, foot length, 50% power frequency-RD, 95% power frequency-RD, 50% power frequency-AP, total power-ML, 95% power frequency-ML, centroidal frequency-RD, frequency dispersion-AP, and frequency dispersion-AP showed significant differences between the Non-Fall Risk and Fall Risk groups. The description of general participant characteristics and statistical analysis of the CoP indices are shown in Tables A1 and 1, respectively.

Table 1. Description of general participant characteristics by the fall risk group.

	Total	Non-Fall Risk	Fall Risk	p-Value Means Difference Test
	n = 76	n = 47	n = 29	
Sex [women] n (%)	60 (78.94)	33 (70.21)	27 (93.10)	0.017 *
Age [years]	71.3 ± 6.4	71.7 ± 6.5	70.6 ± 6.3	0.486
Height [cm]	157.2 ± 8.1	158.2 ± 9.1	155.5 ± 5.9	0.124
Weight [kg]	63.1 ± 8.4	63.6 ± 8.2	62.2 ± 8.6	0.477
BMI [kg/m^2]	25.5 ± 2.9	25.4 ± 2.9	25.6 ± 2.9	0.760
Foot length [cm]	22.6 ± 1.3	22.9 ± 1.2	22.0 ± 1.3	0.006 *
Polypharmacy	2.3 ± 1.6	2.3 ± 1.4	2.3 ± 1.8	0.707
Fall in the last year	0.9 ± 5.9	-	2.4 ± 9.5	-

* p-value < 0.05.

The CoP index with the best level of predictive validity according to its AUC is frequency dispersion-AP (AUC = 0.591). Table 2 shows the Top 5 CoP indices with the highest AUC and the full results are shown in Table A1.

Table 2. Statistical analysis of the CoP indices with the best level of predictive validity according to their AUC.

CoP Index	Total	Non-Fall Risk	Fall Risk	KS Test	MD Test	HL Test	AUC (95% CI)
	n = 181	n = 94	n = 87	p-Value	p-Value	p-Value	
Frequency dispersion-AP [-]	7.27 ± 1.06	7.13 ± 1.09	7.42 ± 1.01	0.000 *	0.034 *	0.400	0.591 (0.508–0.674)
Total power-ML [mm^2/Hz]	63.14 ± 114.63	45.52 ± 32.64	82.17 ± 160.14	0.000 *	0.048 *	0.996	0.585 (0.501–0.668)
Total power-RD [mm^2/Hz]	32.63 ± 56.53	25.7 ± 18.25	40.12 ± 78.86	0.000 *	0.097	0.908	0.571 (0.487–0.655)
Range-ML [mm]	27.29 ± 13.28	25.66 ± 9.35	29.06 ± 16.39	0.000 *	0.119	0.029 *	0.567 (0.482–0.651)
Range [mm]	28.50 ± 13.39	26.97 ± 9.75	30.15 ± 16.34	0.000 *	0.146	0.276	0.562 (0.478–0.647)

n = sample size, KS = Kolmogorov–Smirnov, MD = mean difference, HL = Hosmer–Lemeshow, CI = confidence interval, * p-value < 0.05.

The SA algorithm was executed to identify the optimal feature combination, beginning with n = 11 (refer to Section 2.3). The process continued until adding more features no longer resulted in a decrease in the cost function for at least three consecutive dimensions. It was observed that after incorporating n = 32 features, the performance of the classifier began to decline (see the full content in Table A2 and the dictionary features in Table A3). Through all the iterations, sex, BMI, total length-AP, covariance-ML, and 95% power frequency-AP were the most frequent in feature selection, as shown in Figure 1.

Table 3 shows the optimal Bayesian classification models obtained using feature combinations selected by the SA algorithm. The 31-feature model (Top 1) demonstrated the highest mean AUC of 0.815 ± 0.110 for hold-out validation, though this value decreased by 8% under bootstrap aggregation validation. Conversely, the 15-feature model (Top 4) exhibited the lowest variability between sets at 0.780 ± 0.055. These features maintained their robustness more effectively, showing only a 0.7% decrease. Figure 2 illustrates the selected features comprising these top-performing classifiers.

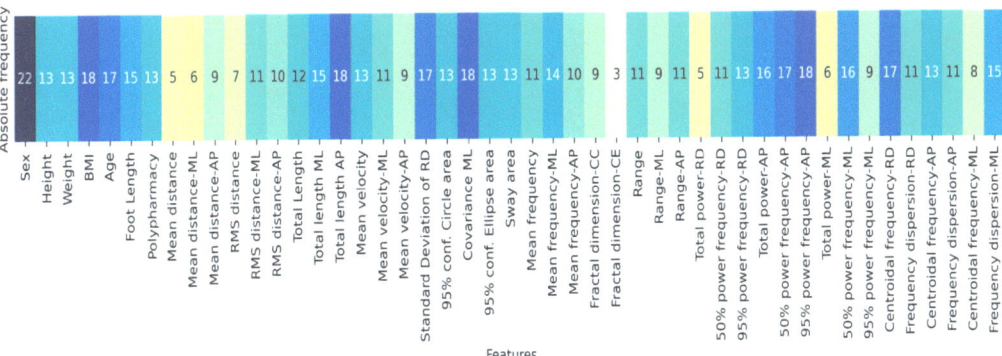

Figure 1. Absolute frequencies of the features selected by SA through all dimensions (*n* = 11 to 35). The colors refer to a gradient bar associated with the frequency of use of the features.

Table 3. List of best-performance results in feature selection.

	Top	n	Train			Test			Validation			Train–Test–Validation
			SE	SP	AUC	SE	SP	AUC	SE	SP	AUC	AUC (Mean ± Std)
Hold-out	1	31	0.92	0.96	0.94	0.72	0.78	0.75	0.70	0.78	0.74	0.815 ± 0.110
	2	29	0.92	0.91	0.91	0.72	0.68	0.70	0.64	0.89	0.77	0.797 ± 0.109
	3	24	0.88	0.91	0.89	0.66	0.73	0.70	0.70	0.78	0.74	0.782 ± 0.102
	4	15	0.80	0.85	0.83	0.94	0.63	0.78	0.70	0.73	0.72	0.780 ± 0.055
	5	30	0.92	0.80	0.86	0.83	0.63	0.73	0.64	0.84	0.74	0.780 ± 0.072
Bootstrap	1	31	0.94	0.98	0.96	0.33	0.84	0.58	0.33	0.84	0.65	0.734 ± 0.200
	2	29	0.90	1.00	0.95	0.16	0.89	0.53	0.16	0.89	0.58	0.690 ± 0.228
	3	24	0.94	0.96	0.95	0.38	0.84	0.61	0.38	0.84	0.53	0.702 ± 0.220
	4	15	0.82	0.85	0.84	0.77	0.68	0.73	0.77	0.82	0.85	0.773 ± 0.059
	5	30	0.92	0.89	0.90	0.50	0.73	0.61	0.50	0.73	0.56	0.698 ± 0.183

n = features dimension, SE = sensitivity, SP = specificity, AUC = Area Under the Curve.

Features such as standard deviation RD, total power AP, and sex consistently appear in all selected optimal combinations. Regarding the sex variable, it was necessary to study its possible influence given the difference in the proportion of women with respect to men in the study sample. Therefore, a mean difference analysis was performed (see results in Table 4) showing that 8 of the 14 predictor variables show a statistically significant difference between sexes.

This finding suggests that the disproportionality in the sample could introduce a bias in the generalization of the classifier's results. However, it is pertinent to note that it has previously been suggested [41] that sex could be a relevant predictor to characterize the fall risk. In the context of the Bayesian paradigm, the conditional and marginal probabilities associated with sex could significantly contribute to the precise discrimination of fall risk classes. Nevertheless, to study the true influence of sex, it is necessary to increase the dataset heterogeneously, which underscores the importance of generating new public stabilometric datasets in biomedical research.

On the other hand, Figure 3 shows the performance of the SA algorithm of the AUC mean value concerning the size of the dimensions, where no general trend is observed. This is confirmed by a correlation coefficient value of −0.083. However, the performance of the classifier was inversely correlated with the solution space, with a value of −0.303.

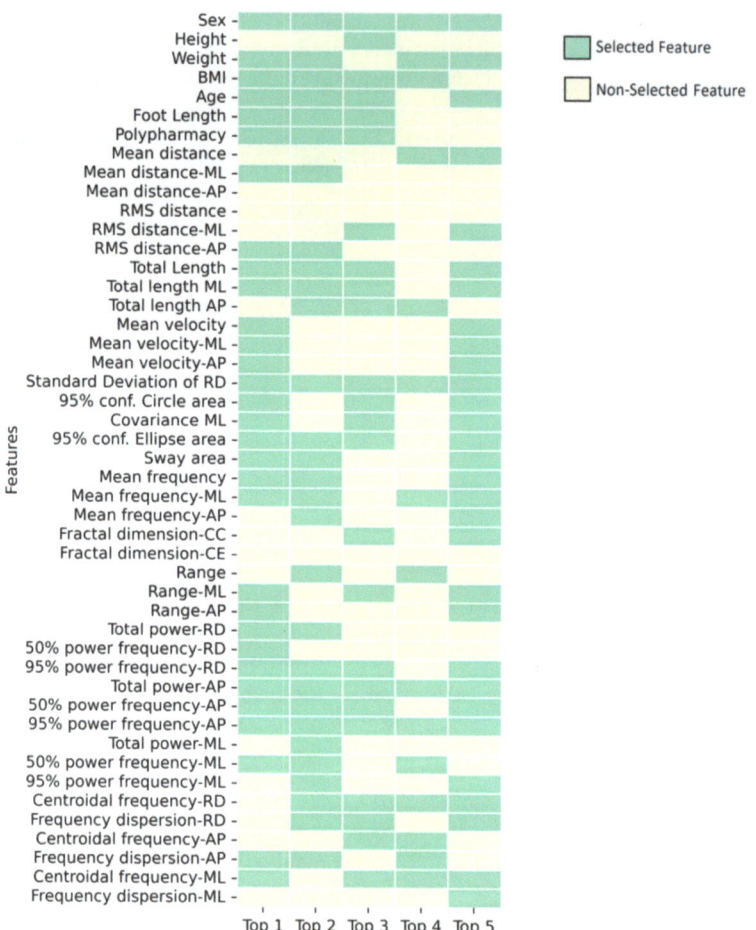

Figure 2. Set of features that integrate the best-performance results in feature selection.

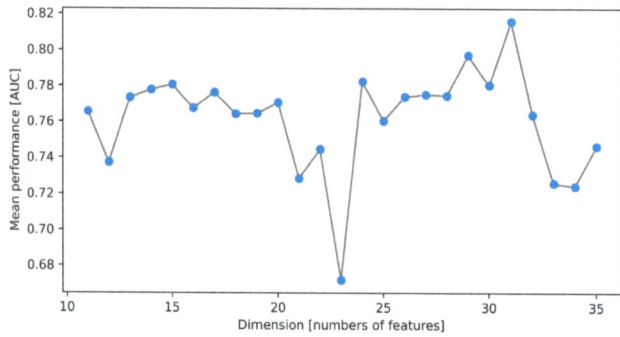

Figure 3. Performance of the SA algorithm based on the AUC value with respect to the dimension size.

Table 4. Descriptive analysis of the Top 4 predictor variables by sex.

	Total	Male	Female	p-Value Means Difference Test
	n = 181	n = 34	n = 147	
Weight [kg]	62.99 ± 8.4	67.89 ± 7.05	61.86 ± 8.3	0.000 *
BMI [kg/m^2]	25.55 ± 2.9	24.3 ± 1.89	25.83 ± 3.02	0.000 *
Mean distance [mm]	5.17 ± 2.45	6.87 ± 3.87	4.78 ± 1.79	0.004 *
Total length AP [mm]	324.71 ± 158.25	411.47 ± 215.79	304.64 ± 134.88	0.009 *
Standard deviation of RD [mm]	2.95 ± 1.48	3.93 ± 2.49	2.72 ± 1.01	0.009 *
Mean frequency-ML [Hz]	4.55 ± 1.81	4.1 ± 1.22	4.65 ± 1.92	0.040 *
Range [mm]	28.5 ± 13.39	37.35 ± 23.01	26.45 ± 8.89	0.010 *
Total power-AP [mm^2/Hz]	22.43 ± 19.49	35.03 ± 24.25	19.51 ± 17.03	0.001 *
95% power frequency-AP [Hz]	9.83 ± 2.5	9.47 ± 2.98	9.91 ± 2.38	0.418
50% power frequency-AP [Hz]	2.66 ± 1.96	2.51 ± 2.08	2.69 ± 1.94	0.458
Centroidal frequency-RD [Hz]	7.08 ± 2.05	6.56 ± 1.55	7.2 ± 2.13	0.101
Centroidal frequency-AP [Hz]	5.42 ± 1.57	5.21 ± 1.83	5.47 ± 1.51	0.390
Frequency dispersion-ML [-]	5.88 ± 1.55	5.4 ± 1.7	5.98 ± 1.5	0.847
Centroidal frequency-ML [Hz]	7.4 ± 0.89	7.43 ± 0.91	7.39 ± 0.89	0.074

* p-value < 0.05.

Moreover, the univariate logistic regression models generated for each feature presented a maximum performance for the centroidal frequency-RD CoP index, with AUC's mean and standard deviation of 0.623 ± 0.107 for train, test, and validation sets. The complete results of the logistic regressions are available in Table A4.

4. Discussion

There are clinical tools that are able to predict the fall risk with the help of expert evaluators' judgments based on extensive questionnaires to which elderly patients often do not know how to respond with certainty, and may also involve the execution of physical tests that may generate stress or fear, so previous factors alter the reliability of the results [42–46]. On the other hand, the use of stabilometry allows for a CoP index calculation that provides quantitative data to obtain more objective results, which, in combination with patient descriptive variables and heuristic search methods, can be useful for fall risk prediction based on computational classifier models.

The predictive capacity of classifiers based on Machine Learning benefits from feature selection, which aims at extracting the most explanatory data of the phenomenon to be predicted, and eliminating irrelevant and redundant data to reduce the dimensionality (number of features to be used) of the classifiers [47]. SA is a metaheuristic search algorithm analogously inspired by the statistical physics of heating and cooling annealing processes in metals, which can find an optimal cost function value in a large solution space. Its performance and relative ease of application have made it one of the most popular techniques for solving combinatorial problems, including feature selection [39,48,49].

Feature selection methods can be divided into filter, wrapper, and embedded methods. Filter methods perform the selection based on statistical tests such as correlations, goodness of fit, significance of coefficients, etc. On the other hand, wrapper methods select the best features by optimizing the performance of a previously chosen classification algorithm, as in the case of the Bayesian classifier optimized by SA. On the contrary, in embedded methods, feature selection is integrated in the classifier algorithm, since during the training step, its parameters are adjusted by determining the importance of each feature to produce the best diagnostic capacity [47]. Previous findings suggest that wrapper methods perform best in identifying fall risk using Machine Learning and/or statistical models [20].

This study used 47 features, of which 7 were related to participant information and 40 CoP indices, including time, frequency, and hybrid domain metrics. These were used to generate classification models based on Bayesian techniques optimized by SA, which were subsequently compared with feature selection techniques based on filter methods and univariate logistic regression models.

The best performance of the univariate logistic regression models was the centroidal frequency-RD index, which matched the selection of the Hosmer–Lemeshow goodness-of-fit methods and the mean difference test; however, its performance was poor (maximum mean AUC and standard deviation of 0.623 ± 0.107 for the training, test, and validation sets). Comparatively, the SA algorithm showed the ability to automatically identify the set of descriptor characteristics for fall risk, maximizing the diagnostic capability. Although the highest performance was presented when the algorithm selected 31 characteristics (Top 1), the results that presented less variability in the phenomenon to be predicted were given when the algorithm selected 15 characteristics (Top 4). Among these selection proposals, there was a difference of 0.035 between the diagnostic capabilities given by their AUC means.

Compared to previous studies, the predictive model proposed in Top 1 demonstrates an AUC performance improvement of at least 6.5%. Table 5 provides a detailed comparison with other works that have used static stabilometry to classify fall risk through computational or statistical methods.

Table 5. State-of-the-art performance of classifiers for fall risk detection, balance alteration, and fall history.

Work (Year)	Technology	Stabilometric Test	Dataset	Sample Size	Pre-Processing	Algorithm	Label	Validation Method	Performance
Top 1 (This work)	Force platform (OPT400600-1000) 100 Hz	Static test with open eyes	[26]	76 older adults	Compute CoP indices	BC and SA	Fall risk (FH + FES score)	60-20-20 hold-out	AUC: 0.815 SE: 0.783 SP: 0.847
Top 4 (This work)	Force platform (OPT400600-1000) 100 Hz	Static test with open eyes	[26]	76 older adults	Compute CoP indices	BC and SA	Fall risk (FH + Short FES-I)	60-20-20 hold-out	AUC: 0.780 SE: 0.818 SP: 0.741
[23] (2021)	Force platform (OPT400600-1000) 100 Hz	Static test with open and close eyes on soft and hard surface	[26]	76 older adults	Empirical Mode DeComposition, and compute CoP indices	RF	Fall risk (FH + Short FES-I e)	80-20 hold-out	SE: 0.760 SP: 0.860 ACC: 0.820
[15] (2016)	Wii Balance Board 25 Hz	Static test with open and close eyes	Own	80 older adults	Compute CoP indices	Raking Forest	FH	70-30 hold-out	AUC: 0.750
[20] (2019)	Force platform (OPT400600-1000) 100 Hz	Static test with open and close eyes on soft and hard surface	[26]	76 older adults	Compute CoP indices	MLP SVM NB K-NN and Feature selection	Fall risk (FH + Short FES-I)	80-20 hold-out	AUC: 0.710 ACC: 0.800
[50] (2018)	Force platform (OPT400600-1000) 100 Hz	Static test with open and close eyes on soft and hard surface	[26]	163 people between 18 and 85 years old	Compute CoP indices	K-NN DTs MLP NB RF SVM	Fall risk (HF + MiniBEST)	10-Fold	ACC: 0.649
[24] (2021)	Force platform (AccuSway) 120 Hz	Static test with open and close eyes	Own	126 older women with osteoporosis	Compute CoP indices, and data balancing	NB SVM AdaBoost K-NN	FH	10-Fold	SE: 0.810 SP: 0.190
[17] (2016)	Force platform (Advenced Mechanical Technology) 100 Hz	Static test with open and close eyes	Own	76 older adults	Compute CoP indices	LR	FH	None	AUC: 0.900
[51] (2022)	Wii Balance Board 50 Hz	Static test with open and close eyes	Own	46 older adults	Compute CoP indices	LR	Balance deficit (4-stage balance)	None	AUC: 0.770 SE: 0.930 SP: 0.620

Table 5. Cont.

Work (Year)	Technology	Stabilometric Test	Dataset	Sample Size	Pre-Processing	Algorithm	Label	Validation Method	Performance
[52] (2013)	Force platform (Tecnobody) 20 Hz	Static test with open and close eyes	Own	100 older adults	Compute CoP indices	LR	FH	None	SE: 0.880 SP: 0.670
[21] (2018)	Force platform (EMG system do Brasil) 100 Hz	Unipodal static test	Own	170 older adults	Compute CoP indices	ROC	FH	None	AUC: 0.720 SE: 0.660 SP: 0.680
[16] (2021)	Wii Balance Board 50 Hz	Static test with open and close eyes	Own	497 older adults	Compute CoP indices	LR	Balance alteration (4-stage balance)	None	AUC: 0.710 SE: 0.490 SP: 0.830
[19] (2015)	Wii Balance Board	Static test with open eyes	Own	73 older adults	Compute CoP indices	LR	FH	None	AUC: 0.71
[18] (2017)	Wii Balance Board 100 Hz	Static test with open and close eyes	Own	100 older adults	Compute CoP indices	Discriminant analysis	FH	None	SE: 0.710 SP: 0.570
[53] (2020)	Force platform (SmartScale-Zibro) 60 Hz	Static test with open eyes	Own	412 older adults	Compute CoP indices	ROC	FH	None	AUC: 0.640 SE: 0.640 SP: 0.590

For algorithm: BC = Bayesian classifier, SA = Simulated Annealing, RF = Random Forest, MLP = Multi-Layer Perceptron, SVM = Support Vector Machine, NB = Naïve Bayes, KNN = K-Nearest Neighbor, DTs = Decision Trees, LR = Logistic Regression, ROC = Receiver Operating Characteristic analysis. For labels: FH = fall history, Short FES-I = Short Falls Efficacy Scale-International, MiniBEST = Mini-Balance Evaluation Systems Test. For performance: SE = sensitivity, SP = specificity, AUC = Area Under the Curve, ACC = accuracy.

Features such as sex, weight, BMI, mean distance, total length AP, standard deviation of RD, mean frequency-ML, range, total power-AP, 95% power frequency-AP, 50% power frequency-ML, centroidal frequency-RD, centroidal frequency-AP, frequency dispersion-AP, and centroidal frequency-ML compose the optimal combination (Top 4). Of these, only the features sex, weight, BMI, and total length-AP were included in the initial proposed solution based on the state of the art. This demonstrates the ability of the SA algorithm to overcome local optima by selecting features that maximize the cost function.

On the other hand, in our previous findings [51], the range, total power-AP, and standard deviation of RD indices were included among the 10 CoP indices with the highest AUC for identifying balance alterations in older adults with a high prevalence of poor physical performance identifying the optimal cut-off point, while the total power-AP, 95% power frequency-AP, and centroidal frequency-AP indices were associated with the prediction of balance alterations in healthy older adults [16]. This supports 9 of the 15 characteristics selected by the SA algorithm, and with the inclusion of the 6 complementary ones, new evidence is provided for the understanding of the fall risk phenomenon in older adults. Furthermore, the current research suggests that frequency and hybrid CoP indices have equal or better descriptive power than time domain indices. However, their use is not as widespread in the state of the art, since due to the computational power, they need to be calculated, and most commercial systems are limited to providing CoP indicators in the time domain.

In other findings, an inverse correlation was observed between the size of the search space and the ability to select an optimal combination of the SA algorithm. In the present problem, the maximum search space was given by 5.38258×10^{11} of possible combinations corresponding to 21 dimensions, but as shown in Figure 3, as the SA algorithm approached this maximum and the number of dimensions increased, its performance decreased. This trend continued only up to 24 dimensions (Top 3), where the solution space was reduced to 3.53697×10^{11}. The performance of the cost function continued to improve as features were added to the classifier, from 24 up to 31. However, although the solution space kept decreasing for higher dimensions, the performance of the Bayesian classifier was affected.

This suggests the occurrence of the so-called "curse of dimensionality" starting from 31 or more features in this dataset.

A limitation of the present study was the use of CoP indices derived only from stabilometric tests under conditions of a firm surface and open eyes; however, this dataset was analyzed because it comes from a test that is simpler and faster to perform and may be generalizable not only to people of different ages, but also with different cognitive and physical abilities. In this context, to avoid a disproportionate increase in the solution space affecting the performance of the SA algorithm, the number of features was limited to the 47 commonly analyzed in the stabilometric domain. Based on the performance observed in the Top 4, it would be important to highlight that future studies could incorporate new nonlinear-type experimental features and apply advanced feature extraction techniques, such as Deep Learning, Genetic Programming, and Codebook-based approaches, which have been shown to perform well in other biomedical areas, such as gait analysis [27] and heart rate variability [54], among others. Another limitation of the study lies in the data sample analyzed, since it is relatively small and has a bias influenced by the predominance of the female ratio in the sample under study, with only 21.06% corresponding to information from men.

The observation of statistically significant sex differences in Top 4 predictor variables underscores the need to apply sex-stratified analyses in future research, provided that a more complete dataset is available. Such stratification could reveal sex-specific patterns that would otherwise be hidden in general analyses. Furthermore, these potential approaches could substantially improve both the predictive accuracy and clinical utility of fall risk assessment tools.

5. Conclusions

The results suggest that the SA algorithm is a useful tool to perform feature selection in Bayesian classifiers for the diagnosis of fall risk from CoP indices and patient descriptive variables. This is advantageous because it provides an alternative or complementary and generalized resource with an acceptable level of fall risk assessment for people for whom the physical activities involved in clinical tools may be challenging.

Supplementary Materials: Supporting information about the database, result tables, and source code can be downloaded from the public repository (https://github.com/enriquehdez98/Fall-Risk-Diagnosis-) on GitHub.

Author Contributions: Conceptualization, E.H.-L., Á.G.E.-P., L.M.S.-F. and L.P.-R.; methodology, E.H.-L., Á.G.E.-P., L.M.S.-F. and L.P.-R.; software, E.H.-L., Á.G.E.-P. and L.M.S.-F.; validation, L.M.S.-F. and L.P.-R.; formal analysis, E.H.-L., Á.G.E.-P. and L.M.S.-F.; investigation, E.H.-L. and Á.G.E.-P.; resources, E.H.-L., Á.G.E.-P. and L.P.-R.; data curation, E.H.-L. and L.M.S.-F.; writing—original draft preparation, E.H.-L., Á.G.E.-P., L.M.S.-F. and L.P.-R.; writing—review and editing, E.H.-L., Á.G.E.-P., L.M.S.-F. and L.P.-R.; visualization, E.H.-L. and Á.G.E.-P.; supervision, L.M.S.-F. and L.P.-R.; project administration, E.H.-L. and Á.G.E.-P.; funding acquisition, Á.G.E.-P. All authors have read and agreed to the published version of the manuscript.

Funding: The publication of this paper was supported by Universidad Autónoma del Estado de México, Mexico.

Institutional Review Board Statement: Not applicable.

Informed Consent Statement: Not applicable.

Data Availability Statement: Databases are anonymized and available as Supplementary Material.

Acknowledgments: We would like to extend our sincere gratitude to Lilyam Lizette Olmos García-Rojas for her invaluable support in the initial stage of the algorithm's programming. Her commitment and dedication were instrumental in the development of this research. In addition, we thank the "Sistemas Mecatrónicos y Computacionales Aplicados, UAEMéx-UAPT" academic team and its leader M.C.V.E., for providing the infrastructure to carry out this research.

Conflicts of Interest: The authors declare no conflicts of interest.

Appendix A

Table A1. Statistical analysis of the CoP indices.

CoP Index	Total $n = 181$	Non-Fall Risk $n = 94$	Fall Risk $n = 87$	KS Test p-Value	MD Test p-Value	HL Test p-Value	AUC (95% CI)
Mean distance [mm]	5.16 ± 2.45	4.95 ± 2.02	5.39 ± 2.83	0.000 *	0.322	0.828	0.542 (0.457–0.627)
Mean distance-ML [mm]	4.00 ± 2.15	3.84 ± 1.83	4.17 ± 2.44	0.000 *	0.339	0.515	0.541 (0.456–0.625)
Mean distance-AP [mm]	2.46 ± 1.18	2.35 ± 0.98	2.57 ± 1.36	0.000 *	0.430	0.824	0.534 (0.449–0.618)
RMS distance [mm]	5.96 ± 2.83	5.71 ± 2.29	6.23 ± 3.31	0.000 *	0.318	0.503	0.543 (0.458–0.627)
RMS distance-ML mm]	5.00 ± 2.65	4.78 ± 2.16	5.24 ± 3.09	0.000 *	0.303	0.43	0.544 (0.459–0.628)
RMS distance-AP [mm]	3.08 ± 1.42	2.97 ± 1.24	3.2 ± 1.59	0.000 *	0.448	0.448	0.532 (0.447–0.617)
Total Length [mm]	713.92 ± 333.48	694.21 ± 269.03	735.22 ± 391.93	0.000 *	0.607	0.116	0.477 (0.391–0.564)
Total length ML [mm]	563.81 ± 272.52	536.17 ± 217.65	593.67 ± 320.13	0.000 *	0.943	0.015 *	0.503 (0.414–0.591)
Total length AP [mm]	324.71 ± 158.24	330.34 ± 141.11	318.62 ± 175.51	0.000 *	0.161	0.026 *	0.439 (0.355–0.524)
Mean velocity [mm/s]	11.89 ± 5.55	11.57 ± 4.48	12.25 ± 6.53	0.000 *	0.607	0.116	0.477 (0.391–0.564)
Mean velocity-ML [mm/s]	9.39 ± 4.54	8.93 ± 3.62	9.89 ± 5.33	0.000 *	0.943	0.015 *	0.503 (0.414–0.591)
Mean velocity-AP [mm/s]	5.41 ± 2.63	5.5 ± 2.35	5.31 ± 2.92	0.000 *	0.161	0.026 *	0.439 (0.355–0.524)
Standard deviation of RD [mm]	2.94 ± 1.47	2.82 ± 1.13	3.08 ± 1.77	0.000 *	0.267	0.465	0.547 (0.463–0.632)
95% conf. Circle area [mm^2]	38.79 ± 55.95	33.49 ± 31.05	44.52 ± 73.8	0.000 *	0.276	0.586	0.547 (0.462–0.631)
Covariance ML [mm^2]	0.01 ± 0.87	0.11 ± 0.84	-0.09 ± 0.9	0.000 *	0.214	0.848	0.446 (0.362–0.53)
95% conf. Ellipse area [mm^2]	31.48 ± 37.62	27.33 ± 23.57	35.97 ± 48.19	0.000 *	0.214	0.15	0.553 (0.468–0.638)
Sway area [mm^2/s]	2.01 ± 2.35	1.78 ± 1.46	2.26 ± 3.02	0.000 *	0.619	0.46	0.521 (0.435–0.607)
Mean frequency [Hz]	3.90 ± 1.43	3.97 ± 1.37	3.82 ± 1.51	0.000 *	0.181	0.299	0.442 (0.357–0.527)
Mean frequency-ML [Hz]	4.54 ± 1.81	4.55 ± 1.75	4.53 ± 1.89	0.000 *	0.718	0.597	0.484 (0.399–0.569)
Mean frequency-AP [Hz]	4.19 ± 1.70	4.39 ± 1.72	3.96 ± 1.67	0.000 *	0.079	0.427	0.424 (0.34–0.508)
Fractal dimension-CC [-]	17.04 ± 1.18	17.12 ± 1.15	16.95 ± 1.22	0.027 *	0.205	0.028 *	0.445 (0.36–0.53)

Table A1. *Cont.*

CoP Index	Total	Non-Fall Risk	Fall Risk	KS Test	MD Test	HL Test	AUC (95% CI)
	$n = 181$	$n = 94$	$n = 87$	p-Value	p-Value	p-Value	
Fractal dimension-CE [-]	17.29 ± 1.13	17.38 ± 1.05	17.2 ± 1.21	0.025 *	0.092	0.217	0.427 (0.342–0.512)
Range [mm]	28.50 ± 13.39	26.97 ± 9.75	30.15 ± 16.34	0.000 *	0.146	0.276	0.562 (0.478–0.647)
Range-ML [mm]	27.29 ± 13.28	25.66 ± 9.35	29.06 ± 16.39	0.000 *	0.119	0.029 *	0.567 (0.482–0.651)
Range-AP [mm]	16.82 ± 7.23	16.51 ± 6.89	17.15 ± 7.61	0.000 *	0.723	0.248	0.515 (0.43–0.6)
Total power-RD [mm^2/Hz]	32.63 ± 56.53	25.7 ± 18.25	40.12 ± 78.86	0.000 *	0.097	0.908	0.571 (0.487–0.655)
50% power frequency-RD [Hz]	3.21 ± 1.86	3.45 ± 1.88	2.94 ± 1.8	0.000 *	0.023 *	0.78	0.402 (0.319–0.485)
95% power frequency-RD [Hz]	14.10 ± 4.05	14.61 ± 3.75	13.54 ± 4.29	0.002 *	0.032 *	0.044 *	0.407 (0.323–0.492)
Total power-AP [mm^2/Hz]	22.42 ± 19.49	21.6 ± 18.89	23.31 ± 20.19	0.000 *	0.727	0.452	0.515 (0.43–0.599)
50% power frequency-AP [Hz]	2.65 ± 1.96	2.91 ± 2.09	2.38 ± 1.77	0.000 *	0.039 *	0.077	0.411 (0.328–0.494)
95% power frequency-AP [Hz]	9.82 ± 2.50	9.91 ± 2.44	9.73 ± 2.57	0.200	0.639	0.191	0.48 (0.395–0.565)
Total power-ML [mm^2/Hz]	63.14 ± 114.63	45.52 ± 32.64	82.17 ± 160.14	0.000 *	0.048 *	0.996	0.585 (0.501–0.668)
50% power frequency-ML [Hz]	2.61 ± 1.80	2.8 ± 1.84	2.41 ± 1.74	0.000 *	0.056	0.425	0.417 (0.334–0.501)
95% power frequency-ML [Hz]	10.99 ± 2.76	11.38 ± 2.57	10.57 ± 2.9	0.200	0.048 *	0.24	0.442 (0.357–0.526)
Centroidal frequency-RD [Hz]	7.08 ± 2.04	7.37 ± 1.94	6.75 ± 2.11	0.028 *	0.017 *	0.172	0.396 (0.313–0.48)
Frequency dispersion-RD [-]	7.32 ± 0.61	7.27 ± 0.65	7.38 ± 0.56	0.005 *	0.188	0.628	0.556 (0.472–0.64)
Centroidal frequency-AP [Hz]	5.41 ± 1.57	5.61 ± 1.6	5.2 ± 1.51	0.013 *	0.090	0.054	0.427 (0.343–0.51)
Frequency dispersion-AP [-]	7.27 ± 1.06	7.13 ± 1.09	7.42 ± 1.01	0.000 *	0.034 *	0.400	0.591 (0.508–0.674)
Centroidal frequency-ML [Hz]	5.87 ± 1.54	6.12 ± 1.45	5.6 ± 1.6	0.200	0.022 *	0.081	0.418 (0.334–0.502)
Frequency dispersion-ML [-]	7.39 ± 0.89	7.35 ± 0.89	7.44 ± 0.89	0.000 *	0.371	0.088	0.538 (0.453–0.623)

n = sample size, KS = Kolmogorov–Smirnov, MD = mean difference, HL = Hosmer–Lemeshow, CI = confidence interval, * p-value < 0.05

Table A2. Bayesian classifier performance results using Simulated Annealing.

n	Combination of Optimal Features	Train			Test			Validation		
		SE	SP	AUC	SE	SP	AUC	SE	SP	AUC
11	1, 2, 15, 19, 20, 21, 36, 37, 43, 44, 45	0.769	0.75	0.759	0.888	0.736	0.812	0.764	0.684	0.724
12	1, 2, 4, 10, 16, 17, 23, 30, 34, 37, 42, 47	0.75	0.821	0.785	0.777	0.631	0.704	0.705	0.736	0.721
13	1, 4, 5, 16, 17, 18, 22, 29, 30, 37, 42, 44, 47	0.865	0.75	0.807	0.833	0.631	0.732	0.823	0.736	0.78
14	1, 3, 4, 8, 12, 16, 18, 22, 35, 36, 37, 42, 44, 47	0.788	0.803	0.796	0.888	0.684	0.786	0.764	0.736	0.75
15	1, 3, 4, 8, 16, 20, 26, 30, 36, 38, 40, 42, 44, 45, 46	0.807	0.857	0.832	0.944	0.631	0.788	0.705	0.736	0.721
16	1, 2, 4, 6, 7, 12, 13, 16, 17, 20, 22, 27, 32, 38, 42, 43	0.846	0.803	0.824	0.722	0.736	0.729	0.705	0.789	0.747
17	1, 2, 4, 5, 7, 9, 13, 17, 22, 27, 30, 35, 37, 38, 40, 43, 47	0.884	0.821	0.853	0.666	0.736	0.701	0.705	0.842	0.773
18	1, 3, 4, 6, 7, 8, 11, 19, 20, 24, 27, 28, 30, 34, 36, 38, 40, 42	0.711	0.857	0.784	0.777	0.736	0.757	0.764	0.736	0.75
19	2, 4, 5, 6, 7, 9, 10, 11, 13, 14, 16, 20, 32, 33, 34, 36, 40, 42, 47	0.788	0.892	0.84	0.666	0.684	0.675	0.764	0.789	0.777
20	1, 3, 4, 6, 7, 10, 11, 14, 15, 18, 20, 22, 24, 31, 34, 35, 37, 42, 44, 47	1	0.696	0.848	0.722	0.631	0.676	0.941	0.631	0.786
21	1, 2, 4, 5, 6, 11, 14, 15, 16, 20, 21, 22, 23, 24, 35, 36, 37, 39, 40, 41, 45	0.826	0.75	0.788	0.777	0.631	0.704	0.647	0.736	0.691
22	1, 2, 3, 5, 12, 16, 20, 21, 22, 25, 26, 27, 28, 30, 31, 34, 38, 40, 44, 45, 46, 47	0.903	0.714	0.809	0.722	0.684	0.703	0.705	0.736	0.721
23	1, 2, 6, 9, 10, 11, 13, 14, 15, 16, 18, 23, 26, 29, 32, 34, 38, 39, 40, 41, 42, 45, 47	0.634	0.714	0.674	0.666	0.684	0.675	0.647	0.684	0.665
24	1, 2, 4, 5, 6, 7, 12, 14, 15, 16, 20, 21, 22, 23, 28, 31, 35, 36, 37, 38, 42, 43, 44, 46	0.884	0.91	0.897	0.666	0.736	0.701	0.705	0.789	0.747
25	1, 3, 5, 10, 12, 16, 17, 18, 19, 20, 21, 22, 23, 24, 25, 26, 28, 32, 35, 36, 38, 41, 42, 44, 45	0.826	0.839	0.833	0.722	0.789	0.755	0.647	0.736	0.691
26	1, 2, 3, 5, 7, 9, 10, 12, 15, 18, 20, 21, 22, 24, 25, 26, 27, 31, 32, 34, 37, 38, 40, 44, 46, 47	0.98	0.75	0.865	0.777	0.631	0.704	0.764	0.736	0.75
27	2, 3, 5, 6, 12, 13, 15, 16, 17, 20, 21, 22, 23, 24, 25, 26, 27, 30, 33, 35, 36, 37, 38, 40, 42, 43, 47	0.846	0.839	0.842	0.666	0.736	0.701	0.823	0.736	0.78
28	1, 2, 4, 5, 6, 7, 10, 12, 13, 14, 15, 16, 17, 22, 25, 26, 27, 28, 31, 32, 33, 35, 37, 38, 40, 41, 42, 43	0.961	0.785	0.873	0.777	0.631	0.704	0.647	0.842	0.744
29	1, 3, 4, 5, 6, 7, 9, 13, 14, 15, 16, 20, 23, 24, 25, 26, 27, 30, 33, 35, 36, 37, 38, 39, 40, 41, 42, 43, 45	0.923	0.91	0.916	0.722	0.684	0.703	0.647	0.894	0.77
30	1, 3, 5, 8, 12, 14, 15, 17, 18, 19, 20, 21, 22, 23, 24, 25, 26, 27, 28, 31, 32, 35, 36, 37, 38, 41, 42, 43, 46, 47	0.923	0.803	0.863	0.833	0.631	0.732	0.647	0.842	0.744
31	1, 3, 4, 5, 6, 7, 9, 13, 14, 15, 17, 18, 19, 20, 21, 22, 23, 24, 25, 26, 31, 32, 33, 34, 35, 36, 37, 38, 40, 45, 46	0.923	0.964	0.943	0.722	0.789	0.755	0.705	0.789	0.747
32	2, 4, 5, 6, 7, 8, 11, 13, 15, 16, 17, 18, 19, 21, 22, 23, 24, 25, 26, 28, 32, 36, 37, 38, 40, 41, 42, 43, 44, 45, 46, 47	1	0.785	0.892	0.722	0.684	0.703	0.705	0.684	0.695
33	1, 3, 4, 5, 6, 7, 10, 12, 14, 15, 16, 17, 18, 19, 21, 22, 23, 24, 25, 26, 27, 30, 34, 35, 36, 37, 38, 39, 40, 41, 44, 45, 47	0.769	0.785	0.777	0.777	0.631	0.704	0.705	0.684	0.695
34	1, 4, 5, 6, 10, 11, 12, 14, 15, 16, 17, 19, 20, 21, 22, 23, 24, 25, 26, 28, 30, 31, 32, 34, 36, 37, 38, 39, 40, 42, 43, 44, 45, 47	0.807	0.857	0.832	0.611	0.684	0.647	0.647	0.736	0.691
35	1, 3, 4, 5, 6, 7, 13, 14, 15, 16, 17, 18, 19, 20, 21, 22, 23, 24, 26, 28, 29, 30, 31, 32, 34, 35, 36, 38, 39, 40, 41, 43, 44, 46, 47	0.865	0.821	0.843	0.722	0.684	0.703	0.647	0.736	0.691

n = features dimension, SE = sensitivity, SP = specificity, AUC = Area Under the Curve.

Table A3. Dictionary Bayesian classifier performance results using Simulated Annealing.

Feature	Label Meaning
1	Sex
2	Height [cm]
3	Weight [kg]
4	BMI [kg/m^2]
5	Age [years]
6	Foot length [cm]
7	Polypharmacy
8	Mean distance [mm]
9	Mean distance-ML [mm]
10	Mean distance-AP [mm]
11	RMS distance [mm]
12	RMS distance-ML [mm]
13	RMS distance-AP [mm]
14	Total Length [mm]
15	Total length ML [mm]
16	Total length AP [mm]
17	Mean velocity [mm/s]
18	Mean velocity-ML [mm/s]
19	Mean velocity-AP [mm/s]
20	Standard deviation of RD [mm]
21	95% conf. circle area [mm^2]
22	Covariance ML [mm^2]
23	95% conf. ellipse area [mm^2]
24	Sway area [mm^2/s]
25	Mean frequency [Hz]
26	Mean frequency-ML [Hz]
27	Mean frequency-AP [Hz]
28	Fractal dimension-CC [-]
29	Fractal dimension-CE [-]
30	Range [mm]
31	Range-ML [mm]
32	Range-AP [mm]
33	Total power-RD [mm^2/Hz]
34	50% power frequency-RD [Hz]
35	95% power frequency-RD [Hz]
36	Total power-AP [mm^2/Hz]
37	50% power frequency-AP [Hz]
38	95% power frequency-AP [Hz]
39	Total power-ML [mm^2/Hz]
40	50% power frequency-ML [Hz]
41	95% power frequency-ML [Hz]
42	Centroidal frequency-RD [Hz]
43	Frequency dispersion-RD [-]
44	Centroidal frequency-AP [Hz]
45	Frequency dispersion-AP [-]
46	Centroidal frequency-ML [Hz]
47	Frequency dispersion-ML [-]

Table A4. Logistic regression performance.

Feature	Train			Test			Validation		
	SE	SP	AUC	SE	SP	AUC	SE	SP	AUC
Sex	0.903	0.303	0.603	1.000	0.210	0.605	0.941	0.368	0.654
Height [cm]	0.538	0.553	0.546	0.333	0.473	0.403	0.294	0.526	0.410
Weight [kg]	0.480	0.642	0.561	0.222	0.368	0.295	0.411	0.684	0.547
BMI [kg/m^2]	0	1	0.5	0	1	0.5	0	1	0.5
Age [years]	0.250	0.821	0.535	0.388	0.789	0.589	0.235	0.894	0.565
Foot length [cm]	0.557	0.66	0.609	0.444	0.526	0.485	0.470	0.789	0.630
Polypharmacy	0.423	0.75	0.586	0.333	0.684	0.508	0.470	0.578	0.524
Mean distance [mm]	0.230	0.821	0.526	0.222	0.842	0.532	0.058	0.789	0.424
Mean distance-ML [mm]	0.250	0.839	0.544	0.111	0.789	0.450	0.294	0.789	0.541
Mean distance-AP [mm]	0.192	0.857	0.524	0.277	0.894	0.586	0.058	0.789	0.424
RMS distance [mm]	0.250	0.839	0.544	0.222	0.842	0.532	0.058	0.789	0.424
RMS distance-ML [mm]	0.250	0.821	0.535	0.111	0.789	0.450	0.235	0.789	0.512
RMS distance-AP [mm]	0.192	0.875	0.533	0.222	0.947	0.584	0.058	0.842	0.450
Total length [mm]	0.307	0.839	0.573	0.166	0.736	0.451	0.117	0.789	0.453
Total length ML [mm]	0.423	0.839	0.631	0.166	0.736	0.451	0.176	0.842	0.509
Total length AP [mm]	0	1	0.5	0	1	0.5	0	1	0.5
Mean velocity [mm/s]	0.307	0.839	0.573	0.166	0.736	0.451	0.117	0.789	0.453
Mean velocity-ML [mm/s]	0.423	0.839	0.631	0.166	0.736	0.451	0.176	0.842	0.509
Mean velocity-AP [mm/s]	0	1	0.5	0	1	0.5	0	1	0.5
Standard deviation of RD [mm]	0.134	0.821	0.478	0.222	0.842	0.532	0.176	0.842	0.509
95% conf. circle area [mm^2]	0.096	0.857	0.476	0.166	0.842	0.504	0.058	0.842	0.45
Covariance ML [mm^2]	0.269	0.803	0.536	0.222	0.789	0.505	0.294	0.789	0.541
95% conf. ellipse area [mm^2]	0.134	0.892	0.513	0.222	0.947	0.584	0.058	0.842	0.450
Sway area [mm^2/s]	0.230	0.857	0.543	0.111	0.947	0.529	0.176	0.894	0.535
Mean frequency [Hz]	0.250	0.839	0.544	0.166	0.684	0.425	0.176	0.789	0.482
Mean frequency-ML [Hz]	0.326	0.767	0.547	0.333	0.473	0.403	0.176	0.736	0.456
Mean frequency-AP [Hz]	0.365	0.660	0.513	0.388	0.789	0.589	0.529	0.631	0.58
Fractal dimension-CC [-]	0.057	0.982	0.519	0	0.947	0.473	0	0.947	0.473
Fractal dimension-CE [-]	0.076	0.982	0.529	0	0.947	0.473	0	0.894	0.447
Range [mm]	0.230	0.821	0.526	0.166	0.789	0.478	0.294	0.842	0.568
Range-ML [mm]	0.326	0.803	0.565	0.222	0.789	0.505	0.235	0.842	0.538
Range-AP [mm]	0.019	0.982	0.5	0	1	0.5	0	1	0.5
Total power-RD [mm^2/Hz]	0.211	0.857	0.534	0.111	0.894	0.502	0.176	0.894	0.535
50% power frequency-RD [Hz]	0.480	0.678	0.579	0.444	0.631	0.538	0.647	0.473	0.560
95% power frequency-RD [Hz]	0.250	0.892	0.571	0.333	0.894	0.614	0.470	0.842	0.656
Total power-AP [mm^2/Hz]	0.250	0.857	0.553	0.055	0.947	0.501	0.058	0.947	0.503
50% power frequency-AP [Hz]	0.576	0.553	0.565	0.611	0.315	0.463	0.764	0.526	0.645
95% power frequency-AP [Hz]	0.019	1	0.509	0	1	0.5	0	0.947	0.473
Total power-ML [mm^2/Hz]	0.269	0.892	0.581	0.166	0.894	0.53	0.176	0.789	0.482
50% power frequency-ML [Hz]	0.480	0.642	0.561	0.444	0.736	0.59	0.588	0.526	0.557
95% power frequency-ML [Hz]	0.365	0.714	0.539	0.333	0.631	0.482	0.411	0.684	0.547
Centroidal frequency-RD [Hz]	0.384	0.732	0.558	0.444	0.684	0.564	0.705	0.789	0.747
Frequency dispersion-RD [-]	0.250	0.732	0.491	0.444	0.789	0.616	0.529	0.631	0.58
Centroidal frequency-AP [Hz]	0.423	0.714	0.568	0.444	0.578	0.511	0.588	0.684	0.636
Frequency dispersion-AP [-]	0.538	0.553	0.546	0.555	0.473	0.514	0.647	0.421	0.534
Centroidal frequency-ML [Hz]	0.403	0.678	0.541	0.388	0.684	0.536	0.529	0.578	0.554
Frequency dispersion-ML [-]	0.192	0.875	0.533	0.222	0.947	0.584	0.294	0.789	0.541

SE = sensitivity, SP = specificity, AUC = Area Under the Curve.

References

1. World Health Organization: Falls. Available online: https://www.who.int/news-room/fact-sheets/detail/falls (accessed on 24 March 2024).
2. Talbot, L.A.; Musiol, R.J.; Witham, E.K.; Metter, E.J. Falls in Young, Middle-Aged and Older Community Dwelling Adults: Perceived Cause, Environmental Factors and Injury. *BMC Public Health* **2005**, *5*, 86. [CrossRef] [PubMed]
3. WHO. *WHO Global Report on Falls Prevention in Older Age*; WHO Library Cataloguing-in-Publication Data: Geneva, Switzerland, 2008; ISBN 978 92 4 156353 6.

4. Sun, R.; Sosnoff, J.J. Novel Sensing Technology in Fall Risk Assessment in Older Adults: A Systematic Review. *BMC Geriatr.* **2018**, *18*, 14. [CrossRef] [PubMed]
5. Fabre, J.M.; Ellis, R.; Kosma, M.; Wood, R.H. Falls Risk Factors and a Compendium of Falls Risk Screening Instruments. *J. Geriatr. Phys. Ther.* **2010**, *33*, 184–197. [CrossRef] [PubMed]
6. Mancini, M.; Horak, F.B. The Relevance of Clinical Balance Assessment Tools to Differentiate Balance Deficits. *Eur. J. Phys. Rehabil. Med.* **2010**, *46*, 239. [PubMed]
7. Cho, H.Y.; Heijnen, M.J.H.; Craig, B.A.; Rietdyk, S. Falls in Young Adults: The Effect of Sex, Physical Activity, and Prescription Medications. *PLoS ONE* **2021**, *16*, e0250360. [CrossRef]
8. Gallouj, K.; Altintas, E.; El Haj, M. "I Remember the Fall": Memory of Falls in Older Adults. *Clin. Gerontol.* **2023**, *46*, 695–703. [CrossRef]
9. Paillard, T.; Noé, F. Techniques and Methods for Testing the Postural Function in Healthy and Pathological Subjects. *BioMed Res. Int.* **2015**, *2015*, 891390. [CrossRef]
10. Clark, R.A.; Mentiplay, B.F.; Pua, Y.H.; Bower, K.J. Reliability and Validity of the Wii Balance Board for Assessment of Standing Balance: A Systematic Review. *Gait Posture* **2018**, *61*, 40–54. [CrossRef]
11. Hernandez-Laredo, E.; Parra-Rodríguez, L.; Estévez-Pedraza, Á.G.; Martínez-Méndez, R. A Low-Cost, IoT-Connected Force Platform for Fall Risk Assessment in Older Adults. In Proceedings of the XLVI Mexican Conference on Biomedical Engineering; Flores Cuautle, J.D.J.A., Benítez-Mata, B., Salido-Ruiz, R.A., Alonso-Silverio, G.A., Dorantes-Méndez, G., Zúñiga-Aguilar, E., Vélez-Pérez, H.A., et al., Eds.; Springer Nature: Cham, Switzerland, 2024; pp. 374–385.
12. Terekhov, Y. Stabilometry as a Diagnostic Tool in Clinical Medicine. *Can. Med. Assoc. J.* **1976**, *115*, 631–633.
13. Palmieri, R.M.; Ingersoll, C.D.; Stone, M.B.; Krause, B.A. Center-of-Pressure Parameters Used in the Assessment of Postural Control. *J. Sport Rehabil.* **2002**, *11*, 51–66. [CrossRef]
14. Prieto, T.E.; Myklebust, J.B.; Hoffmann, R.G.; Lovett, E.G.; Myklebust, B.M. Measures of Postural Steadiness: Differences between Healthy Young and Elderly Adults. *IEEE Trans. Biomed. Eng.* **1996**, *43*, 956–966. [CrossRef] [PubMed]
15. Audiffren, J.; Bargiotas, I.; Vayatis, N.; Vidal, P.P.; Ricard, D. A Non Linear Scoring Approach for Evaluating Balance: Classification of Elderly as Fallers and Non-Fallers. *PLoS ONE* **2016**, *11*, e0167456. [CrossRef] [PubMed]
16. Estévez-Pedraza, Á.G.; Parra-Rodríguez, L.; Martínez-Méndez, R.; Portillo-Rodríguez, O.; Ronzón-Hernández, Z. A Novel Model to Quantify Balance Alterations in Older Adults Based on the Center of Pressure (CoP) Measurements with a Cross-Sectional Study. *PLoS ONE* **2021**, *16*, e0256129. [CrossRef] [PubMed]
17. Fino, P.C.; Mojdehi, A.R.; Adjerid, K.; Habibi, M.; Lockhart, T.E.; Ross, S.D. Comparing Postural Stability Entropy Analyses to Differentiate Fallers and Non-Fallers. *Ann. Biomed. Eng.* **2016**, *44*, 1636. [CrossRef]
18. Howcroft, J.; Lemaire, E.D.; Kofman, J.; McIlroy, W.E. Elderly Fall Risk Prediction Using Static Posturography. *PLoS ONE* **2017**, *12*, e0172398. [CrossRef]
19. Kwok, B.C.; Clark, R.A.; Pua, Y.H. Novel Use of the Wii Balance Board to Prospectively Predict Falls in Community-Dwelling Older Adults. *Clin. Biomech. Bristol Avon* **2015**, *30*, 481–484. [CrossRef]
20. Reilly, D.Ó. Feature Selection for the Classification of Fall-Risk in Older Subjects: A Combinational Approach Using Static Force-Plate Measures. *bioRxiv* **2019**. bioRxiv:807818. [CrossRef]
21. Oliveira, M.R.; Vieira, E.R.; Gil, A.W.O.; Fernandes, K.B.P.; Teixeira, D.C.; Amorim, C.F.; Silva, R.A.D. One-Legged Stance Sway of Older Adults with and without Falls. *PLoS ONE* **2018**, *13*, e0203887. [CrossRef]
22. Silva, J.; Madureira, J.; Tonelo, C.; Baltazar, D.; Silva, C.; Martins, A.; Alcobia, C.; Sousa, I. Comparing Machine Learning Approaches for Fall Risk Assessment. In Proceedings of the 10th International Conference on Bio-Inspired Systems and Signal Processing, Porto, Portugal, 26 July 2024; pp. 223–230.
23. Liao, F.-Y.; Wu, C.-C.; Wei, Y.-C.; Chou, L.-W.; Chang, K.-M. Analysis of Center of Pressure Signals by Using Decision Tree and Empirical Mode Decomposition to Predict Falls among Older Adults. *J. Healthc. Eng.* **2021**, *2021*, 6252445. [CrossRef]
24. Cuaya-Simbro, G.; Perez-Sanpablo, A.-I.; Morales, E.-F.; Quiñones Uriostegui, I.; Nuñez-Carrera, L. Comparing Machine Learning Methods to Improve Fall Risk Detection in Elderly with Osteoporosis from Balance Data. *J. Healthc. Eng.* **2021**, *2021*, 8697805. [CrossRef]
25. Sahoo, A.K.; Pradhan, C.; Das, H. Performance Evaluation of Different Machine Learning Methods and Deep-Learning Based Convolutional Neural Network for Health Decision Making. In *Nature Inspired Computing for Data Science*; Rout, M., Rout, J.K., Das, H., Eds.; Springer International Publishing: Cham, Switzerland, 2020; pp. 201–212. ISBN 978-3-030-33820-6.
26. Bailly, A.; Blanc, C.; Francis, É.; Guillotin, T.; Jamal, F.; Wakim, B.; Roy, P. Effects of Dataset Size and Interactions on the Prediction Performance of Logistic Regression and Deep Learning Models. *Comput. Methods Programs Biomed.* **2022**, *213*, 106504. [CrossRef] [PubMed]
27. Fatima, R.; Khan, M.H.; Nisar, M.A.; Doniec, R.; Farid, M.S.; Grzegorzek, M. A Systematic Evaluation of Feature Encoding Techniques for Gait Analysis Using Multimodal Sensory Data. *Sensors* **2024**, *24*, 75. [CrossRef] [PubMed]
28. Ruchinskas, R. Clinical Prediction of Falls in the Elderly. *Am. J. Phys. Med. Rehabil.* **2003**, *82*, 273–278. [CrossRef] [PubMed]
29. Piirtola, M.; Era, P. Force Platform Measurements as Predictors of Falls among Older People–A Review. *Gerontology* **2006**, *52*, 1–16. [CrossRef]

30. Quijoux, F.; Vienne-Jumeau, A.; Bertin-Hugault, F.; Zawieja, P.; Lefèvre, M.; Vidal, P.P.; Ricard, D. Center of Pressure Displacement Characteristics Differentiate Fall Risk in Older People: A Systematic Review with Meta-Analysis. *Ageing Res. Rev.* **2020**, *62*, 101117. [CrossRef]
31. Santos, D.A.; Duarte, M. A Public Data Set of Human Balance Evaluations. *PeerJ* **2016**, *4*, e2648. [CrossRef]
32. Stel, V.S.; Smit, J.H.; Pluijm, S.M.F.; Lips, P. Balance and Mobility Performance as Treatable Risk Factors for Recurrent Falling in Older Persons. *J. Clin. Epidemiol.* **2003**, *56*, 659–668. [CrossRef]
33. Pajala, S.; Era, P.; Koskenvuo, M.; Kaprio, J.; Törmäkangas, T.; Rantanen, T. Force Platform Balance Measures as Predictors of Indoor and Outdoor Falls in Community-Dwelling Women Aged 63-76 Years. *J. Gerontol. A Biol. Sci. Med. Sci.* **2008**, *63*, 171–178. [CrossRef]
34. Thapa, P.B.; Gideon, P.; Brockman, K.G.; Fought, R.L.; Ray, W.A. Clinical and Biomechanical Measures of Balance as Fall Predictors in Ambulatory Nursing Home Residents. *J. Gerontol. A. Biol. Sci. Med. Sci.* **1996**, *51*, M239–M246. [CrossRef]
35. Berg, K.O.; Maki, B.E.; Williams, J.I.; Holliday, P.J.; Wood-Dauphinee, S.L. Clinical and Laboratory Measures of Postural Balance in an Elderly Population. *Arch. Phys. Med. Rehabil.* **1992**, *73*, 1073–1080.
36. Park, M.W.; Kim, Y.D. A Systematic Procedure for Setting Parameters in Simulated Annealing Algorithms. *Comput. Oper. Res.* **1998**, *25*, 207–217. [CrossRef]
37. Parthasarathy, S.; Rajendran, C. An Experimental Evaluation of Heuristics for Scheduling in a Real-Life Flowshop with Sequence-Dependent Setup Times of Jobs. *Int. J. Prod. Econ.* **1997**, *49*, 255–263. [CrossRef]
38. Duda, R.O.; Hart, P.E.; Stork, D.G. *Pattern Classification*; John Wiley & Sons: Hoboken, NJ, USA, 2012; ISBN 978-1-118-58600-6.
39. Kirkpatrick, S.; Gelatt, C.D.; Vecchi, M.P. Optimization by Simulated Annealing. *Science* **1983**, *220*, 671–680. [CrossRef] [PubMed]
40. Knox, S.W. *Machine Learning: A Concise Introduction*; John Wiley & Sons: Hoboken, NJ, USA, 2018; ISBN 978-1-119-43919-6.
41. Kubo, Y.; Fujii, K.; Hayashi, T.; Tomiyama, N.; Ochi, A.; Hayashi, H. Sex Differences in Modifiable Fall Risk Factors. *J. Nurse Pract.* **2021**, *17*, 1098–1102. [CrossRef]
42. Ambrose, A.F.; Paul, G.; Hausdorff, J.M. Risk Factors for Falls among Older Adults: A Review of the Literature. *Maturitas* **2013**, *75*, 51–61. [CrossRef]
43. Moylan, K.C.; Binder, E.F. Falls in Older Adults: Risk Assessment, Management and Prevention. *Am. J. Med.* **2007**, *120*, 493.e1–493.e6. [CrossRef]
44. Oliver, D.; Daly, F.; Martin, F.C.; McMurdo, M.E.T. Risk Factors and Risk Assessment Tools for Falls in Hospital In-Patients: A Systematic Review. *Age Ageing* **2004**, *33*, 122–130. [CrossRef]
45. Oliver, D. Falls Risk-Prediction Tools for Hospital Inpatients. Time to Put Them to Bed? *Age Ageing* **2008**, *37*, 248–250. [CrossRef]
46. Vassallo, M.; Poynter, L.; Sharma, J.C.; Kwan, J.; Allen, S.C. Fall Risk-Assessment Tools Compared with Clinical Judgment: An Evaluation in a Rehabilitation Ward. *Age Ageing* **2008**, *37*, 277–281. [CrossRef]
47. Pudjihartono, N.; Fadason, T.; Kempa-Liehr, A.W.; O'Sullivan, J.M. A Review of Feature Selection Methods for Machine Learning-Based Disease Risk Prediction. *Front. Bioinforma.* **2022**, *2*, 72. [CrossRef]
48. Debuse, J.C.W.; Rayward-Smith, V.J. Feature Subset Selection within a Simulated Annealing Data Mining Algorithm. *J. Intell. Inf. Syst.* **1997**, *9*, 57–81. [CrossRef]
49. Nikolaev, A.G.; Jacobson, S.H. Simulated Annealing. In *Handbook of Metaheuristics*; Gendreau, M., Potvin, J.-Y., Eds.; International Series in Operations Research & Management Science; Springer: Boston, MA, USA, 2010; pp. 1–39. ISBN 978-1-4419-1665-5.
50. Giovanini, L.H.F.; Manffra, E.F.; Nievola, J.C. Discriminating Postural Control Behaviors from Posturography with Statistical Tests and Machine Learning Models: Does Time Series Length Matter? In Proceedings of the Computational Science–ICCS 2018; Shi, Y., Fu, H., Tian, Y., Krzhizhanovskaya, V.V., Lees, M.H., Dongarra, J., Sloot, P.M.A., Eds.; Springer International Publishing: Cham, Switzerland, 2018; pp. 350–357.
51. Estévez-Pedraza, Á.G.; Hernandez-Laredo, E.; Millan-Guadarrama, M.E.; Martínez-Méndez, R.; Carrillo-Vega, M.F.; Parra-Rodríguez, L. Reliability and Usability Analysis of an Embedded System Capable of Evaluating Balance in Elderly Populations Based on a Modified Wii Balance Board. *Int. J. Environ. Res. Public. Health* **2022**, *19*, 11026. [CrossRef] [PubMed]
52. Prosperini, L.; Fortuna, D.; Giannì, C.; Leonardi, L.; Pozzilli, C. The Diagnostic Accuracy of Static Posturography in Predicting Accidental Falls in People with Multiple Sclerosis. *Neurorehabil. Neural Repair* **2013**, *27*, 45–52. [CrossRef] [PubMed]
53. Forth, K.E.; Wirfel, K.L.; Adams, S.D.; Rianon, N.J.; Lieberman Aiden, E.; Madansingh, S.I. A Postural Assessment Utilizing Machine Learning Prospectively Identifies Older Adults at a High Risk of Falling. *Front. Med.* **2020**, *7*, 591517. [CrossRef]
54. Montalvo-Jaramillo, C.I.; Pliego-Carrillo, A.C.; Peña-Castillo, M.Á.; Echeverría, J.C.; Becerril-Villanueva, E.; Pavón, L.; Ayala-Yáñez, R.; González-Camarena, R.; Berg, K.; Wessel, N.; et al. Comparison of Fetal Heart Rate Variability by Symbolic Dynamics at the Third Trimester of Pregnancy and Low-Risk Parturition. *Heliyon* **2020**, *6*, e03485. [CrossRef]

Disclaimer/Publisher's Note: The statements, opinions and data contained in all publications are solely those of the individual author(s) and contributor(s) and not of MDPI and/or the editor(s). MDPI and/or the editor(s) disclaim responsibility for any injury to people or property resulting from any ideas, methods, instructions or products referred to in the content.

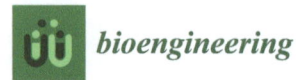

Article

Differential Back Muscle Flexion–Relaxation Phenomenon in Constrained versus Unconstrained Leg Postures

Yi-Lang Chen [1,*] and Ying-Hua Liao [1,2]

1. Department of Industrial Engineering and Management, Ming Chi University of Technology, New Taipei 243303, Taiwan; m07218007@mail2.mcut.edu.tw
2. Taiwan Research Institute, New Taipei 251401, Taiwan
* Correspondence: ylchen@mail.mcut.edu.tw

Abstract: Previous studies examining the flexion–relaxation phenomenon (FRP) in back muscles through trunk forward flexion tests have yielded inconsistent findings, primarily due to variations in leg posture control. This study aimed to explore the influence of leg posture control and individual flexibility on FRP in back and low limb muscles. Thirty-two male participants, evenly distributed into high- and low-flexibility groups, were recruited. Activities of the erector spinae, biceps femoris, and gastrocnemius muscles, alongside the lumbosacral angle (LSA), were recorded as participants executed trunk flexion from 0° to 90° in 15° increments, enabling an analysis of FRP and its correlation with the investigated variables. The findings highlighted significant effects of all examined factors on the measured responses. At a trunk flexion angle of 60°, the influence of leg posture and flexibility on erector spinae activities was particularly pronounced. Participants with limited flexibility exhibited the most prominent FRP under constrained leg posture, while those with greater flexibility and unconstrained leg posture displayed the least FRP, indicated by their relatively larger LSAs. Under constrained leg posture conditions, participants experienced an approximate 1/3 to 1/2 increase in gastrocnemius activity throughout trunk flexion from 30° to 90°, while biceps femoris activity remained relatively constant. Using an inappropriate leg posture during back muscle FRP assessments can overestimate FRP. These findings offer guidance for designing future FRP research protocols.

Keywords: trunk flexion; flexion–relaxation phenomenon; leg posture; flexibility; muscle activity

1. Introduction

Musculoskeletal injuries often arise from repetitive tasks, improper force application, and awkward postures [1]. Notably, physical injuries can be linked to factors such as frequent exposure of the upper body to deep trunk flexion postures or prolonged stooping [2]. While there has been advocacy for squatting over stooping in the past, on-site field surveys reveal that workers commonly favor trunk flexion for its perceived efficiency [3–6].

Lower back pain (LBP) associated with trunk posture has been attributed to the flexion–relaxation phenomenon (FRP) in back muscles occurring during forward trunk bending [7]. FRP manifests when lumbar spinal muscles are supplanted by passive tissues of the spine, such as posterior spinal ligaments, to counterbalance trunk torque on the lumbar spine [8]. Excessive stretching of these passive tissues during FRP may result in increased lower back loads, as these tissues possess viscoelastic properties and are susceptible to creep deformation under sustained load [9–11], potentially resulting in cross-link rupture [12]. Zwambag and Brown [13] emphasized the significant role of passive tissues over back muscles in FRP, underlining its importance in understanding LBP mechanisms. To quantitatively evaluate the extent of FRP, the flexion–relaxation ratio was introduced, which measures the decrease in back muscle activity over a specific range of trunk flexion [14]. This approach allows for the comparison of FRPs across various controlled conditions.

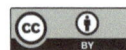

Comprehending back muscle FRP has become pivotal for grasping LBP. Previous FRP studies have primarily focused on trunk forward flexion angle [15,16], individual flexibility [4,17], pelvic movement [18,19], and the presence of LBP [20,21]. During FRP experiments, participants typically execute forward trunk bending. However, control of the lower limbs and pelvic posture can also influence FRP during trunk flexion. Gupta [22] explored the relationship between FRP and lumbopelvic motion, discovering that restricting pelvic rotation led to early FRP occurrence due to reduced spinal stability and increased passive tissue tension. Furthermore, wearing tight jeans constrains pelvic and hip movement. Yoo and Yoo [23] observed significant limitations in hip movement caused by tight jeans, resulting in increased lumbar spine movement to complete trunk flexion, potentially altering FRP patterns [19]. Chen et al. [24] highlighted how jeans restrict pelvic activity, affecting bending and lifting mechanics. Previous findings suggest that pelvic movement affects the occurrence of the FRP. However, a systematic evaluation of how leg posture impacts FRP remains lacking. When standing with knees fully extended, leg muscles, including the lower leg flexor muscles, contribute to maintaining ankle torque [25]. These muscles play a crucial role in maintaining human body balance, thereby influencing FRP during deep trunk flexion. Therefore, in addition to the lumbar erector spinae (LES), several specific muscle groups in the lower limbs related to leg movements are typically examined based on the research purpose. These include the biceps femoris (BF) [4,17,26–29] and the gastrocnemius (GAS) [4,30,31]. Other muscles associated with the pelvis and lower limbs were also evaluated to determine their roles during trunk flexion. However, the BF and GAS are generally considered the primary muscles for assessing hip extension, knee flexion, and knee stabilization [32].

The relationship between lower limb posture and the lumbar spine can evidently impact back muscle FRP. Some studies limit lower limb or pelvic movement during FRP assessment [16,17,19,22,33–35], while others solely control trunk flexion [15,21,36–38]. The critical disparity lies in the constrained leg condition, precisely controlling trunk position (including lower limb and pelvic influences), whereas the unconstrained condition evaluates FRP during trunk forward bending in a natural leg posture. These variations in experimental control variables may impact results, complicating comparisons between studies when examining FRP differences.

This study aimed to elucidate how different lower limb control conditions affect back muscle FRP, potentially leading to varied FRP patterns. It was hypothesized that limiting lower limb movement would prompt distinct FRP patterns in back muscles due to postural balance requirements and increased lower limb muscle activity, given the interconnectedness of the lower limbs, pelvis, and lumbar spine. These findings would offer valuable insights for practical applications in research contexts.

2. Materials and Methods

To explore the influence of lower limb postural control on back muscle FRP, we enlisted 32 male participants and conducted an FRP experiment. Trunk movements were recorded from upright (0°) to forward bending at 15° intervals up to 90°, under two leg postures (constrained and unconstrained). Muscle activities of the LES, BF, and GAS, as well as the lumbosacral angle (LSA), were measured. Notably, the long and medial heads of the BF and GAS muscles were specifically chosen for the test. All procedures adhered to the 2013 World Medical Association Declaration of Helsinki, and informed consent was obtained from all participants.

2.1. Participants

This study involved 32 male university students, aged 19–24 years, all with right-hand and right-leg dominance, and no history of musculoskeletal injuries or back/leg pain. Participants' dominance was verified by referring to previous studies [39,40]. All participants received compensation of approximately USD 50 for their participation. They were instructed to avoid strenuous activities and late nights during the experimental period to ensure their body was in normal condition during the experiment. Prior to commencing the experiment, participants were required to self-report and confirm their adherence to these guidelines. Participants were categorized into low- and high-flexibility groups (16 participants each) using the toe-touch flexibility test, adapted from Shin et al. [4] and Ayala et al. [41]. In this test, participants bent forward from a standing position and attempted to touch the ground with their fingertips (Figure 1). Those who reached 3 cm or more below the floor baseline were placed in the high-flexibility group, while those who did not reach the floor baseline by 3 cm or more were placed in the low-flexibility group. Initially, 48 candidates were screened, as illustrated in Figure 2. After the toe-touch test, 17 individuals met the low-flexibility criteria, and 19 met the high-flexibility criteria. To ensure balanced participant characteristics between the two test groups, a total of 32 individuals (16 in each flexibility level) ultimately participated in the FRP experiment. This approach was primarily intended to avoid potential interference from those with middle flexibility on the research results.

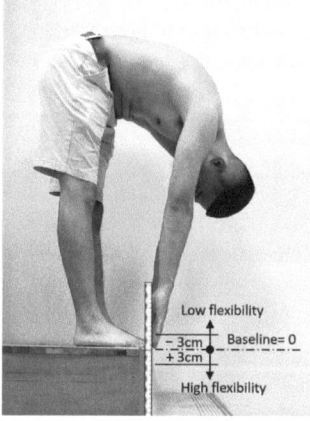

Figure 1. Schematic of criteria for determining individual flexibility.

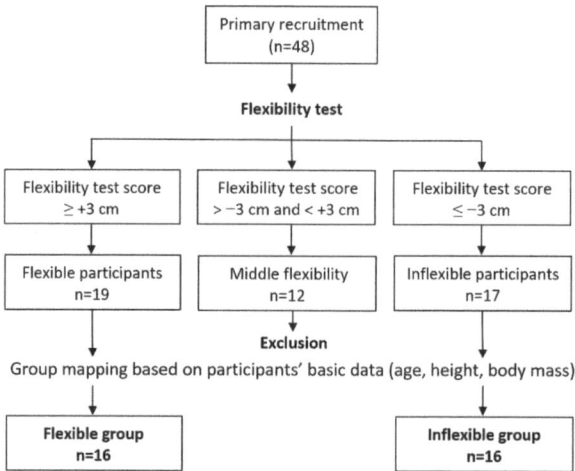

Figure 2. Flowchart depicting the selection process for the two test groups enrolled in the study.

Table 1 presents the anthropometric data for each group. An independent t-test showed no significant differences between the groups in any variable ($p > 0.05$) except flexibility. The mean (standard deviation) flexibility values were −12.1 cm (8.3 cm) for the low-flexibility group and 9.2 cm (5.9 cm) for the high-flexibility group, with an average difference of 21.3 cm between the groups. Anthropometric data, particularly heights such as acromial, hip, and knee height, which were indistinguishable between the two flexibility groups, helped prevent interference in the test data caused by differences in body size.

Table 1. Fundamental data of the two test participant groups distinguished by flexibility levels.

Items	Low Flexibility (n = 16)		High Flexibility (n = 16)	
	Mean (SD)	Range	Mean (SD)	Range
Age (years)	21.6 (1.4)	19–24	21.6 (1.5)	20–24
Height (cm)	172.8 (4.7)	166–180	173 (4.5)	161–178
Body mass (kg)	67 (7.8)	52–77	68.1 (7.5)	49–78
Acromial height (cm)	142 (4.7)	135–150	141.9 (4.2)	135–151
Hip height (cm)	88.4 (4.6)	78–95	87.0 (3.6)	79–93
Knee height (cm)	47.8 (2.4)	44–52	47.5 (1.8)	44–50
Flexibility (cm)	−12.1 (8.3)	−3–−34	9.2 (5.9)	3–25

Note: Data were presented in mean (standard deviation, SD).

2.2. Electromyography

The TeleMyo 2400, an electromyography (EMG) device from Noraxon (Scottsdale, AZ, USA), was used to measure the activation of the LES, BF, and GAS muscles on each participant's dominant side. The procedures for EMG testing, which included skin preparation, electrode placement, and fixation, as well as data acquisition and processing, adhered to the Surface Electromyography for the Non-Invasive Assessment of Muscles (SENIAM) guidelines [42]. Ag/AgCl surface electrodes, with a 10×10 mm^2 lead-off area and a center-to-center distance of approximately 20 mm, were placed parallel to the muscles. Before electrode application, skin impedance was minimized by shaving excess body hair (if necessary), gently abrading the skin with fine-grade sandpaper, and wiping the skin with alcohol swabs, following SENIAM guidelines. According to SENIAM protocols, the placements of electrodes for the investigated muscles in this study were as follows: (1) LES muscle: the electrodes were positioned 2 finger widths lateral to the spinal process of L1; (2) BF muscle: the electrodes were placed at 50% on the line between the ischial tuberosity and the lateral epicondyle of the tibia; and (3) GAS muscle: the electrodes were placed on the most prominent bulge, aligned with the direction of the leg. In the test, the reference electrode was placed around the ankle.

Prior to EMG data collection, participants engaged in standardized muscle-specific maximum voluntary contraction (MVC) exercises to normalize the EMG data for each trial. The MVC testing protocols were based on Vera-Garcia et al. [43]. For the LES muscles, participants lay prone on a bench with their torsos supported and legs hanging off, exerting maximal effort to extend their lower trunk and hips against manual resistance. For the BF muscles, participants lay prone with knees flexed at 30°, applying maximum effort against manual resistance. For the GAS muscles, participants performed an isometric contraction against resistance in the direction of ankle plantar flexion. Strong verbal encouragement was provided throughout each MVC measurement. Each participant performed three MVC trials per muscle, maintaining each contraction for at least 5 s, with a 3 min rest period between trials. The highest EMG amplitude for each muscle, calculated using a 0.5 s moving average window [43], was used as the MVC value for subsequent analysis [44].

Afterward, the electrical signals from both the MVC tests and experimental trials were filtered using an analog band-pass filter set between 20 and 600 Hz, and then sampled at a rate of 1200 Hz [42]. To obtain integrated EMG (IEMG) data, the sampled signals were fully rectified and processed. A normalization process was then performed to compare IEMG data from the experimental trials with MVC IEMG data over an identical 5 s interval. All muscle activation values were expressed as percentages of the MVC IEMG data (i.e., %MVC).

2.3. Lumbar Spine Curvature Measurements

Participants' spinal curvature was evaluated by measuring the LSA as they stood upright and flexed their trunk in 15° increments from 0° to 90°. The trunk angle was calculated using the line from the acromial shelf to the hip relative to the vertical axis. Before data collection, four adhesive reflective markers were affixed to specific body joints (shoulder, hip, knee, and ankle), along with two stick markers on the skin over the first lumbar and first sacral spinous processes (see Figure 3). The external LSA (ELSA), recorded for each trial using stick markers at S1 and L1, was utilized to estimate the internal LSA using prediction models developed by Chen and Lee [45] and employed in prior studies by Chen et al. [16,17]. Each participant's ELSA at a specific trunk position was subsequently used as a reference to calculate the internal LSA. The models are expressed as follows:

$$IL_1 = 0.988 \times SL_1 + 3.627 \ (R^2 = 0.968)$$

$$IS_1 = 0.734 \times SS_1 + 29.678 \ (R^2 = 0.916)$$

where SL_1 and SS_1 represent the respective angles of the external stick markers L_1 and S_1, and IL_1 and IS_1 represent the internal angles. The internal LSA can be obtained by determining the angle between IL_1 and IS_1 [45].

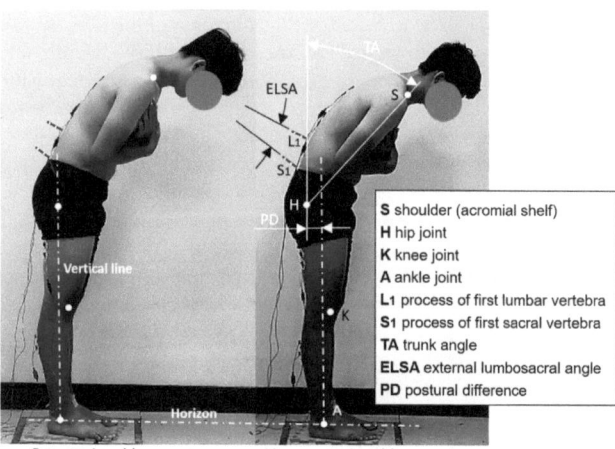

Figure 3. Schematic illustration demonstrating the testing posture, body angles during trunk flexion, and positions of markers and stickers on the participant's body.

2.4. Experimental Design and Procedure

This study evaluated the muscle activities in participants' lower back and legs, as well as the LSA, during trunk flexion at various angles. Prior to the experiment, participants were briefed on and familiarized with the procedures. Each participant performed the tests under both constrained and unconstrained leg postures, as illustrated in Figure 3. Trunk flexion angles ranged from 0° to 90° in 15° increments. Throughout the experiment, participants were instructed to flex their trunk from an upright position to six specific angles while maintaining straight knees and keeping their hands crossed on their chests. Each participant repeated each test combination twice for reliability, and the mean values were used for further analysis. Static EMG and LSA data were collected for each participant across 28 test combinations (2 leg postures × 7 trunk flexion positions × 2 repetitions). The order of these 28 combinations was randomized for each participant to minimize experimental error.

During the test, a MacReflex motion analysis system (Qualisys, Göteborg, Sweden) was set up approximately 5 m to the right-lateral side of the participant and perpendicular to their sagittal plane to capture the 2D marker positions (resolution = 1:30,000 in the camera field of view at 120 Hz, with signals being low-pass filtered at 6 Hz). In this study, when the leg posture was restricted, participants needed to maintain an upright leg posture, with the hip and ankle joints aligned vertically. When the leg posture was not restricted, participants adopted a free leg posture. The postural difference between the two leg conditions is visually illustrated as PD in Figure 3. During the static-posture test, participants were instructed to flex their trunk naturally, following the method used by Chen et al. [16]. To ensure accuracy, the experimenter confirmed that the participant's trunk line (connecting the shoulder and hip markers) and leg line (connecting the hip and ankle markers, when in a constrained leg condition) matched the preset lines on the feedback monitor of the motion analysis system. Participants were verbally guided by the experimenter to flex their trunk until they achieved the desired position with either a constrained or unconstrained leg posture. During the test, participants were instructed to bend their trunks from an upright position to the specified angles as slowly as possible to minimize the impact of movement speed [15].

Upon assuming the required trunk flexion and leg posture, a trigger signal initiated the simultaneous collection of motion and EMG data to ensure synchronization. Participants maintained each posture for at least 5 s [19], with data collected for the full 5 s duration of each position for analysis. A minimum rest period of 3 min was enforced between successive trials to minimize potential muscle fatigue and passive tissue creep, and no participant underwent testing for more than 1.5 h in total.

2.5. Statistical Analysis

Statistical analyses were performed using SPSS version 22.0 (SPSS, Inc., Chicago, IL, USA), with a significance level set at $\alpha = 0.05$. Normal distribution of numerical variables was assessed using the Kolmogorov–Smirnov test, while homogeneity of variances was evaluated using Levene's test to ensure robustness of the analysis. A three-way repeated-measures analysis of variance (ANOVA) was conducted to explore the effects of individual flexibility, leg posture, and trunk flexion on the dependent variables (muscle activations and LSA). Each participant was treated as a block and underwent all treatment combinations in a randomized order. Flexibility was considered a between-subject factor, while trunk angle and leg posture variables served as within-subject factors. Post hoc comparisons were conducted using the Duncan multiple-range test (MRT). Additionally, the independent t-test was employed to assess statistically significant differences in muscle activations and LSA between the two flexibility groups or between the two leg postures for each trunk flexion position.

3. Results

The results of the three-way ANOVA indicated a significant impact of independent variables on all measured responses, as outlined in Table 2. When averaged across other variables (i.e., leg posture and trunk flexion angle), the main effects revealed that greater flexibility was associated with heightened muscle activities of the LES (8.0 %MVC) and BF (6.6 %MVC), but decreased GAS activity (6.1 %MVC), and increased LSA (13.6°), compared to lower flexibility (all $p < 0.01$; 7.3%, 5.9%, 7.2 %MVC, and 11.3°, respectively). Similarly, when participants adopted a constrained leg posture, LES activities (7.1 %MVC vs. 8.3 %MVC; $p < 0.001$) and LSA (11.0° vs. 14.0°; $p < 0.001$) were significantly lower compared to when using an unconstrained leg posture. Conversely, higher BF (6.6 %MVC vs. 5.9 %MVC; $p < 0.01$) and GAS activities (8.0 %MVC vs. 5.3 %MVC; $p < 0.001$) were observed in leg constrained conditions.

Table 2. Results of the three-way analysis of variance (ANOVA) indicating the impact of independent variables on related muscle activations and lumbosacral angle.

Variables	Responses	DF	SS	MS	F	p	Power
Flexibility	Lumbar erector spinae	1	66	66	7.2	<0.01	0.763
	Biceps femoris	1	45	45	8.6	<0.01	0.835
	Gastrocnemius	1	119	119	9.5	<0.01	0.869
	Lumbosacral angle	1	506	506	9.7	<0.01	0.876
Leg posture	Lumbar erector spinae	1	107	107	11.6	<0.001	0.926
	Biceps femoris	1	45	45	8.5	<0.01	0.830
	Gastrocnemius	1	759	759	60.7	<0.001	1.000
	Lumbosacral angle	1	901	901	17.3	<0.001	0.986
Trunk angle	Lumbar erector spinae	6	2007	335	36.4	<0.001	1.000
	Biceps femoris	6	1646	274	52.6	<0.001	1.000
	Gastrocnemius	6	2625	437	35.0	<0.001	1.000
	Lumbosacral angle	6	234,761	39,127	753.3	<0.001	1.000
Flexibility × Leg posture	Lumbar erector spinae	1	4	4	0.4	0.505	0.102
	Biceps femoris	1	<1	<1	<0.1	0.995	0.050
	Gastrocnemius	1	2	2	0.2	0.687	0.069
	Lumbosacral angle	1	41	41	0.8	0.374	0.144
Flexibility × Trunk angle	Lumbar erector spinae	6	37	6	0.7	0.668	0.270
	Biceps femoris	6	43	7	1.4	0.222	0.539
	Gastrocnemius	6	19	3	0.3	0.956	0.120
	Lumbosacral angle	6	105	18	0.3	0.917	0.146
Leg posture × Trunk angle	Lumbar erector spinae	6	116	19	2.1	<0.05	0.757
	Biceps femoris	6	17	3	0.6	0.770	0.221
	Gastrocnemius	6	226	38	3.0	<0.01	0.907
	Lumbosacral angle	6	479	80	1.5	0.165	0.593
Flexibility × Leg posture × Trunk angle	Lumbar erector spinae	6	7	1	0.1	0.992	0.083
	Biceps femoris	6	3	1	0.1	0.996	0.076
	Gastrocnemius	6	9	2	0.1	0.994	0.080
	Lumbosacral angle	6	104	17	0.3	0.920	0.144

As presented in Table 2, the interactions of leg posture × trunk angle significantly affected both LES ($p < 0.05$) and GAS activities ($p < 0.01$). Figures 4 and 5 illustrate the cross-analyses for the LES and leg muscle activities under different test combinations, respectively. In the unconstrained leg position, the LES activity was notably higher when the trunk flexed forward at 60° compared to when the legs were constrained. This difference was statistically significant for both the high-flexibility group ($p < 0.01$) and the low-flexibility group ($p < 0.05$). Except for standing with the trunk upright, the GAS activity was notably lower when the legs were unconstrained compared to when they were constrained. Conversely, BF activity exhibited a slight increase in the constrained leg posture during trunk flexion.

Tables 3 and 4 demonstrate the LSA changes (Duncan MRT) under various trunk angles for different flexibility and leg posture groups, respectively, when averaged across the other variable. The effect of the flexibility variable on LSA was statistically significant when the trunk flexed at 30° and 45° ($p < 0.05$), while the effect of leg posture on LSA was significant during trunk flexion at 45° ($p < 0.01$), 60° ($p < 0.01$), and 75° ($p < 0.05$). Figure 6 visually presents the comparative analysis of LSAs across different test combinations at varying trunk angles.

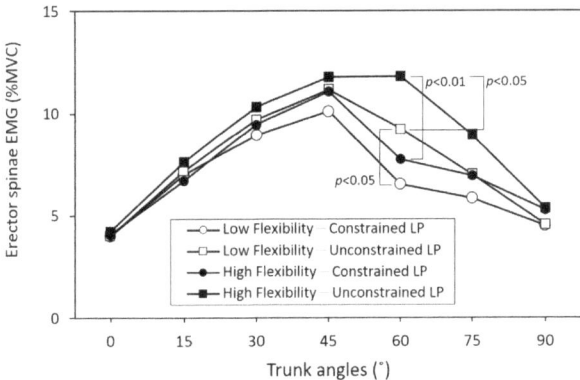

Figure 4. Lumbar erector spinae (LES) activities across different trunk flexion angles, with comparisons using independent t-tests between two leg postures (LP) for each flexibility group.

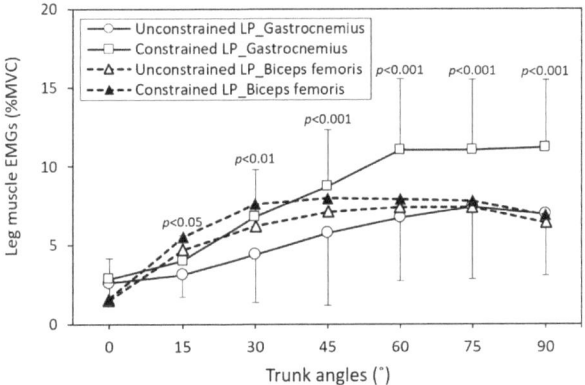

Figure 5. Leg muscle activities across various trunk flexion angles between the two leg postures (LP), with comparisons using independent t-tests for gastrocnemius electromyography.

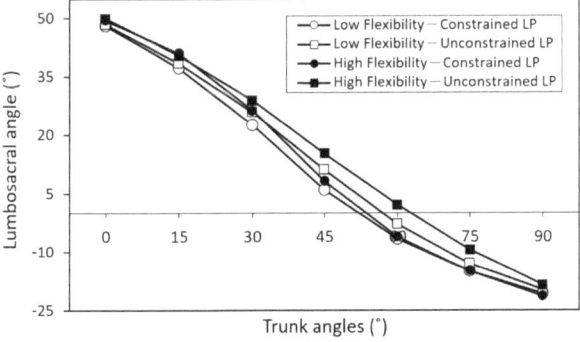

Figure 6. Comparisons of lumbosacral angles (LSAs) for four test combinations comprising two flexibility levels and two leg postures (LP).

Table 3. Lumbosacral angle categorized into Duncan groups across two flexibility levels (unit: °, n = 32).

Trunk Angle (°)	Low Flexibility	Duncan Groups	High Flexibility	Duncan Groups	Difference
0	48.1 (5.8)	A	49.6 (8.3)	A	1.5
15	37.8 (6.5)	B	40.6 (7.3)	B	2.8
30	24.2 (6.8)	C	27.6 (7.0)	C	3.4 *
45	8.5 (6.6)	D	11.7 (6.5)	D	3.2 *
60	−4.8 (7.0)	E	−2.0 (8.7)	E	2.8
75	−14.0 (6.1)	F	−12.2 (7.6)	F	1.8
90	−20.3 (7.1)	G	−20.0 (7.4)	G	0.3

Note: Data in mean (standard deviation) with the same letter do not differ in Duncan's test; * $p < 0.05$.

Table 4. Lumbosacral angle categorized into Duncan groups across different leg postures (unit: °, n = 32).

Trunk Angle (°)	Constrained Leg Posture	Duncan Groups	Unconstrained Leg Posture	Duncan Groups	Difference
0	48.7 (7.4)	A	49.0 (6.9)	A	0.3
15	39.1 (7.9)	B	39.4 (6.1)	B	0.3
30	24.4 (7.3)	C	27.3 (6.8)	C	2.9
45	7.1 (8.0)	D	13.1 (7.6)	D	6.0 **
60	−6.4 (7.4)	E	−0.4 (7.4)	E	6.0 **
75	−14.9 (6.3)	F	−11.1 (7.1)	F	3.8 *
90	−21.1 (6.8)	G	−19.2 (7.6)	G	1.9

Note: Data in mean (standard deviation) with the same letter do not differ in Duncan's test; * $p < 0.05$, ** $p < 0.01$.

4. Discussion

This study delved into the effects of the two leg postures (natural or constrained) on back muscle FRP, a topic not previously explored. From an ergonomic and practical standpoint, investigating various trunk forward bending angles when FRP occurs holds relevance for on-site operations or task design. It highlights how the interconnected movements between the trunk and lower limbs influence FRP, particularly its occurrence and magnitude. This diverges from the clinical application of FRP as an indicator for diagnosing patients' LBP, which typically focuses on maximum or near-maximum trunk forward flexion [20,21,46,47]. The primary contribution of this study lies in clarifying that when leg posture is constrained, as expected, it may lead to an overestimation of the degree of FRP in the back muscles compared to the natural leg posture. The study findings provide reference points for subsequent research on FRP-related topics.

The ANOVA results revealed that all independent variables had a significant main effect on the measured responses (Table 2). Constraining the leg posture resulted in a more pronounced FRP of the LES muscle. Figure 4 illustrates the LES activities for four combinations of flexibility and leg posture at different trunk flexion angles. It is evident from the figure that when the trunk was bent forward at 45°, constraining the leg posture reduced LES activity, irrespective of whether it was in the high-flexibility ($p < 0.01$) or low-flexibility group ($p < 0.05$). Notably, when the high-flexibility group adopted a natural leg posture, FRP might even be delayed until the trunk flexed at 60°, a significant difference compared to the low-flexibility group ($p < 0.05$). Previous studies have indicated that individuals with low flexibility exhibit earlier onset of FRP [16,17,37] and lower BF muscle activity [24] than those with high flexibility, a phenomenon observed in this study as well. Table 2 also indicates that the interaction of leg posture and trunk angle significantly influenced LES activity ($p < 0.05$). As depicted in Figure 4, when trunk forward flexion is less than 45°, LES activities remain relatively constant (when averaged across data from high- and low-flexibility groups). However, within trunk forward flexion angles of 45° to 75°, there is a significant difference in LES activities between the two leg postures, particularly at 60°, where constrained and unconstrained LES activities are 7.1 %MVC and 10.5 %MVC, respectively, with a difference of 3.4 %MVC. Considering the flexibility variable, this difference increases to 5.3 %MVC.

Nordin et al. [48] discovered that when the knees are straight and the trunk is flexed forward, the initial 50–60° of trunk flexion primarily involves lumbar spine movement, followed by forward pelvic rotation to complete the flexion action. Solomonow et al. [8], through a combination of movement and EMG measurements, determined that the onset of FRP in the back muscles of healthy subjects typically occurs around 45–50° of trunk forward bending, consistent with the findings of this study. However, some studies have reported earlier occurrences of FRP [49]. Figure 6 illustrates the change in LSAs at different trunk flexion angles. The collective effect of leg posture and individual flexibility on LSA remains relatively consistent, wherein larger LSAs correspond to higher LES activities, suggesting a relatively lower degree of FRP. In real-world material handling operations, previous studies have noted that trunk forward flexion angles typically fall within the range of 30° to 60° [50,51]. Therefore, assessing FRP characteristics within this trunk flexion range holds particular significance. This study revealed that the influence of leg posture on FRP predominantly manifests within this range, highlighting the crucial connection between the leg posture variable and actual working postures.

This study is subject to several limitations. Firstly, despite the participation of 32 young individuals in the experiment, the grouping resulted in only 16 individuals in each group. The relatively small sample size represents a primary limitation of this study, and its findings may not be broadly applicable, particularly to the female population, considering potential gender differences in flexibility [52]. Future studies could enhance their validity by increasing the number of participants and including individuals with diverse demographic characteristics for more comprehensive generalization. Additionally, this study did not include males with middle flexibility (scores between ±3 cm, as shown in Figures 1 and 2); instead, it focused on recruiting two extreme flexibility groups. Shin et al. [4] employed a mid-flexibility group in addition to low- and high-flexibility groups, noting that LES FRP in mid-flexibility participants fell proportionally between the two extremes, especially at a trunk flexion angle of 90°. Furthermore, this study revealed that FRP is based on the specific and non-continuous trunk angles examined. In our study, we measured the activities of the LES, BF, and GAS muscles. Instead of focusing on muscle activity, this study attempted to use changes in lumbar lordosis to evaluate how pelvic movement influences FRP. Further investigation is needed to understand the impact of other muscle groups in the lower limbs, especially those involved in pelvic movement, on FRP-related tests.

5. Conclusions

This study examined the activities of lower back and leg muscle groups, along with changes in lumbar lordosis, across different trunk angles and leg postures. The findings revealed that when trunk flexion was not considered in conjunction with leg posture, the degree of FRP in back muscles decreased, and FRP onset could be delayed in individuals with high flexibility. Conversely, when leg posture was constrained, back muscle FRP tended to be overestimated, with LES activities closely associated with the measured LSAs. These results suggest that when applying back muscle FRP to on-site manual work evaluations, caution is needed, as laboratory protocols that control leg posture may lead to an overestimation of the FRP degree. Therefore, careful interpretation of the results is warranted.

Author Contributions: Conceptualization, Y.-L.C.; methodology, Y.-L.C. and Y.-H.L.; software, Y.-H.L.; validation, Y.-L.C.; formal analysis, Y.-H.L.; investigation, Y.-L.C. and Y.-H.L.; resources, Y.-L.C.; data curation, Y.-H.L.; writing—original draft preparation, Y.-H.L.; writing—review and editing, Y.-L.C.; visualization, Y.-L.C.; supervision, Y.-L.C.; project administration, Y.-L.C.; funding acquisition, Y.-L.C. All authors have read and agreed to the published version of the manuscript.

Funding: This research was funded by the National Science and Technology Council (NSTC), Taiwan, grant number 107-2221-E-131-021-MY3 and the APC was also funded by the NSTC.

Institutional Review Board Statement: The study was conducted in accordance with the Declaration of Helsinki and approved by the Research Ethics Committee of National Taiwan University in Taiwan (protocol code: NTU-REC 201712EM014 and date of approval: 16 January 2018).

Informed Consent Statement: Informed consent was obtained from all participants involved in the study.

Data Availability Statement: The data are available upon reasonable request to the corresponding author.

Acknowledgments: The authors would like to thank all participants for their contributions to the study.

Conflicts of Interest: The authors declare no conflicts of interest.

References

1. Keyserling, W.M. Workplace risk factors and occupational musculoskeletal disorders, part 1: A review of biomechanical and psychophysical research on risk factors associated with low-back pain. *Am. Ind. Hyg. Assoc. J.* **2000**, *61*, 39–50. [CrossRef]
2. Shin, G.; D'souza, C.; Liu, Y.H. Creep and fatigue development in the low back in static flexion. *Spine* **2009**, *34*, 1873–1878. [CrossRef] [PubMed]
3. Baril-Gingras, G.; Lortie, M. The handling of objects other than boxes: Univariate analysis of handling techniques in a large transport company. *Ergonomics* **1995**, *38*, 905–925. [CrossRef] [PubMed]
4. Shin, G.; Shu, Y.; Li, Z.; Jiang, Z.; Mirka, G. Influence of knee angle and individual flexibility on the flexion–relaxation response of the low back musculature. *J. Electromyogr. Kinesiol.* **2004**, *14*, 485–494. [CrossRef] [PubMed]
5. Plamondon, A.; Delisle, A.; Bellefeuille, S.; Denis, D.; Gagnon, D.; Larivière, C.; IRSST MMH Research Group. Lifting strategies of expert and novice workers during a repetitive palletizing task. *Appl. Ergon.* **2014**, *45*, 471–481. [CrossRef] [PubMed]
6. Kamat, S.R.; Zula, N.M.; Rayme, N.S.; Shamsuddin, S.; Husain, K. The ergonomics body posture on repetitive and heavy lifting activities of workers in aerospace manufacturing warehouse. *IOP Conf. Ser. Mater. Sci. Eng.* **2017**, *210*, 012079. [CrossRef]
7. Floyd, W.F.; Silver, P.H.S. Function of erector spinae in flexion of the trunk. *Lancet* **1951**, *257*, 133–134. [CrossRef]
8. Solomonow, M.; Baratta, R.V.; Banks, A.; Freudenberger, C.; Zhou, B.H. Flexion-relaxation response to static lumbar flexion in males and females. *Clin. Biomech.* **2003**, *18*, 273–279. [CrossRef] [PubMed]
9. McGill, S.M.; Brown, S. Creep responses of the lumbar spine to prolonged full flexion. *Clin. Biomech.* **1992**, *7*, 43–46. [CrossRef]
10. Shin, G.; Mirka, G.A. An in vivo assessment of the low back response to prolonged flexion: Interplay between active and passive tissues. *Clin. Biomech.* **2007**, *22*, 965–971. [CrossRef]
11. Kang, S.H.; Mirka, G.A. Creep deformation of viscoelastic lumbar tissue during sustained submaximal trunk flexion postures. *J. Biomech.* **2023**, *115*, 111647. [CrossRef] [PubMed]
12. Depalle, B.; Qin, Z.; Shefelbine, S.J.; Buehler, M.J. Influence of cross-link structure, density and mechanical properties in the mesoscale deformation mechanisms of collagen fibrils. *J. Mech. Behav. Biomed. Mater.* **2015**, *52*, 1–13. [CrossRef]
13. Zwambag, D.P.; Brown, S.H. Experimental validation of a novel spine model demonstrates the large contribution of passive muscle to the flexion relaxation phenomenon. *J. Biomech.* **2020**, *102*, 109431. [CrossRef] [PubMed]
14. Gouteron, A.; Tabard-Fougere, A.; Bourredjem, A.; Casillas, J.M.; Armand, S.; Genevay, S. The flexion relaxation phenomenon in nonspecific chronic low back pain: Prevalence, reproducibility and flexion–extension ratios. A systematic review and meta-analysis. *Eur. Spine J.* **2022**, *31*, 136–151. [CrossRef]
15. Alessa, F.; Ning, X. Changes of lumbar posture and tissue loading during static trunk bending. *Hum. Mov. Sci.* **2018**, *57*, 59–68. [CrossRef]
16. Chen, Y.L.; Lin, W.C.; Liao, Y.H.; Lin, C.J. Effect of individual flexibility and knee posture on the back muscle flexion-relaxation phenomenon. *Int. J. Ind. Ergon.* **2018**, *68*, 82–88. [CrossRef]
17. Chen, Y.L.; Lin, W.C.; Liao, Y.H.; Chen, Y.; Kang, P.Y. Changing the pattern of the back-muscle flexion–relaxation phenomenon through flexibility training in relatively inflexible young men. *PLoS ONE* **2021**, *16*, e0259619. [CrossRef]
18. Olson, M.; Solomonow, M.; Li, L. Flexion–relaxation response to gravity. *J. Biomech.* **2006**, *39*, 2545–2554. [CrossRef] [PubMed]
19. Eungpinichpong, W.; Buttagat, V.; Areeudomwong, P.; Pramodhyakul, N.; Swangnetr, M.; Kaber, D.; Puntumetakul, R. Effects of restrictive clothing on lumbar range of motion and trunk muscle activity in young adult worker manual material handling. *Appl. Ergon.* **2013**, *44*, 1024–1032. [CrossRef]
20. Shamsi, M.; Ahmadi, A.; Mirzaei, M.; Jaberzadeh, S. Effects of static stretching and strengthening exercises on flexion relaxation ratio in patients with LBP: A randomized clinical trial. *J. Bodyw. Mov. Ther.* **2022**, *30*, 196–202. [CrossRef]
21. Gouteron, A.; Tabard-Fougère, A.; Moissenet, F.; Bourredjem, A.; Rose-Dulcina, K.; Genevay, S.; Laroche, D.; Armand, S. Sensitivity and specificity of the flexion and extension relaxation ratios to identify altered paraspinal muscles' flexion relaxation phenomenon in nonspecific chronic low back pain patients. *J. Electromyogr. Kinesiol.* **2023**, *68*, 102740. [CrossRef] [PubMed]
22. Gupta, A. Analyses of myo-electrical silence of erectors spinae. *J. Biomech.* **2001**, *34*, 491–496. [CrossRef] [PubMed]
23. Yoo, I.G.; Yoo, W.G. Effects of the wearing of tight jeans on lumbar and hip movement during trunk flexion. *J. Phys. Ther. Sci.* **2012**, *24*, 659–661. [CrossRef]

24. Chen, Y.L.; Lin, W.C.; Chen, Y.; Wen, Y.W.; Tsai, T.L.; Yan, S.Q. Effect of wearing jeans on the back muscle flexion-relaxation phenomenon. *Int. J. Ind. Ergon.* **2020**, *76*, 102938. [CrossRef]
25. Pollock, C.L.; Ivanova, T.D.; Hunt, M.A.; Garland, S.J. Motor unit recruitment and firing rate in medial gastrocnemius muscles during external perturbations in standing in humans. *J. Neurophysiol.* **2014**, *112*, 1678–1684. [CrossRef] [PubMed]
26. Behm, D.G.; Burry, S.M.; Greeley, G.E.; Poole, A.C.; MacKinnon, S.N. An unstable base alters limb and abdominal activation strategies during the flexion relaxation response. *J. Sports Sci. Med.* **2006**, *5*, 323–332. [PubMed Central]
27. Descarreaux, M.; Lafond, D.; Cantin, V. Changes in the flexion-relaxation response induced by hip extensor and erector spinae muscle fatigue. *BMC Musculoskel. Dis.* **2010**, *11*, 112. [CrossRef]
28. Kim, M.H.; Yoo, W.G. Comparison of the hamstring muscle activity and flexion-relaxation ratio between asymptomatic persons and computer work-related low back pain sufferers. *J. Phys. Ther. Sci.* **2013**, *25*, 535–536. [CrossRef] [PubMed]
29. Ulrey, B.L.; Fathallah, F.A. Effect of a personal weight transfer device on muscle activities and joint flexions in the stooped posture. *J. Electromyogr. Kinesiol.* **2013**, *23*, 195–205. [CrossRef]
30. Nikzad, S.; Pirouzi, S.; Taghizadeh, S.; Hemmati, L. Relationship between hamstring flexibility and extensor muscle activity during a trunk flexion task. *J. Chiropr. Med.* **2020**, *19*, 21–27. [CrossRef]
31. Shamsi, M.; Mirzaei, M.; Hopayian, K. A controlled clinical trial investigating the effects of stretching and compression exercises on electromyography of calf muscles in chronic LBP patients with a deep gluteal syndrome. *BMC Sports Sci. Med. Rehabil.* **2024**, *16*, 12. [CrossRef] [PubMed]
32. Netter, F.H. *Atlas of Human Anatomy*; Elsevier Health Sciences: Amsterdam, The Netherlands, 2014.
33. Laird, R.A.; Keating, J.L.; Kent, P. Subgroups of lumbo-pelvic flexion kinematics are present in people with and without persistent low back pain. *BMC Musculoskel. Dis.* **2018**, *19*, 309. [CrossRef] [PubMed]
34. Shahvarpour, A.; Preuss, R.; Sullivan, M.J.; Negrini, A.; Larivière, C. The effect of wearing a lumbar belt on biomechanical and psychological outcomes related to maximal flexion-extension motion and manual material handling. *Appl. Ergon.* **2018**, *69*, 17–24. [CrossRef] [PubMed]
35. Mackey, S.; Barnes, J.; Pike, K.; De Carvalho, D. The relation between the flexion relaxation phenomenon onset angle and lumbar spine muscle reflex onset time in response to 30 min of slumped sitting. *J. Electromyogr. Kinesiol.* **2021**, *58*, 102545. [CrossRef] [PubMed]
36. Ippersiel, P.; Preuss, R.; Fillion, A.; Jean-Louis, J.; Woodrow, R.; Zhang, Q.; Robbins, S.M. Inter-joint coordination and the flexion-relaxation phenomenon among adults with low back pain during bending. *Gait Posture* **2021**, *85*, 164–170. [CrossRef] [PubMed]
37. Ramezani, M.; Kordi Yoosefinejad, A.; Motealleh, A.; Ghofrani-Jahromi, M. Comparison of flexion relaxation phenomenon between female yogis and matched non-athlete group. *BMC Sports Sci. Med. Rehabil.* **2022**, *14*, 14. [CrossRef]
38. Li, Y.; Pei, J.; Li, C.; Wu, F.; Tao, Y. The association between different physical activity levels and flexion-relaxation phenomenon in women: A cross-sectional study. *BMC Sports Sci. Med. Rehabil.* **2023**, *15*, 62. [CrossRef] [PubMed]
39. Jung, H.S.; Jung, H.S. Hand dominance and hand use behaviour reported in a survey of 2437 Koreans. *Ergonomics* **2009**, *52*, 1362–1371. [CrossRef] [PubMed]
40. Schorderet, C.; Hilfiker, R.; Allet, L. The role of the dominant leg while assessing balance performance. A systematic review and meta-analysis. *Gait Posture* **2021**, *84*, 66–78. [CrossRef]
41. Ayala, F.; de Baranda, P.S.; Croix, M.D.S.; Santonja, F. Reproducibility and criterion-related validity of the sit and reach test and toe touch test for estimating hamstring flexibility in recreationally active young adults. *Phys. Ther. Sport* **2012**, *13*, 219–226. [CrossRef]
42. Stegeman, D.; Hermens, H. *Standards for Surface Electromyography: The European Project Surface EMG for Noninvasive Assessment of Muscles (SENIAM)*; Roessingh Research and Development: Enschede, The Netherlands, 2007; pp. 108–112.
43. Vera-Garcia, F.J.; Moreside, J.M.; McGill, S.M. MVC techniques to normalize trunk muscle EMG in healthy women. *J. Electromyogr. Kinesiol.* **2010**, *20*, 10–16. [CrossRef] [PubMed]
44. Mathiassen, S.E.; Winkel, J.; Hägg, G.M. Normalization of surface EMG amplitude from the upper trapezius muscle in ergonomic studies—A review. *J. Electromyogr. Kinesiol.* **1995**, *5*, 197–226. [CrossRef] [PubMed]
45. Chen, Y.L.; Lee, Y.H. A noninvasive protocol for the determination of lumbosacral vertebral angle. *Clin. Biomech.* **1997**, *12*, 185–189. [CrossRef]
46. Colloca, C.J.; Hinrichs, R.N. The biomechanical and clinical significance of the lumbar erector spinae flexion-relaxation phenomenon: A review of literature. *J. Manip. Physiol. Ther.* **2005**, *28*, 623–631. [CrossRef]
47. Murillo, C.; Martinez-Valdes, E.; Heneghan, N.R.; Liew, B.; Rushton, A.; Sanderson, A.; Falla, D. High-density electromyography provides new insights into the flexion relaxation phenomenon in individuals with low back pain. *Sci. Rep.* **2019**, *9*, 15938. [CrossRef] [PubMed]
48. Nordin, M.; Weiner, S.S.; Lindh, M. Biomechanics of the Lumbar Spine. In *Basic Biomechanics of the Musculoskeletal System*; Nordin, M., Frankel, V., Eds.; Lippincott Williams and Wilkins: Baltimore, MD, USA, 2001; pp. 256–284.
49. Schultz, A.B.; Hadespeck-Grib, K.; Sinkora, G.; Warwick, D.N. Quantitative studies of flexion–relaxation phenomenon in the back muscles. *J. Orthop. Res.* **1985**, *3*, 189–197. [CrossRef]
50. Porta, M.; Pau, M.; Orrù, P.F.; Nussbaum, M.A. Trunk flexion monitoring among warehouse workers using a single inertial sensor and the influence of different sampling durations. *Int. J. Environ. Res. Public Health* **2020**, *17*, 7117. [CrossRef] [PubMed]

51. Skals, S.; Bláfoss, R.; Andersen, M.S.; de Zee, M.; Andersen, L.L. Manual material handling in the supermarket sector. Part 1: Joint angles and muscle activity of trapezius descendens and erector spinae longissimus. *Appl. Ergon.* **2021**, *92*, 103340. [CrossRef]
52. Cornbleet, S.L.; Woolsey, N.B. Assessment of hamstring muscle length in school-aged children using the sit-and-reach test and the inclinometer measure of hip joint angle. *Phys. Ther.* **1996**, *76*, 850–855. [CrossRef]

Disclaimer/Publisher's Note: The statements, opinions and data contained in all publications are solely those of the individual author(s) and contributor(s) and not of MDPI and/or the editor(s). MDPI and/or the editor(s) disclaim responsibility for any injury to people or property resulting from any ideas, methods, instructions or products referred to in the content.

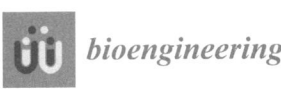

Article

The Efficacy of Body-Weight Supported Treadmill Training and Neurotrophin-Releasing Scaffold in Minimizing Bone Loss Following Spinal Cord Injury

Michael Weiser [1], Lindsay Stoy [2], Valerie Lallo [2], Sriram Balasubramanian [1] and Anita Singh [3,*]

1. School of Biomedical Engineering, Science and Health Systems, Drexel University, Philadelphia, PA 19104, USA
2. Biomedical Engineering, Widener University, Chester, PA 19103, USA
3. Bioengineering, Temple University, Philadelphia, PA 19122, USA
* Correspondence: anitausingh@gmail.com; Tel.: +1-(313)-595-5660

Abstract: Spinal cord injury (SCI) can lead to significant bone loss below the level of the lesion increasing the risk of fracture and increased morbidity. Body-weight-supported treadmill training (BWSTT) and transplantation strategies using neurotrophins have been shown to improve motor function after SCI. While rehabilitation training including BWSTT has also been effective in reducing bone loss post-SCI, the effects of transplantation therapies in bone restoration are not fully understood. Furthermore, the effects of a combinational treatment strategy on bone post-SCI also remain unknown. The aim of this study was to determine the effect of a combination therapy including transplantation of scaffold-releasing neurotrophins and BWSTT on the forelimb and hindlimb bones of a T9-T10 contused SCI animals. Humerus and tibia bones were harvested for Micro-CT scanning and a three-point bending test from four animal groups, namely injury, BWSTT (injury with BWSTT), scaffold (injury with scaffold-releasing neurotrophins), and combinational (injury treated with scaffold-releasing neurotrophins and BWSTT). BWSTT and combinational groups reported higher biomechanical properties in the tibial bone (below injury level) and lower biomechanical properties in the humerus bone (above injury level) when compared to the injury and scaffold groups. Studied structural parameters, including the cortical thickness and bone volume/tissue volume (BV/TV) were also higher in the tibia and lower in the humerus bones of BWSTT and combinational groups when compared to the injury and scaffold groups. While no significant differences were observed, this study is the first to report the effects of a combinational treatment strategy on bone loss in contused SCI animals and can help guide future interventions.

Keywords: spinal cord injury; neurotrophins; spine rehabilitation; biomechanics; bone

Citation: Weiser, M.; Stoy, L.; Lallo, V.; Balasubramanian, S.; Singh, A. The Efficacy of Body-Weight Supported Treadmill Training and Neurotrophin-Releasing Scaffold in Minimizing Bone Loss Following Spinal Cord Injury. *Bioengineering* 2024, 11, 819. https://doi.org/10.3390/bioengineering11080819

Academic Editors: William Zev Rymer and Philippe Gorce

Received: 18 May 2024
Revised: 30 July 2024
Accepted: 6 August 2024
Published: 12 August 2024

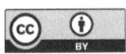

Copyright: © 2024 by the authors. Licensee MDPI, Basel, Switzerland. This article is an open access article distributed under the terms and conditions of the Creative Commons Attribution (CC BY) license (https://creativecommons.org/licenses/by/4.0/).

1. Introduction

Spinal cord injury (SCI) is a common cause of morbidity with a prevalence of 302,000 cases with an incidence of 18,000 new cases annually in the United States [1]. In addition to sensory and motor deficits, SCI also leads to bone loss below the level of lesion, resulting in an increased risk of fracture and greater morbidity [2]. The degree of bone loss is greater in complete SCI as compared to incomplete SCI, with the latter being more common [1,2]. Greater bone loss in complete SCI could be attributed to the increased immobility-related loss of mechanical stimuli, which has a strong influence on bone integrity and structure. Reported changes in the skeletal structure include changes in the cortical and trabecular regions of the bones following SCI [3]. Furthermore, the reported loss of bone mineral density (BMD) has been reported to stem primarily from the degradation of trabecular bone [4,5].

Current treatment for SCI includes rehabilitation therapy such as body-weight-supported treadmill training (BWSTT). Through BWSTT, synapses and motor tasks can be recovered below an incomplete SCI [6]. However, recovery of motor function following a complete SCI has not been demonstrated [7]. Furthermore, expected motor recovery following incomplete SCI is directly related to the number of spared descending pathways [7]. Several clinical and animal studies support the role of BWSTT in restoring motor function while reducing muscle atrophy and bone loss with improvement in BMD [8–10]. Giangregorio et al. (2005) studied five human participants with SCI who underwent BWSTT over 6–8 months and noted a range of increased muscle cross-sectional areas from 3.8% to 56.9%. While BMD was reduced in all participants' lower limbs ranging from -1.2% to -26.7%, the participant displaying the greatest ambulatory function demonstrated the smallest reduction in BMD, and the participant who completed the fewest BWSTT sessions demonstrated the greatest reduction in BMD [8]. In another study, Shields et al. (2006) studied the effects of unilateral electrical stimulation of soleus muscles, simulating training response, in patients with SCI. Stimulation delivering a compressive force of 1.5 times the body weight on the tibia for three years resulted in a 31% increase in trabecular BMD at the distal tibia of trained limbs compared to untrained limbs [11]. Thus, the role of BWSTT in improving bone morphology and strength after SCI along with motor and muscle functions is evident.

In addition to rehabilitation therapy, transplantation strategies is another investigational treatment modality that aims to promote neuroprotection and regeneration post-SCI. Bioengineering transplantation strategies including biomaterials such as polyethylene glycol (PEG) loaded with neurotrophins including brain-derived neurotropic factor (BDNF) and neurotrophin-3 (NT3) have reported promising outcomes [12–14]. After the initial insult to the spinal cord, a cascade of secondary events leads to an acute inflammatory response that induces further tissue damage. Targeting these secondary events to prevent additional tissue damage represents a promising strategy to improve patient outcomes. BDNF and NT3 are known to play a key role in minimizing secondary injury while promoting regeneration and sprouting of injured axons [6,15]. Piantino et al. (2006) studied axonal rewiring in rats that underwent spinal cord hemisection and implantation with NT3 delivered via hydrogels. They noted significant increases in motor function studied using BBB scores for NT3-treated animals (16.43 ± 0.86) compared to controls (13.75 ± 0.72) supported by significantly more axonal sprouting ($p < 0.01$) in the NT3 animals [15]. Another study demonstrated increased recovery of fine motor control in a cervical dorsolateral funiculotomy animal model when transplanted with neurotrophins loaded PNIPAAM-g-PEG versus PNIPAAM-g-PEG alone [16]. These available studies support the role of neurotrophins-loaded scaffolds in promoting motor recovery and regeneration of fibers post-SCI. However, no study has related the effects of these transplantation approaches on bone loss post-SCI. Since neuroprotection and regeneration post-transplantation of neurotrophins results in improved motor function, it can be hypothesized that the improved motor function will reduce bone atrophy. It remains unknown if the motor function improvements post-transplantation therapy are significant enough to reduce bone loss following SCI. Furthermore, the promising outcomes of BWSTT, the current standard of care for SCI subjects, and transplantation strategies holding the most promise in treating SCI warrant additional studies that investigate the effects of combinational treatment strategies combining these two strategies in treating SCI-related bone loss. The current study fills this critical gap and aims to determine the effects of a combinational therapy using transplantation of biomaterials loaded with neurotrophins at the SCI site in conjunction with BWSTT on structural and biomechanical properties of the forelimb (unaffected) and the hindlimb (affected) bones in a thoracic contusion SCI animal model. We hypothesize that the combination of these therapies will reduce bone loss below the level of the lesion (affected hind limb) when compared to no treatment and alone treatments. Furthermore, the combinational intervention will also result in reduced over-compensation of the unaffected limb when compared to no treatment and alone treatments.

2. Methods

Thirty-two adult female Sprague Dawley rats (body weight: 200–250 g) were used in the current study. Female rats were used due to our previous experience in handling them while performing treadmill training experiments. Animals were assigned to one of the four groups (n = 8 per group, power of 0.8, alpha and effect size of 0.05) listed in Table 1. The power analysis was performed based on a previously reported study by Tom et al. [7]. Group 1 (injury) was an injury group that received a T9/10 contusion SCI and no treatment. Group 2 (BWSTT) was the body-weight-supported treadmill training alone group that received contusion SCI and BWSTT as treatment. Group 3 (scaffold) was the transplantation alone group that received contusion SCI and an injection of polyethylene glycol (PNIPAAM-g-PEG) loaded with BDNF+NT3 neurotrophins as treatment. Finally, Group 4 (combinational) was the combinatorial group that received a contusion SCI followed by both transplantation (PNIPAAM-g-PEG releasing BDNF+NT3) followed by BWSTT as treatment. Group 2 and Group 3 received their therapies (BWSTT or transplant) one week post-contusion injury, while Group 4 received the transplant surgery one week post-contusion injury and then began BWSTT one week post-transplant surgery. Eight weeks after the surgery or last intervention in each group, the humerus and tibia bones were harvested from the fore and hind limbs of all animals, respectively (Table 2). The use of laboratory animals and all procedures were in accordance with the National Institute of Health and approved by the Institutional Animal Use and Care Committee. All efforts were made to minimize animal suffering during all procedures. Steps taken for animal care and to minimize pain throughout the study are included in the relevant sections below.

Table 1. Animal groups and sample size details.

Groups (n = 8 Each)	Description
Injury (Gr 1)	Injured (SCI + No Treatment)
BWSTT (Gr 2)	BWSTT (SCI + BWSTT)
Scaffold (Gr 3)	PNIPAAM-g-PEG+BDNF+NT3 (SCI + Scaffold releasing Neurotrophins)
Combinational (Gr 4)	Combinational (SCI + Scaffold releasing Neurotrophins + BWSTT)

Table 2. Study timeline including the injury, treatment type and harvest time-point details for each group.

Groups (n = 8)	Week 0	Week 1	Week 2	Week 8	Week 9	Week 10
Injury (Gr 1)				Harvest		
BWSTT (Gr 2)	T9/10 Contusion SCI	BWSTT			Harvest	
Scaffold (Gr 3)		Transplant surgery			Harvest	
Combinational (Gr 4)		Transplant surgery	BWSTT			Harvest

2.1. Spinal Cord Contusion Injury and Animal Care

A moderate contusion SCI at the T9/10 level was induced in all animals per the previously reported studies that have established BWSTT protocols for an animal in a bipedal position. The animals were anesthetized using a ketamine (76 mg/kg, Fort Dodge Animal Health, Fort Dodge, IA, USA), xylazine (7.6 mg/kg, Ben Venue 49 Laboratories, Bedford, OH, USA), and acepromazine maleate (0.6 mg/kg, Boehringer Ingelheim Vetmedica, Inc., St. Joseph, MO, USA) mixture by intraperitoneal injection. Once deeply sedated, the animals were then prepared for a T9-T11 laminectomy. The dura mater was exposed from the laminectomy procedure, an NYU impact device was used to induce a moderate spinal cord contusion injury by dropping a 10 g, 2 mm diameter rod from 25 mm above the dura mater. Subcutaneous fat was then placed on top of the injury site to prevent adherence. The back muscles were sutured and secured by wound clips, and the animals were then set on heating pads and observed until they regained consciousness. The rats' water bottles were substituted with H_2O hydrogels and long-stemmed water bottles, and their food was placed directly into the cage to accommodate for their decreased mobility. For the two weeks after injury, the animals were injected subcutaneously with 3–5 mL of saline twice a day, and ampicillin (0.1 cc, 22.7 mg/mL) once a day. Two to three weeks post-surgery, the rats' bladders were manually expressed three times a day, and urine assessments were performed using urine strips to ensure the animals were recovering well and remained healthy. Animals that presented signs of abnormalities or infection were treated or removed from the study per the approved protocol.

2.2. Biomaterial Scaffold Transplantation Surgery

One week post-contusion SCI, animals in the scaffold group (Gr 3) and combinational group (Gr 4) received a second surgery for the transplantation of poly (N-isopropylacrylamide) grafted with polyethylene glycol (8000 g/mol) (PNIPAAM-PEG) loaded with neurotrophins (BDNF+NT3). Combinational treatment of BDNF+NT3 was chosen based on previously reported studies that have shown motor improvements post-this transplantation approach [12–14]. For this surgery, the animals (in Gr 3 and Gr 4) underwent another T9-T11 laminectomy to expose the dura mater around the original injury. The site of the injury was identified and an injection of a 5 µL solution of PNIPAAM-g-PEG loaded with co-dissolved BDNF ($0.5 \times 10^6/5$ µL) and NT3 ($0.5 \times 10^6/5$ µL) was injected by using a positive displacement pipette. Because of the thermosensitive properties of poly (N-isopropylacrylamide), the solution was kept on ice to ensure it maintained its liquid state; once injected, the solution became an elastic gel. The animals' surgical sites were then closed using the same methods as the initial surgery and the animals received the same aftercare.

2.3. Behavioral Analysis

All animals were tested in an open field to measure their hindlimb function using the Basso, Beattie and Bresnahan (BBB) scale. Animals were allowed to move freely for 4 min each in an enclosure and then scored based on their hindlimb joint movements (hip, knee and ankle) from 0 (no movement of any joints) to 21 (normal movement of all three joints). The BBB tests were conducted before the injury (baseline), 2–3 days after injury, and then each week thereafter until the last time-point by two trained and blinded observers.

2.4. Body Weight Supported Treadmill Training (BWSTT)

One week after the initial contusion injury and one week after the transplantation, animals in Group 2 and Group 4 began BWSTT, respectively. These animals were placed in a vest that was attached to a body-weight support arm by Velcro. The arm was positioned over a treadmill and supported 75% of the animal's body weight. Each animal in these groups walked 1000 steps per day at a speed of 7 cm/s, five days per week for eight weeks [6].

2.5. Bone Harvest

Eight weeks after injury (Gr 1) or the last intervention (Groups 2–4), all the animals were euthanized per the approved protocol and the humerus and tibia bones were harvested from the fore and hind limbs, respectively. For Group 1, the bones were harvested at Week 8. For the BWSTT (Gr 2) and scaffold (Gr 3) groups, the bones were harvested at Week 9 because these animals had the intervention (BWSTT or transplant) starting one week after the initial injury. For the combinational (Gr 4) group, the bones were harvested at Week 10 because these animals had two interventions, the last one (BWSTT) beginning two weeks post-initial contusion injury. During euthanasia, the animals were injected with 1 mL of Euthasol (Virbac AH, Fort Worth, TX, USA). The humerus and tibia bones were then removed from the fore and hind limbs, respectively. Harvested bones were stored in a freezer at −20 degrees Celsius until further scanning and biomechanical testing were performed.

2.6. Micro-CT Scanning

Before scanning, the bones were wrapped in parafilm and placed in a low-density plastic tube filled with PBS solution. The lid was secured with parafilm, and a specialized nut was used to secure the tube into the Micro-CT machine (Skyscan 1172 Micro-CT, Bruker Corporation, Billerica, MA, USA). The entire length of the humerus bone was scanned at a voltage and current value of 80 kV and 124 µA, respectively, with a resolution of 4000×2664 µm^2 and a magnification of 3.48 µm. The entire length of the tibia bone was scanned at a voltage and current value of 65 kV and 156µA, respectively, with a resolution of 2000×1000 µm^2 and a magnification of 4.9 µm. An aluminum 0.5 mm filter was used for both the humerus and tibia scans.

2.7. Micro-CT Analysis

After scanning, the images were reconstructed using NRecon Software (Microphotonics Inc., Allentown, PA, USA) [17]. Bone scan quality was improved by removing defects such as ring artifacts and beam hardening. After reconstruction, the diaphyseal regions were defined to draw the regions of interest (ROIs) in each area. ROIs were drawn on each image in the designated region to create volumes of interest (VOIs) using CTan Software (Bruker Corporation, Billerica, MA, USA). The humeral diaphyseal region was characterized as 1.5 mm above and below the midpoint of the bone (3 mm in total) (Figure 1). The tibial diaphyseal region was 2 mm above and below the midpoint of the bone (4 mm in total) (Figure 2). Once the VOIs were created, CTan Software (Bruker Corporation, Billerica, MA, USA) was utilized to run 2D and 3D binary analysis on the images to quantify the bone parameters including bone volume to total volume ratio (BV/TV) and the cortical thickness.

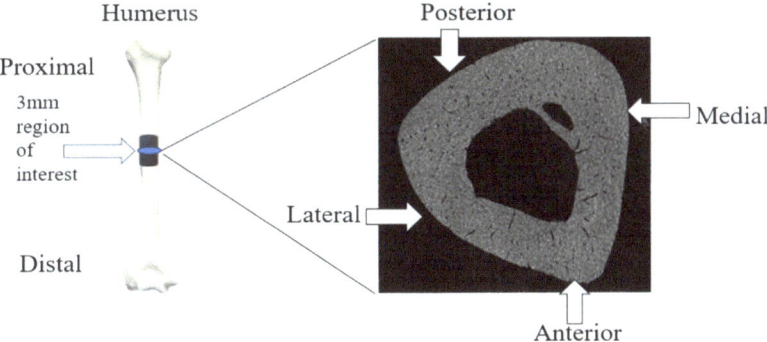

Figure 1. Region of interest (ROI) of humeral diaphysis and representative cross-sectional CT image.

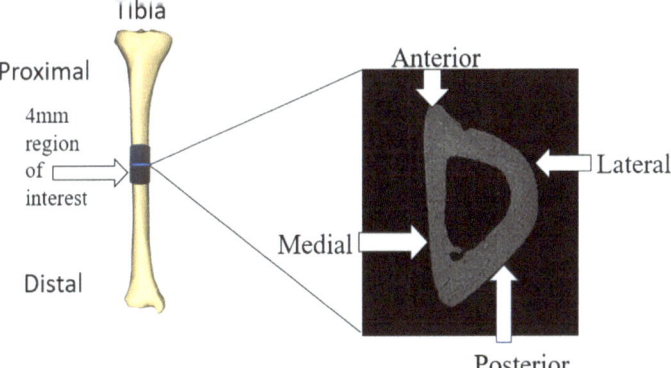

Figure 2. Region of interest (ROI) of tibial diaphysis and representative cross-sectional CT image.

2.8. Three-Point Bending Biomechanical Testing and Analysis

After Micro-CT scanning, the bones underwent three-point bending biomechanical testing (Figure 3). Bones were tested until failure at a rate of 5 mm/min while the load–displacement data were acquired. To account for any rotation of bones during the test, videos (front and side/cross-sectional view) were captured to determine the specific bending axis when the bones failed [18,19]. These axes were used to calculate the bone-specific Moment of Inertia (MOI), which measures the capacity of a cross-section to resist bending, using the Micro-CT images and BoneJ Software (V7.0.19) [20] (Figure 4). The stress–strain parameters were then calculated using a customized MATLAB code (R2023a, MathWorks, Natick, MA, USA), and the obtained plots were used to determine each bone's ultimate stress, strain at ultimate stress, ultimate load, and energy to maximum force, which was measured as the area under the load–displacement curve at maximum force [21,22].

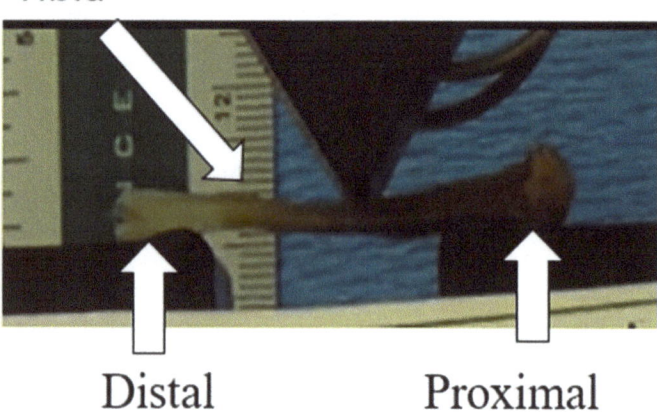

Figure 3. Three-point bending setup.

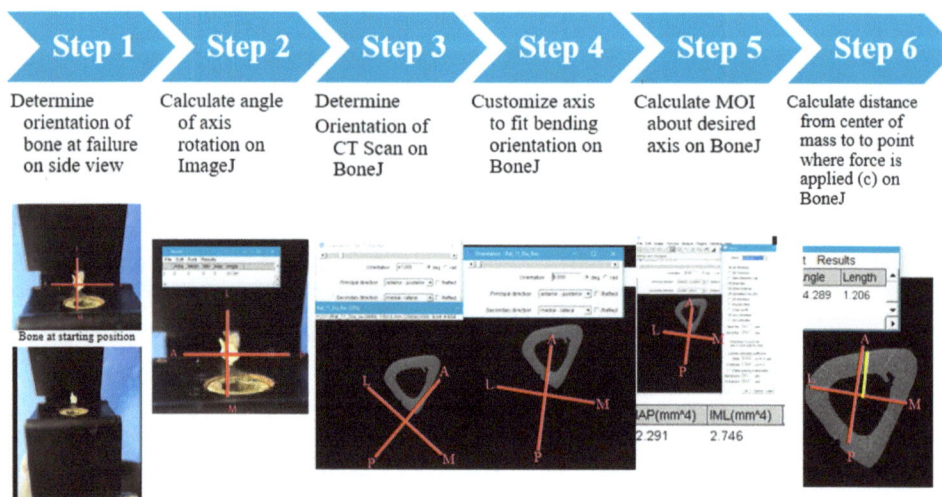

Figure 4. Detailed steps utilized to calculate MOI for each tested bone sample. Red lines are the orientation axis. Yellow line is the distance from the center of mass to th the point where force is applied as mentioned in Step 6.

2.9. Statistical Analysis

Statistical analysis was performed using SPSS (Version 11.5, IBM, Chicago, IL, USA), and significance was determined using a p-value of <0.05. The dataset was analyzed for distribution and the obtained normally distributed data was analyzed using two-way ANOVA for each studied parameter. A post hoc Bonferroni test was performed for multiple comparisons between groups. All values are expressed as mean ± standard deviation.

3. Results
3.1. Behavioral Test: BBB

Scores obtained from the two scorers were averaged. No significant differences in BBB scores were observed in any study groups post-injury.

3.2. Structural Parameters Obtained from Micro-CT Images
Cortical Thickness

For the tibia, both the BWSTT (Gr 2) and combinational (Gr 4) groups had a greater diaphyseal cortical thickness than the injury (Gr 1) and scaffold (Gr 3) groups. The combinational group had the greatest overall cortical thickness, which aligns with our hypothesis that the extent of bone loss was expected to be minimal in the combinational group when compared to the no-treatment or alone-treatment groups (Figures 5 and 6). For humeri, the scaffold group had the greatest cortical thickness. Both the combinational and BWSTT groups demonstrated less cortical thickness than the injury and scaffold groups, supporting our hypothesis of increased forelimb compensation in the injured and scaffold-alone SCI animals (Figures 5 and 6). However, no observed differences were statistically significant.

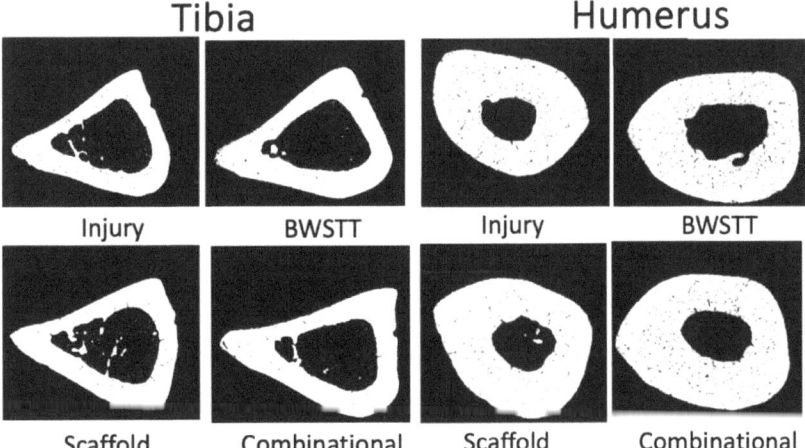

Figure 5. Exemplar Micro-CT images of the diaphyseal region of the tibia and humerus bones from each group.

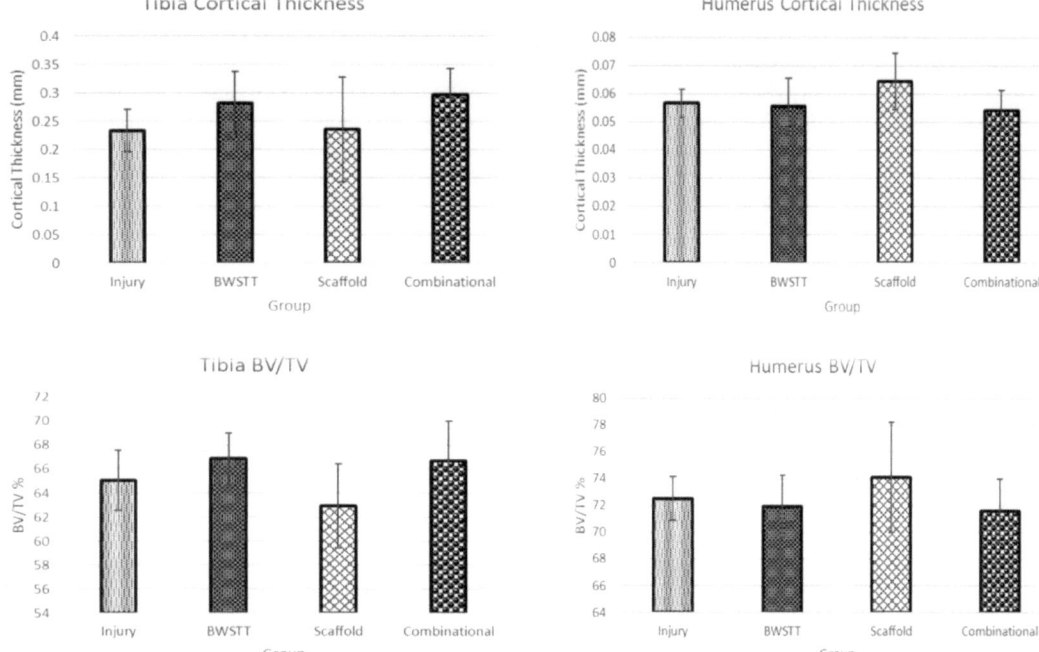

Figure 6. Structural parameters (cortical thickness and BV/TV) of tibia and humerus bones obtained from Micro-CT images. All values are expressed as mean ± SD. No significant differences were observed in any parameters between groups for both tibia and humerus bones ($p > 0.05$).

3.3. Bone Volume to Total Volume Ratio (BV/TV)

For the tibia, the group with the greatest BV/TV was the BWSTT (Gr 2) followed by the combinational (Gr 4) group. Both groups demonstrated greater BV/TV when compared to the injury (Gr 1) and scaffold (Gr 3) groups. The observed BV/TV was lowest in the scaffold group (Figure 6). For humeri, the scaffold group had the highest BV/TV followed by the injury group. The lowest BV/TV was reported in the combinational group, indicating the lowest degree of forelimb compensation (Figure 6). However, no observed differences were statistically significant.

3.4. Biomechanical Parameters Obtained from Three-Point Bending Test
Moment of Inertia (MOI)

For tibia, the group with the greatest MOI was the BWSTT (Gr 2) followed by the combinational (Gr 4) group. The scaffold (Gr 3) group and injury (Gr 1) group both were less than the BWSTT and combinational groups (Figure 7). For humeri, very little difference was noted between the four groups with the combinational group having the lowest MOI. This further supports the hypothesis that the combinational group had the lowest degree of forelimb compensation (Figure 7). However, no observed differences were statistically significant.

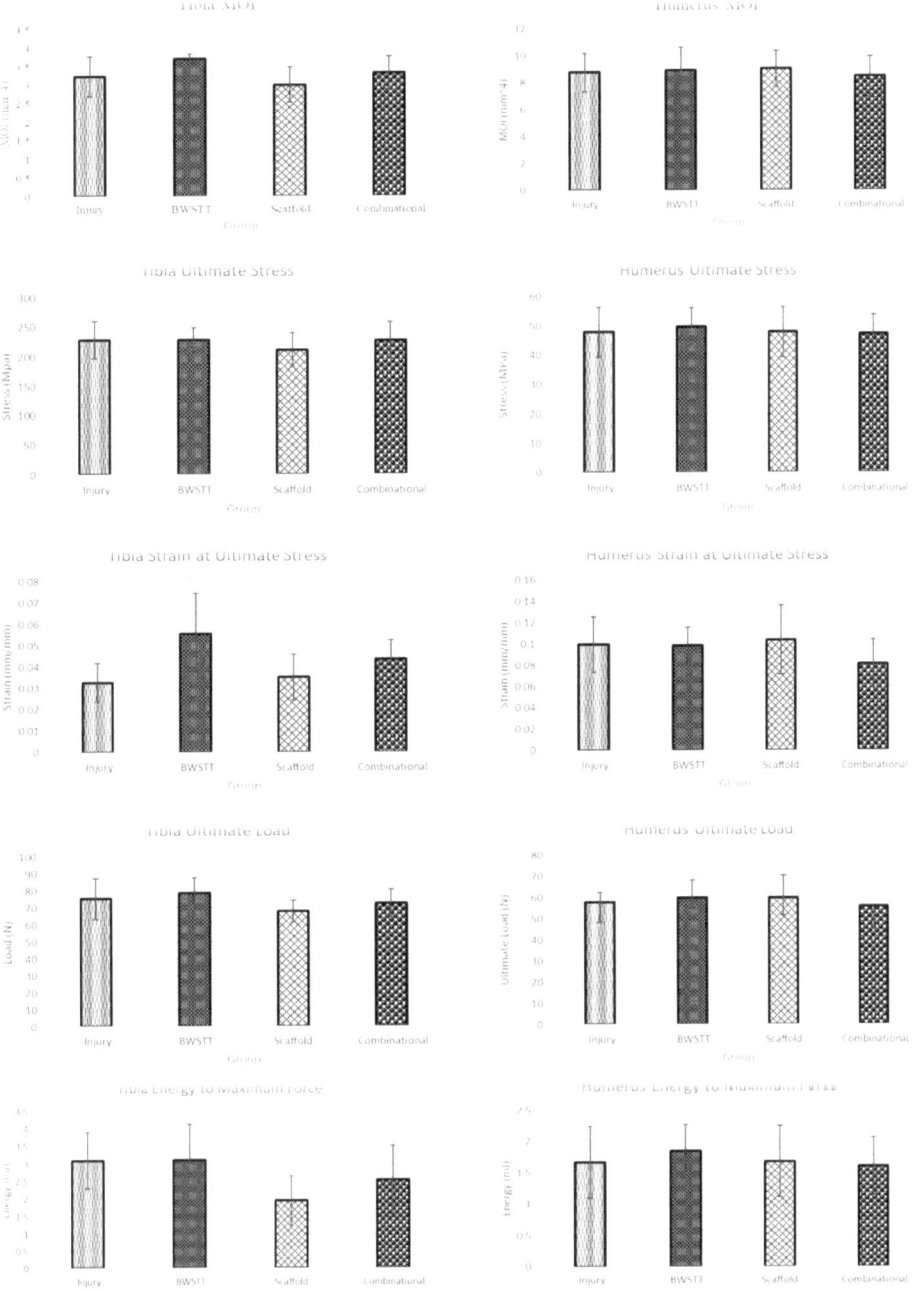

Figure 7. Biomechanical parameters (MOI, ultimate stress, strain at ultimate stress, ultimate load, and energy to maximum force) of tibia and humerus bones when subjected to three-point bending. All values are expressed as mean ± SD. No significant differences were observed in any parameters between groups for both tibia and humerus bones ($p > 0.05$).

3.5. Ultimate Stress

For the tibia, there was very minimal difference in the ultimate stress values between groups except for the scaffold (Gr 3) group, which was the lowest (Figure 7). For humeri, average ultimate stress values were also minimally different from each other (Figure 7). No observed differences were statistically significant.

3.6. Strain at Ultimate Stress

For the tibia, the BWSTT (Gr 2) group had the greatest average ultimate strain, followed by the combinational (Gr 4) group. The injury (Gr 1) group demonstrated the lowest average ultimate strain (Figure 7). For humeri, the combinational group had the lowest average strain at ultimate stress. This suggests less forelimb compensation within this group. The remaining three groups had a minimal difference in ultimate strain (Figure 7). No observed differences were statistically significant.

3.7. Ultimate Load

For the tibia, the BWSTT (Gr 2) group displayed the greatest average ultimate load while the scaffold (Gr 3) group reported the lowest ultimate load (Figure 7). For humeri, the combinational (Gr 4) group reported the lowest average ultimate load. This supports our hypothesis of less forelimb compensation occurring in this group. The remaining three groups were minimally different from each other (Figure 7). No observed differences were statistically significant.

3.8. Energy to Maximum Force

For the tibia, the BWSTT (Gr 2) group was noted to have the greatest energy while the scaffold (Gr 3) group had the lowest energy (Figure 7). For humeri, there was a slight difference in groups with the combinational (Gr 4) group demonstrating the lowest average energy to maximum force (Figure 7). This suggests the combinational group underwent less forelimb compensation. However, no observed differences were statistically significant.

4. Discussion

The aims of this study were to evaluate the structural and biomechanical changes in the hindlimb (tibia) and forelimb (humerus) bones of thoracic contused SCI rats after various treatment approaches, namely BWSTT, transplantation using bioengineering scaffold-releasing neurotrophins, and combinational (including both transplant and BWSTT). Micro-CT imaging of the analyzed bones reported increased cortical thickness and BV/TV in the affected hindlimb bone (tibia), which was below the level of injury, of the combinational and BWSTT groups. Similar findings of active treadmill training improving bone quality have been reported previously in SCI animals. Yarrow et al. (2012) reported that quadrupedal BWSTT slowed the reduction in cortical bone area measured on Micro-CT following SCI [23]. In the current study, the BWSTT and combinational therapies were also effective in reducing forelimb (unaffected limb) overcompensation as evidenced by the lower cortical thickness and BV/TV in the humerus bones of the animals in these groups when compared to animals in the injury and scaffold alone groups. The findings from this study also reported that the transplant of scaffold-releasing neurotrophins alone was not effective in reducing bone loss in the hindlimbs or decreasing overcompensation-induced bone changes in the forelimbs. Previously reported transplantation studies have demonstrated PEG hydrogel loaded with BDNF to be effective in axonal regeneration. Grous et al. (2013) studied the use of PEG and BDNF on rats that underwent SCI and reported improved fine motor skills in addition to regenerating axons [24]. Tom et al. (2018) also reported the beneficial effects of a bioengineered scaffold loaded with neurotrophins and BWSTT in restoring H-reflex responses after SCI. While these studies report the efficacy of transplantation therapy on axonal regeneration, spasticity, and functional performance, they did not investigate the effects of transplantation therapy on bone changes [7]. Findings from the current study are the first to report the effects of transplantation therapy alone and in combination with BWSTT on SCI-induced changes in both the forelimb (unaffected) and hindlimb (affected) bones.

For the studied biomechanical parameters, our results supported the radiographic findings. Correlations between biomechanical and radiographic findings have been reported previously. Voor et al. (2012) reported a 67% loss in the BV/TV and a 50% reduction in the strength of the cancellous bone of contused SCI animals [24]. The beneficial effects of exercise including BWSTT, and other training have been reported to improve bone quality post-SCI. Zamarioli et al. (2013) studied the efficacy of standing frame therapy on maintaining bone biomechanics in rats that underwent SCI. They found that standing frame therapy following SCI attenuated the loss of stiffness in the femur and tibial bones of rats that underwent SCI without therapy [25]. Several other studies have confirmed the beneficial effects of training post-rehabilitation training in SCI subjects [26,27]. The current study confirms these findings. We found that the BWSTT and combinational groups had stronger tibia (affected hindlimb), as evidenced by higher MOI, ultimate stress, strain at ultimate stress, ultimate load, and maximum energy. These therapies also correlated with reduced forelimb overcompensation as the humeri in these groups were noted to exhibit weaker mechanical properties when compared to injury and scaffold alone groups. Also, the scaffold-alone group was not effective in strengthening the tibia, which aligns with our previously discussed results of lower cortical thickness and BV/TV.

Findings from our study confirm the previously reported beneficial effects of BWSTT in bone restoration. This study further provides evidence of combinational therapy including BWSTT and hydrogel-releasing neurotrophins to have a similar beneficial effect and offers promise to serve as a therapy that can minimize bone loss following SCI. Although the combinational group received an additional transplantation therapy of scaffold loaded with neurotrophins, it failed to have any additional benefit when compared to BWSTT alone treatment. We attribute this to the delayed BWSTT in the combinational group. Delayed rehabilitation training has been reported to have a determinantal effect on bone recovery as reported previously [23]. In the combinational group animals, a transplantation therapy was performed seven days post-contusion injury as supported by previously published work that reported the beneficial outcomes of delayed transplant in SCI animals [24–30]. However, this delayed transplantation imposed a longer immobilization period for the combinational group and further delayed (two-week delay) the onset of the BWSTT in this group. The two-week delay in starting the BWSTT in the combinational group animals could have resulted in no further improvement in bone restoration in this group. However, it is noteworthy that despite the delayed training, animals in the combinational group did report improvement in the affected bone quality and reduced overcompensation-based changes in the unaffected forelimb bone. This warrants future studies that include additional injury and sham groups that undergo BWSTT two weeks later thereby mimicking the transplantation surgery in the combinational group and allowing a time-matched comparison of the studied interventions.

The rationale for the current study was to fill the current gap in understanding the effects of combinational treatment strategies in treating SCI-related bone loss. This study offers an understanding of the effects of no, alone and combinational treatment approaches on bone loss in affected and unaffected limb post-moderate SCI. While the findings of this study are novel, there are some major limitations of the current study is that there was no age-matched control group, and only female animals were utilized in this study. Since no sex-related differences have been reported in bone loss studies reported previously [31], we consider the use of female rats that have been extensively used in the published BWSTT and transplantation studies and allowed the discussion of findings from the alone treatment groups of our study to be justified [16,27]. However, an age-matched control would allow investigation of the extent of recovery, with the interventions investigated, when compared to uninjured normal bones. Including an age-matched control group proved to be challenging in this study as the treadmill training alone, transplant alone and combinational group animals had different euthanasia timelines and were sacrificed at

Week 9, Week 10 and Week 11, respectively. An age-matched sham animal group would require 24 additional animals to have a comparative baseline for each group. Based on these findings, we decided to compare all treatment groups to the injury group with the goal of reporting any recovery/improvement and not restoration to a control/sham animal. We also recommend future studies to include a larger sample size to better characterize the efficacy of combinational therapy. For the studied bone micro-structural parameters, the reported p values were >0.685 in the current study. For studied bone biomechanical parameters, the reported p values were >0.716 in the current study. Future studies should carefully account for the sample size and statistical analysis required to confirm the effects of the combinatorial treatment strategy. Overall, despite the lack of statistical significance, this study is the first to report the effects of combinational treatment strategies and serves as a guide for future studies that can further investigate the efficacy of the combinational treatment strategy on bone loss in SCI animal models across various species. Studies should also investigate the timing of interventions (acute versus delayed) and explore the critical windows for intervention post-SCI. Utilizing additional behavioral tests, physiological assessment and biochemical analysis that help evaluate motor function, pain and other functional outcome while elucidating the underlying mechanism of recovery will further support a combinational treatment strategy as a promising treatment modality for curing SCI.

Author Contributions: Contributions: M.W., S.B. and A.S. have provided substantial contributions to research design, the acquisition, analysis, interpretation of data, drafting, and revising of the final version. S.B. and A.S. have also provided the approval of the final version. L.S. and V.L. have provided substantial contributions to research design, the acquisition, analysis, and interpretation of data. All authors have read and agreed to the published version of the manuscript.

Funding: This research was funded by the New Jersey Commission on Spinal Cord Research Exploratory Research Grant # CSCR14ERG001 and the APC did not require any funding.

Institutional Review Board Statement: The animal study protocol was approved by the Institutional Review Board of Rowan University (protocol code 10662 and 25 July 2014–15 July 2015).

Informed Consent Statement: Not applicable.

Data Availability Statement: Data is unavailable due to ethical restrictions but can be made available upon request and approval from the institution.

Acknowledgments: We greatly acknowledge Jennifer Vernengo's lab for providing us with the bioengineering scaffold. We also thank the staff at the vivarium, Brittany King and Karl Dryer for helping with the treadmill setup and animal care.

Conflicts of Interest: The authors declare no conflict of interest.

References

1. NSCISC. Available online: https://www.nscisc.uab.edu/ (accessed on 28 May 2023).
2. Jiang, S.D.; Dai, L.Y.; Jiang, L.S. Osteoporosis after spinal cord injury. *Osteoporos. Int.* **2006**, *17*, 180–192, Erratum in *Osteoporos. Int.* **2006**, *17*, 1278–1281. [CrossRef] [PubMed]
3. Dudley-Javoroski, S.; Shields, R.K. Muscle and bone plasticity after spinal cord injury: Review of adaptations to disuse and to electrical muscle stimulation. *J. Rehabil. Res. Dev.* **2008**, *45*, 283–296. [CrossRef] [PubMed]
4. Modlesky, C.M.; Majumdar, S.; Narasimhan, A.; Dudley, G.A. Trabecular bone microarchitecture is deteriorated in men with spinal cord injury. *J. Bone Miner. Res.* **2004**, *19*, 48–55. [CrossRef]
5. Slade, J.M.; Bickel, C.S.; Modlesky, C.M.; Majumdar, S.; Dudley, G.A. Trabecular bone is more deteriorated in spinal cord injured versus estrogen-free postmenopausal women. *Osteoporos. Int.* **2005**, *16*, 263–272. [CrossRef] [PubMed]
6. Singh, A.; Balasubramanian, S.; Murray, M.; Lemay, M.; Houle, J. Role of spared pathways in locomotor recovery after body-weight-supported treadmill training in contused rats. *J. Neurotrauma* **2011**, *28*, 2405–2416. [CrossRef]
7. Tom, B.; Witko, J.; Lemay, M.; Singh, A. Effects of bioengineered scaffold loaded with neurotrophins and locomotor training in restoring H-reflex responses after spinal cord injury. *Exp. Brain Res.* **2018**, *236*, 3077–3084. [CrossRef] [PubMed]
8. Giangregorio, L.M.; Webber, C.E.; Phillips, S.M.; Hicks, A.L.; Craven, B.C.; Bugaresti, J.M.; McCartney, N. Can body weight supported treadmill training increase bone mass and reverse muscle atrophy in individuals with chronic incomplete spinal cord injury? *Appl. Physiol. Nutr. Metab.* **2006**, *31*, 283–291. [CrossRef] [PubMed]

9. Giangregorio, L.M.; Hicks, A.L.; Webber, C.E.; Phillips, S.M.; Craven, B.C.; Bugaresti, J.M.; McCartney, N. Body weight supported treadmill training in acute spinal cord injury: Impact on muscle and bone. *Spinal Cord.* **2005**, *43*, 649–657. [CrossRef]
10. Sutor, T.W.; Kura, J.; Mattingly, A.J.; Otzel, D.M.; Yarrow, J.F. The Effects of Exercise and Activity-Based Physical Therapy on Bone after Spinal Cord Injury. *Int. J. Mol. Sci.* **2022**, *23*, 608. [CrossRef]
11. Shields, R.K.; Dudley-Javoroski, S. Musculoskeletal plasticity after acute spinal cord injury: Effects of long-term neuromuscular electrical stimulation training. *J. Neurophysiol.* **2006**, *95*, 2380–2390. [CrossRef]
12. Comolli, N.; Neuhuber, B.; Fischer, I.; Lowman, A. In vitro analysis of PNIPAAm-PEG, a novel, injectable scaffold for spinal cord repair. *Acta Biomater.* **2009**, *5*, 1046–1055. [CrossRef] [PubMed]
13. Arvanian, V. Role of neurotrophins in spinal plasticity and locomotion. *Curr. Pharm. Des.* **2013**, *19*, 4509–4516. [CrossRef]
14. Mendell, L.M.; Munson, J.B.; Arvanian, V.L. Neurotrophins and synaptic plasticity in the mammalian spinal cord. *J. Physiol.* **2001**, *533 Pt 1*, 91–97. [CrossRef] [PubMed]
15. Piantino, J.; Burdick, J.A.; Goldberg, D.; Langer, R.; Benowitz, L.I. An injectable, biodegradable hydrogel for trophic factor delivery enhances axonal rewiring and improves performance after spinal cord injury. *Exp. Neurol.* **2006**, *201*, 359–367. [CrossRef] [PubMed]
16. Grous, L.C.; Vernengo, J.; Jin, Y.; Himes, B.T.; Shumsky, J.S.; Fischer, I.; Lowman, A. Implications of poly(N-isopropylacrylamide)-g-poly(ethylene glycol) with codissolved brain-derived neurotrophic factor injectable scaffold on motor function recovery rate following cervical dorsolateral funiculotomy in the rat. *J. Neurosurg. Spine* **2013**, *18*, 641–652. [CrossRef] [PubMed]
17. D'Andrea, C.R.; Alfraihat, A.; Singh, A.; Anari, J.B.; Cahill, P.J.; Schaer, T.; Snyder, B.D.; Elliott, D.; Balasubramanian, S. Part 1. Review and meta-analysis of studies on modulation of longitudinal bone growth and growth plate activity: A macro-scale perspective. *J. Orthop. Res.* **2021**, *39*, 907–918. [CrossRef]
18. Singh, A.; Shaji, S.; Delivoria-Papadopoulos, M.; Balasubramanian, S. Biomechanical Responses of Neonatal Brachial Plexus to Mechanical Stretch. *J. Brachial Plex. Peripher. Nerve Inj.* **2018**, *13*, e8–e14. [CrossRef] [PubMed]
19. Singh, A. Extent of impaired axoplasmic transport and neurofilament compaction in traumatically injured axon at various strains and strain rates. *Brain Inj.* **2017**, *31*, 1387–1395. [CrossRef] [PubMed]
20. Doube, M.; Kłosowski, M.M.; Arganda-Carreras, I.; Cordelières, F.P.; Dougherty, R.P.; Jackson, J.S.; Schmid, B.; Hutchinson, J.R.; Shefelbine, S.J. BoneJ: Free and extensible bone image analysis in ImageJ. *Bone* **2010**, *47*, 1076–1079. [CrossRef]
21. Turner, C.H.; Burr, D.B. Basic biomechanical measurements of bone: A tutorial. *Bone* **1993**, *14*, 595–608. [CrossRef]
22. Singh, A.; Ferry, D.; Balasubramanian, S. Efficacy of Clinical Simulation-Based Training in Biomedical Engineering Education. *J. Biomech. Eng.* **2019**, *141*, 121011. [CrossRef] [PubMed]
23. Yarrow, J.F.; Wnek, R.D.; Conover, C.F.; Reynolds, M.C.; Buckley, K.H.; Kura, J.R.; Sutor, T.W.; Otzel, D.M.; Mattingly, A.J.; Borst, S.E.; et al. Passive Cycle Training Promotes Bone Recovery after Spinal Cord Injury without Altering Resting-State Bone Perfusion. *Med. Sci. Sports Exerc.* **2023**, *55*, 813–823. [CrossRef] [PubMed]
24. Voor, M.J.; Brown, E.H.; Xu, Q.; Waddell, S.W.; Burden, R.L., Jr.; Burke, D.A.; Magnuson, D.S. Bone loss following spinal cord injury in a rat model. *J. Neurotrauma* **2012**, *29*, 1676–1682. [CrossRef] [PubMed]
25. Zamarioli, A.; Battaglino, R.A.; Morse, L.R.; Sudhakar, S.; Maranho, D.A.; Okubo, R.; Volpon, J.B.; Shimano, A.C. Standing frame and electrical stimulation therapies partially preserve bone strength in a rodent model of acute spinal cord injury. *Am. J. Phys. Med. Rehabil.* **2013**, *92*, 402–410. [CrossRef] [PubMed]
26. Sezer, N.; Akkuş, S.; Uğurlu, F.G. Chronic complications of spinal cord injury. *World J. Orthop.* **2015**, *6*, 24–33. [CrossRef] [PubMed]
27. Singh, A.; Murray, M.; Houle, J.D. A training paradigm to enhance motor recovery in contused rats: Effects of staircase training. *Neurorehabil. Neural Repair* **2011**, *25*, 24–34. [CrossRef] [PubMed]
28. Sandrow, H.R.; Shumsky, J.S.; Amin, A.; Houle, J.D. Aspiration of a cervical spinal contusion injury in preparation for delayed peripheral nerve grafting does not impair forelimb behavior or axon regeneration. *Exp. Neurol.* **2008**, *210*, 489–500. [CrossRef] [PubMed]
29. Tom, V.J.; Houle, J.D. Intraspinal microinjection of chondroitinase ABC following injury promotes axonal regeneration out of a peripheral nerve graft bridge. *Exp. Neurol.* **2008**, *211*, 315–319. [CrossRef]
30. Tom, V.J.; Kadakia, R.; Santi, L.; Houlé, J.D. Administration of chondroitinase ABC rostral or caudal to a spinal cord injury site promotes anatomical but not functional plasticity. *J. Neurotrauma* **2009**, *26*, 2323–2333. [CrossRef]
31. Mosley, J.R.; Lanyon, L.E. Growth rate rather than gender determines the size of the adaptive response of the growing skeleton to mechanical strain. *Bone* **2002**, *30*, 314–319. [CrossRef]

Disclaimer/Publisher's Note: The statements, opinions and data contained in all publications are solely those of the individual author(s) and contributor(s) and not of MDPI and/or the editor(s). MDPI and/or the editor(s) disclaim responsibility for any injury to people or property resulting from any ideas, methods, instructions or products referred to in the content.

MDPI AG
Grosspeteranlage 5
4052 Basel
Switzerland
Tel.: +41 61 683 77 34

Bioengineering Editorial Office
E-mail: bioengineering@mdpi.com
www.mdpi.com/journal/bioengineering

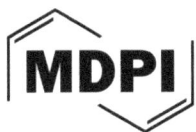

Disclaimer/Publisher's Note: The title and front matter of this reprint are at the discretion of the Guest Editor. The publisher is not responsible for their content or any associated concerns. The statements, opinions and data contained in all individual articles are solely those of the individual Editor and contributors and not of MDPI. MDPI disclaims responsibility for any injury to people or property resulting from any ideas, methods, instructions or products referred to in the content.